Forensic Psychoanalysis

Forensic Psychoanalysis examines the traumatic psychological origins of violence and explores the ways in which such disasters can be prevented and treated.

The book encapsulates Professor Brett Kahr's lengthy career in the field of forensic mental health, investigating all aspects of this vital arena, from the history of criminality to the current-day application of psychoanalysis and psychodynamic psychotherapy to the care of rapists, arsonists, genital exhibitionists, paedophiles, and murderers. This gripping text surveys more than one century of literature on the psychotherapeutic treatment of the criminally insane and provides tremendous insight into how mental health professionals can contribute to the reduction of global violence.

Forensic Psychoanalysis will be crucial for all readers interested in both the prevention of criminality and its psychological treatment.

Professor Brett Kahr has worked in the mental health field for over forty years. He is Senior Fellow at the Tavistock Institute of Medical Psychology in London and, also, Visiting Professor of Psychoanalysis and Mental Health at Regent's University London. A trained historian, Kahr is both an Honorary Fellow as well as the Honorary Director of Research at the Freud Museum London. He is the author of twenty books and series editor of over eighty-five further titles. He serves as Chair of the Scholars Committee of the British Psychoanalytic Council and, additionally, as a Consultant Psychotherapist at The Balint Consultancy. He works with individuals and couples in Central London.

The Forensic Psychotherapy Monograph Series

Series Editor: Professor Brett Kahr

For further information about this series please visit https://www.routledge.com/The-Forensic-Psychotherapy-Monograph-Series/book-series/KARNFPM vast and deep clinical knowledge, as well as his artistry as an historian *par excellence*, we are invited into the extreme end of human experience and its many challenging manifestations in the consulting room. This book deserves your study."

Richard Curen is Chair of the Forensic Psychotherapy Society and a member of the Board of the International Association for Forensic Psychotherapy. A Visiting Lecturer and Supervisor at the Portman Clinic, and a member of the Institute of Psychotherapy and Disability, he works in private practice in London.

"In this truly unique panoply, Professor Brett Kahr has created a book that encompasses the multitudinous arenas of forensic psychotherapy, past, present, and future. His case descriptions are compelling, even astonishing, and cross a spectrum of examples from more traditional forensic cases of incarcerated, dangerous criminals, to vignettes of marital couples and, of especial importance, he also includes so-called "non-forensic" or "sub-clinical" cases whom one might encounter in private practice. Professor Brett Kahr's encyclopaedic knowledge as an historian and as a clinician is further enriched by how compassionately he writes when referring to perpetrators and victims, as well as in his examination of modern thinking about "rehumanising the dehumanised"."

Dr. Carine Minne is the Chair of the Violence Committee of the International Psychoanalytical Association. She is also the Editor-in-Chief of *The International Journal of Forensic Psychotherapy*, and the Past President of the International Association for Forensic Psychotherapy.

"Brett Kahr provides a lively and illuminating introduction to the history and practice of forensic psychotherapy, including illustrations of a range of outpatient treatments with various offenders or near offenders. He brings to life many of the early generations of practitioners who have contributed to this speciality. Brett Kahr's openness about his countertransference, for example fear, disgust, and concern, will aid those embarking on such complex, challenging but also rewarding work."

Dr Cleo Van Velsen is a Consultant Psychiatrist in Forensic Psychotherapy and Consultant Psychiatrist in the Family Trauma Team at the Anna Freud Centre for Children and Families, and, also, a member of the British Psychoanalytical Society.

"This is a work of genius. We are extremely blessed to have Brett Kahr as part of our community. His contributions are truly remarkable in so many different arenas."
Profesora Estela Welldon is Emeritus Consultant Psychiatrist at the Portman Clinic in London and an Honorary Member of the American Psychoanalytic Association as well as the recipient of the Lifetime Achievement Award of the British Psychoanalytic Council. Her many classic books include *Mother, Madonna, Whore: The Idealization and Denigration of Women.*

"Once again, Professor Brett Kahr has given us a rich work about the treatment of all kinds of offenders. He is one of the most experienced practitioners in the field of forensic psychotherapy, and his books never fail to inform and stimulate. He writes with warmth and humanity about what he learned from decades of meeting people for therapy, and his writer's voice is "analytic" in the best sense, going beyond the surface level. There is so much to recommend in this book, especially the chapters on the historical account of the development of forensic psychotherapy and on what Professor Kahr calls the "sub-clinical" patient, describing people with intense feelings of cruelty, hate, and rage who have no history of convictions for violence. The book ends with a plea for more psychotherapy for perpetrators of violence because it can really help people change their minds for the better – a view which I heartily endorse."
Dr. Gwen Adshead is a forensic psychiatrist and psychotherapist at Broadmoor Hospital. She has worked in prisons and secure psychiatric facilities for over thirty years and has published widely on the theory and practice of forensic psychotherapy. Her first book for a general audience, written with Eileen Horne, is called *The Devil You Know.*

"In this engaging book, Professor Kahr combines the intellectual rigour of an academic historian with the acumen and compassion of an experienced clinician. His analysis of the development of forensic psychotherapy is compelling and highlights the remarkable achievements of the discipline to date. Importantly, he also emphasises future roles for forensic psychotherapy in addressing social inequality, prison reform and, also, taking a preventative, public health approach to violence reduction and to "rehumanising the dehumanised"."
Dr. Colin Campbell is a Consultant Forensic Psychiatrist and Associate Medical Director of the South London and Maudsley NHS Foundation Trust, UK, as well as the President of the International Association for Forensic Psychotherapy.

"This is an utterly splendid and extraordinary book for several reasons. Professor Kahr skilfully manages to draw us in and open our eyes to the fascinating field of forensic psychoanalysis through his expert and careful examination. Due to his

Forensic Psychoanalysis

From Sub-Clinical Psychopaths to Serial Killers

Brett Kahr

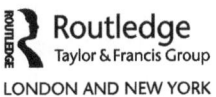
Routledge
Taylor & Francis Group

LONDON AND NEW YORK

Designed cover image: Getty | Charles O'Rear

First published 2025
by Routledge
4 Park Square, Milton Park, Abingdon, Oxon OX14 4RN

and by Routledge
605 Third Avenue, New York, NY 10158

Routledge is an imprint of the Taylor & Francis Group, an informa business

British Library Cataloguing-in-Publication Data
A catalogue record for this book is available from the British Library

ISBN: 9781032901190 (hbk)
ISBN: 9781032901176 (pbk)
ISBN: 9781003546245 (ebk)

DOI: 10.4324/9781003546245

Typeset in Times New Roman
by codeMantra

In Memoriam.
Jeannie Milligan (1949–2021)
A true pioneer of forensic psychoanalysis, and a magnificent friend and colleague, who left us far too soon, and who will be much missed.

Contents

Books by Professor Brett Kahr

D.W. Winnicott: A Biographical Portrait (1996).

Forensic Psychotherapy and Psychopathology: Winnicottian Perspectives, Editor (2001).

Exhibitionism (2001).

The Legacy of Winnicott: Essays on Infant and Child Mental Health, Editor (2002).

Sex and the Psyche (2007).

Who's Been Sleeping in Your Head?: The Secret World of Sexual Fantasies (2008).

Life Lessons from Freud (2013).

Tea with Winnicott (2016).

Coffee with Freud (2017).

New Horizons in Forensic Psychotherapy: Exploring the Work of Estela V. Welldon, Editor (2018).

How to Flourish as a Psychotherapist (2019).

Bombs in the Consulting Room: Surviving Psychological Shrapnel (2020).

Celebrity Mad: Why Otherwise Intelligent People Worship Fame (2020).

On Practising Therapy at 1.45 A.M.: Adventures of a Clinician (2020).

Dangerous Lunatics: Trauma, Criminality, and Forensic Psychotherapy (2020).

Freud's Pandemics: Surviving Global War, Spanish Flu, and the Nazis (2021).

How to Be Intimate with 15,000,000 Strangers: Musings on Media Psychoanalysis (2023).

Hidden Histories of British Psychoanalysis: From Freud's Death Bed to Laing's Missing Tooth (2024).

Expanding Psychoanalysis: The Contributions of Susie Orbach, Editor (2025).

The Holes in Winnicott's Trousers: The Brilliance and Shadows of a Psychoanalyst (2025).

Acknowledgements

I owe my deepest thanks to Ms. Susannah Frearson, our senior Publisher in the fields of mental health and psychoanalysis at the publishers Routledge, part of the Taylor and Francis Group, with whom I have had the great privilege to work. Susannah Frearson could not be a more congenial and professional collaborator, and she always communicates with me in an immensely creative and helpful and supportive manner, for which I extend my warmest appreciation. With her blessing, we managed to transform the "Forensic Psychotherapy Monograph Series" into a joint collaboration between Routledge and the International Association for Forensic Psychotherapy.

Likewise, I extend similar gratitude to Ms. Frearson's long-standing colleague, Ms. Saloni Singhania, for her amazing encouragement and assistance. And I thank Mr. Nick Craggs, the Senior Production Editor of Books for Taylor and Francis, with whom I have had the pleasure and honour of collaborating on a previous project, namely, my recent book on media psychoanalysis (Kahr, 2023a) and, subsequently, my edited book about the contributions of Dr. Susie Orbach (Kahr, 2025a). He has facilitated the publication of this text with his usual reliability and attention to detail. And, as ever, Ms. Pamela Bertram, the copyeditor, who works alongside Nick Craggs, has proved the most splendid of professionals.

Needless to say, I could not have written this book or, indeed, undertaken the work described herein without a lifetime of learning facilitated by my many esteemed forensic teachers and colleagues from whom I have gained so much wisdom and insight across the decades. In particular, I wish to express deepest thanks to a small handful of experienced individuals, not least, Dr. Gwen Adshead, Dr. Anne Aiyegbusi, Dr. Colin Campbell, Mr. Donald Campbell, Ms. Jessica Collier, the late Dr. Alan Corbett, the late Dr. Murray Cox, Mr. Richard Curen, the late Mrs. Sira Dermen, Dr. Ronald Doctor, Dr. Judith Freedman, Professor James Gilligan, the late Dr. Mervin Glasser, Mr. John Gordon, Dr. Elif Gürisik, Dr. Robert Hale, Professor the Baroness Sheila Hollins, the late Dr. Gabriel Kirtchuk, the late Professor Gill McGauley, the late Ms. Jeannie Milligan, Dr. Carine Minne, Ms. Elena Mundici, Dr. Konstantin Nemirovskiy, Ms. Katya Orrell, Ms. Annie Pesskin, Dr. Valerie Sinason, Ms. Pamela Windham Stewart, Dr. Cleo Van Velsen, Dr. Eileen Vizard, C.B.E., Profesora Estela Welldon, Dr. Sarah Wynick, and so many others, as well as all of the members of the Sohn Seminar, sponsored by the British Psychoanalytical Society, from whom I have absorbed so very much over the years.

I wish to extend particular thanks and appreciation to Profesora Estela Welldon and to Dr. Carine Minne, who might best be described, respectively, as the veritable Queen of Forensic Psychotherapy and the Crown Princess of Forensic Psychotherapy! These two deeply brilliant women have taught me so much over the decades and have brought such immense insight and pleasure and hope to my world. I offer my warmest appreciation to Profesora Welldon for all of her iconic work as the founder of modern forensic psychotherapy, which I have described in detail in this book. And I convey extra-special thanks to Dr. Minne, not only for her multitudinous contributions to our field, as Editor-in-Chief of *The International Journal of Forensic Psychotherapy*, as Chair of the Violence Committee of the International Psychoanalytical Association, and as Past President of the International Association for Forensic Psychotherapy, *inter alia*, but, also, for having kindly written a special foreword to this collection of essays with such gracious generosity. I shall never forget the delicious supper that I enjoyed some years ago with Profesora Welldon and Dr. Minne during which we decided to launch *The International Journal of Forensic Psychotherapy*. Dr. Minne deserves great credit for having created a magnificent phrase, now branded on the front cover of each issue of the journal, which encapsulates our work, namely, "rehumanising the dehumanised".

I also owe tremendous appreciation to the much-loved, much-missed Ms. Jeannie Milligan, one of our most esteemed and admired colleagues who, tragically, died in a fire in 2021, and whom we continue to mourn. I have dedicated this volume of essays to the memory of the great Jeannie, one of my very first forensic teachers at the Portman Clinic and, ultimately, a highly admired colleague and friend.

Series Editor's Foreword

In 1801, the English judiciary condemned a thirteen-year-old boy to death and then hanged him on the gallows at Tyburn, in the heart of London. But what crime had he committed? Apparently, this young lad had stolen merely a spoon (Westwick, 1940). Tragically, during the early nineteenth century, such an infraction could actually result in capital punishment.

Throughout much of human history, our ancestors have performed rather poorly when responding to acts of violence. In most cases, our predecessors will either have *ignored* murderousness, as in the case of Graeco-Roman infanticide, which occurred so regularly in the ancient world that it acquired an almost normative status (deMause, 1974; Kahr, 1994a); or they will have *punished* destructible behaviours with retaliatory sadism – a form of unconscious identification with the aggressor. Any history of criminology will readily reveal the cruel punishments inflicted upon prisoners throughout the ages, ranging from beatings and stockades, to more severe forms of torture, culminating in eviscerations, lynchings, beheadings, and electrocutions (e.g., Kahr, 2020b).

Only during the last 100 years have we begun to develop the capacity to respond more intelligently and more humanely to dangerousness and destruction. Since the advent of psychoanalysis, we now have access to a much deeper understanding of both the aetiology of aggressive acts and their treatment; and, fortunately, we need no longer ignore criminals or abuse them – instead, we can offer forensic psychotherapeutic interventions with compassion and containment, as well as conduct research which can help to prevent future acts of violence. By *treating* sadistic patients, rather than by *punishing* them, forward-thinking mental health practitioners now possess the ability to draw upon the new discipline of forensic psychotherapy, designed to understand the causes of violence, in order to help rehumanise the dehumanised.

The discipline of forensic psychotherapy can trace its origins to the very early days of psychoanalysis. On 6th February, 1907, at a meeting of the Wiener Psychoanalytische Vereinigung [Vienna Psycho-Analytical Society], Professor Sigmund Freud bemoaned the often horrible treatment of mentally ill offenders. According to Herr Otto Rank, Freud's secretary at the time, the founder of psychoanalysis expressed his sorrow at the "unsinnige Behandlung dieser Leute" (quoted in Rank, 1907a, p. 101), which translates as the "nonsensical treatment of these people" (quoted in Rank, 1907b, p. 108).

Subsequently, many of the early psychoanalytical practitioners preoccupied themselves with forensic topics. Dr. Hanns Sachs, himself a trained lawyer, and the Princesse Marie Bonaparte, a noted French aristocrat, spoke fiercely against capital punishment. Sachs, one of the first members of Freud's inner circle, regarded the death penalty for offenders as an example of group sadism (Moellenhoff, 1966); while Bonaparte (1927), who had studied various murderers throughout her career, actually campaigned to free the convicted killer Caryl Chessman, during his sentence on Death Row at the California State Prison in San Quentin (Bertin, 1982).

Some years later, Mrs. Melanie Klein (1932a), the Austrian-born, British-based clinician, concluded her first book, the landmark text *Die Psychoanalyse des Kindes* – known in English as *The Psycho-Analysis of Children* (Klein, 1932b) – with a truly memorable clarion call. Mrs. Klein noted that acts of criminality stem invariably from disturbances in childhood, and that if young people could receive psychoanalytical treatment at an early age, then much cruelty would be prevented in later years. As she argued,

> If every child who shows disturbances that are at all severe were to be analysed in good time, a great number of these people who later end up in prisons or lunatic asylums, or who go completely to pieces, would be saved from such a fate and be able to develop a normal life (Klein, 1932b, p. 374).[1]

Shortly after the publication of Klein's transformative book, Atwell Westwick, a Judge of the Superior Court of Santa Barbara, California, published a little-known, though highly inspiring, article on "Criminology and Psychoanalysis" in *The Psychoanalytic Quarterly*. Westwick may well be the first judge to have committed himself in print to the value of psychoanalysis in the study of criminality, arguing that punishment of the forensic patient remains, in fact, a sheer waste of time. With passion, he queried,

> Can we not, in our well nigh hopeless and overwhelming struggle with the problems of delinquency and crime, profit by medical experience with the problems of health and disease? Will we not, eventually, terminate the senseless policy of sitting idly by until misbehavior occurs, often with irreparable damage, then dumping the delinquent into the juvenile court or reformatory and dumping the criminal into prison? (Westwick 1940, p. 281)

Westwick noted that we should, instead, train judges, probation officers, social workers, as well as teachers and parents, in the precepts of psychoanalysis, in order to arrive at a more sensitive, non-punitive understanding of the nature of criminality. As Westwick (1940, p. 281) opined, "When we shall have succeeded in committing society to such a program, when we see it launched definitely upon the venture, as in time it surely will be – then shall we have erected an appropriate memorial to Sigmund Freud."

Although the roots of forensic psychotherapy stem back to the early years of the twentieth century (e.g., Kahr, 2018c, 2022d), the discipline did not become constellated more formally until the 1980s and 1990s, due, in large measure, to the pioneering work of the esteemed forensic psychiatrist and forensic psychotherapist, Dr. Estela Valentina Welldon (1988, 1996, 2002, 2011, 2015), and many of her colleagues; and, thankfully, the profession now boasts a much more robust foundation, with training courses available for young mental health workers in the United Kingdom and beyond. Since the inauguration of the Diploma in Forensic Psychotherapy, created by Dr. Welldon, hosted by the Portman Clinic in London, and sponsored by the British Postgraduate Medical Federation of the University of London, with the support and encouragement of its leader, Professor Sir Michael Peckham (Kahr, 2021e), students can now seek further instruction in the psychodynamic treatment of patients who act out in a dangerous and illegal manner. Dr. Welldon – subsequently Profesora Welldon – created not only the world's first training programme in forensic psychotherapy, but she also launched the International Association for Forensic Psychotherapy in 1991, and hosted its inaugural conference in 1992 at St. Bartholomew's Hospital in London. This passionate and devoted organisation has certainly helped to develop the field globally.

Back in 1997, at the kind invitation of Mr. Cesare Sacerdoti, the owner of H. Karnac (Books) at that time, I had the privilege of commissioning a host of titles for a new book series, designed to promote this growing branch of forensic psychological assessment, treatment, and prevention; and the very first titles appeared several years later (Bloom, 2001; Kahr, 2001a; Saunders, 2001). Over time, this Forensic Psychotherapy Monograph Series, now published by Routledge, part of the Taylor and Francis Group, has endeavoured to produce a regular stream of high-quality titles, written by leading members of the profession, who share their expertise in a concise and practice-orientated fashion. We trust that this collection of books, which, in 2022, became the official monograph series of the International Association for Forensic Psychotherapy, will help to consolidate and to disseminate the knowledge and experience that we have already acquired, and will also provide more creative pathways in the decades to come.

As the new millennium begins to unfold, we now have an opportunity for psychotherapeutically-inclined forensic mental health professionals to work in close conjunction with child psychologists and with infant mental health specialists so that the problems of violence can be tackled not only retrospectively but, also, preventatively. With the growth of the field of forensic psychotherapy, we at last have reason to be hopeful that serious criminality can be forestalled and perhaps, one day, even eradicated.

Professor Brett Kahr
Series Editor, Forensic Psychotherapy Monograph Series, International
Association for Forensic Psychotherapy

Note

1 The original German phrase reads: "Würde jedes Kind, das ernstere Störungen zeigt, rechtzeitig der Analyse unterzogen, dann könnte wohl ein großer Teil jener Menschen, die andernfalls in Gefängnissen und Irrenhäusern landen oder sonst völlig scheitern, vor diesem Schicksal bewahrt bleiben und sich zu normalen Menschen entwickeln" (Klein, 1932a, p. 293).

Special Foreword

In this truly unique panoply, Professor Brett Kahr has created a book that encompasses the multitudinous arenas of forensic psychotherapy, past, present, and future. He manages to cover the history of forensic mental health, provide descriptions of innumerable subtypes of psychopathologies, as well as refer to the creative brainstorming he rightly considers essential for the multidisciplinary professionals in the field, to further our understanding and the interventions that we provide.

Drawing heavily upon his training, not only as a clinician but, also, as an academic historian, and written in his usual, impeccable, scholarly fashion, Kahr provides detailed explorations of the origins of this field and the importance to us all of learning from the wisdom of earlier theoreticians and psychoanalysts. His case descriptions are compelling, even astonishing, and cross a spectrum of examples from more traditional forensic cases of incarcerated, dangerous criminals, to vignettes of marital couples and, of especial importance, he also includes so-called "non-forensic" or "sub-clinical" cases whom one might encounter in private practice. The latter cases are striking in that the author conveys how, in a sense, all cases seen have a "forensic" part, making this book of relevance to all psychotherapy practitioners and not only to those working in forensic psychiatry settings or within the criminal justice system.

Professor Kahr ignites the reader's mind with his reminder of classical psychoanalysis and Freud's genius insights. He explores further the true reality of "castration anxiety" as a leading aetiological factor in both genital exhibitionism and, also, in killing. Some men, with traumatic earlier histories, who feel impotent (and consequently humiliated), can enact their need for greater potency, not only by exposing their genitals publicly but, also, by penetrating unfortunate victims with honorary phalluses such as knives, guns, and even bayonets and missiles.

Notably, Kahr incorporates his very original and much-quoted work on the "infanticidal introject" and the "infanticidal attachment" as well as other forms of unconscious death wishes. Furthermore, he explores a new form of killing – little discussed in the literature – namely, "pet murder", as a symbolic form of neonaticide. Such murderous experiences by parents towards pets can actually function as displaced killings of children, which result in grotesque psychopathological consequences, and are described in this book.

Professor Brett Kahr's encyclopaedic knowledge as an historian and as a clinician is further enriched by how compassionately he writes when referring to perpetrators and victims, as well as in his examination of modern thinking about "rehumanising the dehumanised". This links with the state of hope sounded by the author, who, throughout this brilliant book, provides the momentum for a richer and bolder multidisciplinary forensic psychoanalytical profession.

Dr. Carine Minne
Chair, Violence Committee, International Psychoanalytical Association.
Editor-in-Chief, *The International Journal of Forensic Psychotherapy*.
Past President, International Association for Forensic Psychotherapy

Preamble

Confessions of a Private Forensic Practitioner

Many long decades ago, as a young undergraduate student, I had the great privilege of attending a series of lectures about the discipline known as "psychopathology", namely, the study of what we might refer to as disturbances of the mind or, more colloquially, as "madness". My esteemed teacher – a brilliant clinical psychologist – delivered some magnificently gripping talks about a vast range of nosological categories, including schizophrenia, depression, hysteria, obsessive-compulsive disorder, early infantile autism, and so many more, as well as a plethora of presentations about various treatment options, including psychopharmacology, behavioural therapy and, even, psychoanalysis. I took extensive notes, which I have retained to this very day.

I found those talks to be immensely engaging – utterly captivating, in fact – and I knew that I had made the right decision to study psychology.

My professor did offer one talk on the subject of "psychopathy", namely, a category of mental illness deployed to describe those individuals who suffer from "guiltlessness and lovelessness" and who might, as well, be unkind. Although trained as a clinical psychologist, my teacher had never worked in a high-security institution; hence, despite having made a brief reference to so-called "hardened criminals", he devoted most of the lecture on psychopathy to a discussion of unethical businessmen who lacked fully developed superego structures and who would, therefore, often cheat and lie. To the best of my memory, the professor spoke exclusively about immoral *males*, rather than females. I gained many insights into the way in which psychopathic characters – often dressed in suits and ties – can deceive their colleagues in the workplace. But my fellow students and I learned absolutely nothing about the more extreme variety of psychopathic characters, namely, murderers, paedophiles, rapists, arsonists or, indeed, terrorists.

Thus, by the time I had decided to pursue my postgraduate studies in psychology and psychotherapy, I had certainly learned a very great deal about the subtle symptomatic distinctions between catatonic schizophrenia and paranoid schizophrenia, and about how to make a differential diagnosis between dissociative hysteria and amnesic hysteria, but I knew very little, in fact, about the more extreme forms of criminality. Indeed, back then, in the late 1970s, virtually nobody ever spoke about child abuse, let alone paedophilia. If memory serves me correctly, I had never even heard my professor utter the word "forensic" at all.

Of course, we knew that human beings had committed murders since the very dawn of time, but few mental health professionals had any direct access to such individuals, most of whom would be locked away for life in institutions which might have employed merely one or two psychiatrists, but, certainly, no psychoanalysts or psychotherapists. Hence, the notion of a mental health practitioner interviewing, let alone *treating*, a hardened criminal proved quite a rarity indeed. Consequently, when I first set foot in a psychiatric hospital, I never expected to meet a so-called "forensic patient". I had secretly assumed that, by the time I qualified, I would open up a private psychoanalytical practice and that I would work with zillions of neurotic men and women who struggled with their marriages or with their bosses at the office. I never imagined that I might, in the future, be welcoming hardened criminals into my consulting room.

Of course, nowadays, the fields of forensic psychology, forensic psychiatry, and even forensic psychotherapy have become so much better known and so much more prominent that, had I embarked upon my studies in the twenty-first century, rather than in the twentieth century, I might well have worked with criminals on a full-time basis. But, back then, virtually all of my colleagues regarded offenders as true rarities and, thus, by no means a matter of focus for most mental health practitioners.

Needless to say, it did not take me long to discover that one would not be required to work at Broadmoor Hospital in the village of Crowthorne, in the county of Berkshire – the oldest and most esteemed maximum-security institution on this side of the pond – in order to encounter murderers and paedophiles and arsonists. I soon came to appreciate that violent patients do exist left, right, and centre; and, in due course, I encountered an increasing number of men and women on the back wards of traditional psychiatric hospitals and, also, in seemingly ordinary community mental health clinics, who had committed truly sadistic crimes. And by the time I opened up my private practice in a quiet, leafy mews in the fashionable district of North-West London known as Hampstead, not far from the one-time home of Professor Sigmund Freud, I had the privilege of treating numerous kindly and neurotic individuals; but, to my surprise, some of them confessed that, although they enjoyed rich careers as ethical doctors and lawyers and accountants, many had also perpetrated acts of criminality of one sort or another, even though no one had ever "caught" them before.

By the late 1980s, I had met so many patients, not only those with documentable criminal *histories*, but, also, those with criminal *tendencies* and, also, criminal *fantasies*, that I knew it would be helpful to learn much more about the psychology of human violence. In 1987, I applied to study at the nearby Portman Clinic – a small building located next to the much larger and much more famous Tavistock Clinic – and I then enjoyed the privilege of becoming a disciple of none other than Dr. Estela Valentina Welldon – a remarkable Argentinian-born, British-based forensic psychiatrist and psychotherapist who had just launched a special course for mental health workers of all backgrounds. In view of my relative youth and inexperience at that time, I received much pleasure and, indeed, surprise, when I obtained a place on Dr. Welldon's training, then entitled the "Introductory Course on the Understanding of Sexual and Social Deviance", and, as the lectures unfolded, I learned a very great deal indeed. Welldon had, by this point, already begun to cultivate links with psychoanalytically orientated forensic specialists from around the world, and, in 1991, she created the International Association for Forensic Psychotherapy and, moreover, launched a special Certificate in Forensic Psychotherapy, awarded by the British Postgraduate Medical Federation at the University of London, which I completed, followed by a Diploma in Forensic Psychotherapy, awarded jointly by the British Postgraduate Medical Federation and by the Faculty of Clinical Science at University College in the University of London, which I also came to receive. I felt very honoured indeed to have become one of Dr. Welldon's very first graduates of these various courses, and I owe her much gratitude for having introduced me to a rich network of teachers and supervisors and colleagues from whom I continue to learn so very much.

Eventually, I received an appointment as a Staff Psychotherapist at the Young Abusers Project at the next-door Tavistock Clinic, where I had the enriching experience of working psychotherapeutically with teenage sex offenders who had already committed acts of extreme sexual violence against even younger children. The noted forensic child psychiatrist and psychoanalyst, Dr. Eileen Vizard, had established this pioneering project, in association with the Department of Health, as well as with both the National Children's Home Action for Children and the National Society for the Prevention of Cruelty to Children; and, in true blue-sky fashion, she helped us all to offer psychological interventions, not only as a form of *treatment* for those juvenile paedophiles but, also, as a means of *prevention*. Dr. Vizard knew that if we could begin to provide psychotherapy to such young sex offenders as soon as possible – immediately after those individuals had committed their very first crimes – we had the opportunity to stop such adolescents from becoming full-time, multi-perpetrator career paedophiles. Consequently, by having championed early intervention, Eileen Vizard and the team certainly helped to reduce the number of victims quite significantly.

Likewise, during the 1990s, I also had the privilege to serve on the Mental Handicap Team at the Tavistock Clinic, directed by Mrs. Valerie Sinason (later Dr. Sinason), an esteemed child and adolescent psychotherapist who ultimately became a psychoanalyst as well, and who specialised in providing intensive psychotherapy to patients who struggled with what we then referred to as "mental handicap", namely, learning disabilities or intellectual disabilities. Many of those handicapped patients had also committed crimes of one variety or another, and together with Sinason and some of our pioneering colleagues, we eventually developed the Institute of Psychotherapy and Disability, an organisation which championed the sub-speciality of "*forensic disability psychotherapy*" (Kahr, 2014a, p. xix), namely, working psychoanalytically with highly handicapped patients who often struggled to speak in full sentences and who would enact their long-standing rage and violence, not in words but, rather, in deeds.

Over the years, I have certainly immersed myself in the world of forensic mental health, whether in psychiatric hospitals, public mental health clinics, or community mental health centres. But, unlike many of my forensic colleagues, I have never worked in the field of forensics on a *full-time* basis. During my younger years, I always divided my hours between the clinical work which I undertook in institutions and my own private psychotherapeutic practice, and I also devoted a significant chunk of my working energies to my academic teaching post, to my various research and writing projects, and, also, to the field of media psychology, having spent many years as Resident Psychotherapist at the British Broadcasting Corporation (Kahr, 2005a, 2023a). So, unlike some of my compatriots who had always toiled from Monday to Friday in maximum-security institutions, I enjoyed a *more broad* career – a true pun, literally – rather than a *Broadmoor* career!

Thus, I have often referred to myself as a "part-time forensicist", rather than a full-time one.

Perhaps if I had discovered the forensic mental health field earlier, I might well have embarked upon a different career trajectory, yet, by having immersed myself not only in forensic institutions but, also, in a more traditional private practice and in academia, I have had the opportunity to integrate these seemingly disparate branches of mental health care. For instance, when I ultimately embarked upon my training in couple psychotherapy and couple psychoanalysis at the Tavistock Martial Studies Institute, I suspect that I might not have survived that experience of treating extremely violent spousal couples had I not already graduated from the Portman Clinic some years previously. Indeed, I often found sitting in a room with screaming husbands and wives threatening to murder one another a far scarier experience than occupying a room with a depressed paedophile who could barely speak beyond a whisper.

Over the years, I have endeavoured to introduce basic forensic concepts and insights into the field of general psychotherapy, and, by having taught my students and my supervisees about forensic matters, many of them ultimately succeeded in working with more violent patients in their own private practices, often with very great success. In this regard, I hope that I have helped colleagues to appreciate the prevalence of what I have come to refer to as "Sub-Clinical Psychopathy" (Kahr, 2020e), or as the "*sub-clinical forensic perpetrator*" (Kahr, 2018d, p. 239), namely, a more invisible form of criminality which often emerges only in the complete privacy of the consulting room. In fact, I have worked very hard to remind us that even so-called "'non-forensic'" (Kahr, 2018d, p. 239) patients, who will *never* encounter the police or the courts, have, nonetheless, committed serious acts of violence, often unconsciously so. Hence, in this respect, I hope that I will have made a small contribution to the recognition of the fact that one need not be a forensic patient in order to be a forensic patient!

In the chapters which follow, I have attempted to chronicle some of my experiences of the world of forensic psychotherapy and forensic psychoanalysis, which include clinical encounters, examinations of the research literature, explorations of the history of our profession, and other topics, including a clarion call for the humanisation of treatment and for the advancement of more blue-sky thinking, helping to champion prevention first and foremost in the decades to come.

In the introductory essay on "The Ugly World of Forensic Mental Health", I have endeavoured to provide a brief portrait of the grotesque settings in which forensic patients must live, whether psychiatric hospitals or prisons, drawing upon my own early experiences of having encountered those men and women in urine-soaked wards, as well as upon the reminiscences of "Mike" and "Rob", the stars of the prison podcast *Banged Up*, which has provided us all with an even more shocking portrait of the ugliness of British institutions. Thereafter, in the first section of the book, I offer two essays, one on "'Let the great Axe fall": From Ancient Babylonian Torture to Modern Forensic Psychotherapy", in which I discuss the extraordinary history of our profession, and the other on "Explosive Patients: Surviving Petrifying Psychotherapeutic Experiences", in which I chronicle some of the more terrifying moments of my clinical encounters with violent patients of every variety. As someone who often receives requests from young psychology and psychotherapy students, keen to explore the possibility of a forensic training and yet uncertain what literature they might read, I hope that these introductory chapters about the viscerality of our profession – past and present – might offer some clarification and insight.

I have devoted the second section of this book to a series of case reports about what I have come to encapsulate as "Sexual Forensics", namely, that branch of forensic mental health which explores those patients – mostly male patients, in fact – who commit crimes with their genitalia. In the opening chapter of this portion of the book, "Why Do Men Expose Their Genitals?: The Unconscious Origins of Exhibitionism", I review the basic insights provided by a whole century of psychoanalytical practitioners from Professor Sigmund Freud to the present day. And in the following chapter, "From Penile Trauma to Flashing: A Case of Forensic Disability Psychotherapy", I offer a summation of my own work with an intellectually disabled genital exhibitionist who had endured an attack on his penis during childhood which, in my estimation, contributed hugely to the development of his sexual offences in later years. Thereafter, I provide an account of my very first consultation with a young forensic patient. In this chapter, "Fragile Monster: How to Make a Paedophile Talk", I endeavour to offer a glimpse into how a classical psychoanalytically orientated treatment might actually begin.

Throughout the third section of the book, I explore the huge and horrifying concept of murder, and I share some very particular aspects of this enormous subject, namely, the role of early infanticidal threats and assaults and, moreover, the impact of castration anxiety experiences on the genesis of violence in later life. In the first of these chapters, "When Daddy Kills the Dog: Pet Murder and the Infanticidal Attachment", I examine a wide range of my own clinical cases, which often involved a caregiver (usually a father or a mother) who attacked or murdered a childhood pet or a childhood toy in the shape of a pet. I have argued that all of my patients will have experienced such assaults as deferred acts of infanticide, or as what I have conceptualised as *"psychological infanticide"* (Kahr, 1993, p. 269), which will have contributed to the formation of the "Infanticidal Attachment" (Kahr, 2007c, p. 119). Thereafter, I investigate the topic of "Castration Anxiety in Men Who Murder", based on a study of the early biographies of several well-known, public-figure serial killers, all of whom suffered from genital shaming and genital attacks in childhood, and many of whom then re-enacted those episodes on the bodies of their victims in later life (cf. Kahr, 2024b).

Across the fourth section of this book, I consider the special category of patient that I have come to refer to as the "non-forensic" patient, namely, those individuals who *have* perpetrated violent acts without necessarily having broken the law or, indeed, without having been caught in certain instances. In the first essay on "The Sub-Clinical Psychopath: Committing Crimes Without Breaking the Law", I draw upon a range of cases in order to paint a portrait of the non-forensic individual patient. And then, in the subsequent chapter, "Criminality in the Bedroom: Unconscious Sadism in Non-Forensic Couples", I describe my work as a couple mental health practitioner who has often encountered long-term marital partners who have confined all of their rage and cruelty to the sexual arena. In many respects, this fourth section of the book provides, in my estimation, a portrait of the ways in which even non-forensic psychotherapists or part-time forensic psychotherapists have the potential to make vital contributions to the field, by learning from formal forensic psychoanalytical insights and by applying that knowledge to our daily work in the old-fashioned, traditional consulting room. I hope that these essays, in particular, may underscore the ways in which every one of us – whether we define ourselves as forensicists or not – will have to encounter forensic, criminal patients in one form or another.

I conclude this tome with a brief chapter on "The Future of Forensic Psychoanalysis" in which I summarise some of the findings contained herein and in which I emphasise that, over time, our field has made huge progress and, moreover, harbours the capacity to exert an even greater impact. As a profession, we do possess the capacity to engage with offenders in a more humane manner; we do have the ability to contribute not only to treatment but, also, to prevention; and, above all, we must bear the obligation to share this knowledge as, alas, we continue to inhabit a very forensic world in which even our global leaders will often perpetrate acts of great criminality which must, eventually, be quashed.

Brett Kahr

"Thoſe that in blood ſuch violent pleaſure have,
Seldome deſcend, but bleeding, to their grave."
Ben Jonson, "Murder", in Robert Allot (Ed.), *Englands Parnaſſus or The Choyſeſt Flowers of our Moderne Poets, with their Poeticall compariſons. Deſcriptions of Bewties, Perſonages, Caſtles, Pallaces, Mountaines, Groues, Seas, Springs, Riuers, & c. Whereunto are annexed other various diſcourſes both pleasſaunt and profitable,* 1600.

Introduction

The Ugly World of Forensic Mental Health

Many forensic patients must endure a lifetime in truly run-down, understaffed, deprived, and, even, unhygienic hospitals and clinics. These men and women, many of whom grew up in rather ugly homes, will then spend the rest of their lives in rather ugly institutions.

I shall never forget the very first time I stepped onto the back wards of a battered, bedraggled psychiatric hospital, tucked away on the outskirts of a tiny village in the remote English countryside. As a very young and extremely inexperienced psychology trainee, my knees literally trembled with fear as I walked through the locked doors of the psychogeriatric unit which housed hundreds of chronic, severely mentally ill patients, most of whom had received a diagnosis of schizophrenia. Within seconds, I became nauseous from the horrific odour of the urine-stained and faeces-smeared carpets, not to mention the morbid stench of the omnipresent cigarette butts spattered all about. Unsurprisingly, I began to retch.

The long-serving and somewhat jaded Consultant Psychiatrist – immune to the ghastliness of the physical surroundings – welcomed me warmly into this hellish environment and suggested that I should begin my apprenticeship with a tour of this nineteenth-century institution. Naively, I assumed that my new boss would escort me round personally; instead, he explained that my tour would actually be conducted by none other than "Fred", one of the oldest patients on the ward, who knew the layout of the hospital better than any of the members of staff.

Within moments, Fred appeared, as if by magic, and shook my hand most graciously. He smiled with tremendous enthusiasm: "So, you're the new psychologist. It's a pleasure to meet you." Fred chatted breezily and did not seem to be schizophrenic at all – quite the opposite, in fact. Only 5'1" in height, he struck me as somewhat childlike, especially as he spoke in rather a high-pitched voice. Certainly, from a physical point of view, this patient did not seem frightening in the least.

Fred then marched me through the dank rooms of the cavernous hospital and, afterwards, escorted me into the surprisingly well-maintained gardens. He chirped, "To your left, Brett, well, that's the infirmary, for patients who need medical treatment. And just beyond, to your right, that's the hairdresser's hut, where some of the old ladies go for their curlers. And over there, beyond that tree, that's the gardening shed."

DOI: 10.4324/9781003546245-1

Fred spoke clearly and calmly and with great attention to detail. After an hour, we returned to the ward, whereupon Fred kindly offered me a cup of tea.

Although I had visited psychiatric institutions previously, as part of my training, I had never before met a patient quite as sweet as Fred. He appeared to be incredibly sane and chipper, so much so that I actually wondered whether someone had made a dreadful mistake by having incarcerated him under the Mental Health Act 1959 all those many years ago.

At this point, the Consultant Psychiatrist reappeared and took me into his tiny office, strewn with stacks of dusty files, and asked me whether I had enjoyed my special walking tour. I told him that I had found Fred to be rather informative and, also, extremely charming to boot. The psychiatrist seemed unsurprised by my description. And then, he quizzed me: "So, Brett, if Fred is such a lovely man, why do *you* think he has been a long-stay patient at this hospital?"

Nervously, I spluttered a grossly inadequate reply and expressed my deep uncertainty as to the reason for Fred's incarceration.

The consultant grilled me further: "Is he, in your estimation, a classic schizophrenic?"

"Well," I replied, "I failed to observe any obvious signs of either hallucinations or delusions or, indeed, of disordered thought."

"You are correct," he replied, "Fred is not *obviously* schizophrenic."

"But if he does not meet the diagnostic criteria for schizophrenia," I queried, "what has brought him here as a patient?"

The Consultant Psychiatrist beamed with a certain arrogance, knowing that I would never guess the real reason for Fred's incarceration. He smirked and then explained, "Many years ago, Fred took a handgun and shot his father in the face at close range, and then he shot his mother in the face, also at close range. Would you ever have suspected that such a small and seemingly unthreatening man could have committed the ultimate double murder?"

My jaw dropped in utter astonishment. Although I had spent only a brief time with Fred and had enjoyed our stroll across the hospital grounds, I had not detected any sense of danger or madness. Fred seemed like a kindly old man. Certainly, I would never have supposed him capable of either patricide or matricide.

Evidently, my education in psychology had only just begun. And before long, I came to realise that one cannot always identify a murderer on the basis of physical appearance alone or, indeed, as a result of merely one hour of conversation. Although some killers *do* look completely deranged, with fire in their eyes and spittle drooling from their mouths, others, by contrast, appear quite placid and even gentle. I would have much to learn about the field of forensic mental health, namely, that branch of modern psychology devoted to the study of psychopathologically troubled individuals who perpetrate violence.

Mad people have committed offences – often grotesquely sadistic crimes – since the very dawn of time. Nowadays, we refer to a perpetrator such as Fred as a "forensic patient" – a mentally ill individual who commits an act, or acts, of deep cruelty. But, back in the nineteenth century, physicians would describe such a patient, somewhat more poetically, and, also, more shamingly, as a "dangerous lunatic" (Clarke, 1886, p. 88).

Now, within the very first hour of my very first day of employment, I had met my very first dangerous lunatic. And, as the years unfolded, I would, in due time, come to meet many more: murderers, paedophiles, arsonists, rapists, and thieves.

Given that most of us manage to navigate our entire lives without ever shooting another human being in the face, or raping a child, or burning down a building, or breaking into someone else's home in the middle of the night, why on earth should these dangerous lunatics do so? Perhaps these individuals suffer from some sort of brain disease or, perhaps, they might simply be rotten eggs, cursed by the Devil. What aetiological factors actually contribute to the development of such terrifying forensic illnesses?

And how might we deal with these people once the police have apprehended them? Should they be sentenced to a lifetime in a maximum-security prison? Should they be incarcerated in perpetuity in a special psychiatric hospital? And for those who do become institutionalised, should we permit them simply to rot in their cells or on the wards, or might we dare to offer some sort of humane psychological treatment in the hope of improving their quality of life and thus contribute to the reduction of the possibility of reoffending in future?

Across most of human history, our ancestors have treated perpetrators in the most cruel and disgusting of manners. Our predecessors have tortured and executed violent criminals unceasingly throughout the centuries. And many of these men and women (some guilty, some innocent) will have spent weeks, months, years, and even decades, locked up inside penal institutions.

But how do we, in the twenty-first century, actually treat our prisoners? Certainly, very few penal institutions offer humanising psychotherapy and other forms of psychological intervention.

Although the ward on which I worked boasted very few mental health professionals, none of whom had trained formally in psychotherapy or psychoanalysis, at least "Fred" – this double murderer – had access to mental health services. Sadly, the vast majority of forensic patients will rarely receive transformative psychological treatments and interventions. Most will be left to languish in grotesque and neglected prison settings and other types of institutions.

Let us now investigate what we might learn from two forensic patients, "Mike" and "Rob", both of whom have generously shared their experiences of life in prison by having appeared regularly on an excellent British podcast, *Banged Up*.

In 2013, Mike, a young professional football player, received an invitation from one of his senior teammates at Bristol Rovers to attend a meeting with some businessmen who promised a financial payment if he would agree to "match-fixing". Mike, a twenty-one-year-old man from South London – known to his friends as "Boats" – did, indeed, speak with these people, completely unaware that the National Crime Agency had already launched an investigation into this group of unscrupulous individuals. In due course, the police arrested Mike on charges of conspiracy and sentenced him to sixteen months in prison. Upon his release, the Football

Association banned Mike from playing in a professional context, and, in consequence, he became a drug dealer and, sometime thereafter, he returned to prison.

Another young man, Rob, who had grown up in a "middle-class" household, became involved in illegal activity regarding mobile telephone contracts. One day, several policemen dressed in riot gear arrested him, and he, too, would be sentenced on charges of conspiracy to commit fraud.

Mike and Rob met in prison. Thankfully, these convicted offenders developed a friendship and could thus provide one another with significant emotional support.

After their release, Mike and Rob agreed to speak publicly, with terrific honesty and transparency and generosity, about the challenges, the horrors and, even, the unexpected rewards of serving time in prison. And, in early 2020, these two men became the stars of the highly engaging podcast, *Banged Up*, created by the television production company Goalhanger Films. This podcast, widely available to anyone with a computer or mobile telephone, provides a unique, first-hand insight into the psychology of prison life, and, in my estimation, it deserves to be listened to, and studied with care, by every single mental health practitioner, especially those of us who work in the field of forensic psychotherapy.

I stumbled upon this podcast quite by happenstance and, after having absorbed the first episode of *Banged Up*, I became so deeply entranced that, over the coming weeks, I studied the next thirteen episodes of the first series with great vigilance as Mike and Rob – the two ex-prisoners – have painted an increasingly grim, often horrifying, but deeply engaging portrait of the shocking viscerality of the British prison system (Kahr, 2020c).

In their broadcasts, Mike and Rob have offered detailed accounts of the grotesque lack of hygiene in penal institutions, and we frequently learn about how often inmates must endure the smells of their own excreta and that of their cellmates. These two ex-prisoners reminisced with much honesty and ugliness about floors drenched with urine, walls smeared with faeces, unbearable bodily odours, and a complete and utter lack of privacy, with no curtain around the toilet. One prisoner quipped that, in all likelihood, convicts had probably used one particular toilet at least 3,000 times before anyone had bothered to clean it.

According to Mike and Rob, the stench would sometimes become so unbearable that certain men would have to be removed from their shared cells because, due to lack of washing, they emitted horrid smells which simply could not be tolerated by anyone else in the vicinity.

Prisoners would often treat one another with great thoughtlessness and disrespect, and, even, cruelty. Apparently, many convicted men would dread sleeping in the bottom bunk bed, because all the inmates had traces of urine on their bare feet, and those who climbed onto the top bunk bed would often immerse their feet in pee before stepping onto their cellmate's sheets.

One of the men recalled his incarceration alongside a terrifying cellmate – a physically large person, convicted of murder – who had asked for a haircut. The frightened prisoner obliged, albeit reluctantly, petrified that if he did not provide a sufficiently good head shave then he, too, might be murdered.

Not only did Mike and Rob and their fellow inmates have to navigate bodily odours, urine, faeces, and dangerously unhygienic conditions, and, heartbreakingly, a sense of basic insecurity, but they had to endure tremendous loneliness and boredom as well, often locked up in the same small cell for twenty-three hours per day. The isolation would become so grim that, at times, the highlight of the week would be a brief visit from the prison governor, updating the men about the results of recent football matches.

The filth, the loneliness, and the lack of safety undoubtedly contributed to a sense of deep fear, murderous rage, and, also, the simmering urge to commit even more criminal acts. In fact, the presenters of *Banged Up* have revealed that many of the inmates became quite skilled at selling marijuana and other drugs inside the prison. Some would have filled up condoms with "weed" prior to incarceration, which they then swallowed and would, ultimately, expel rectally; others would encourage their female partners to smuggle marijuana in condoms, inserted into their oral cavities, and then, on a visit, while kissing, the girlfriend or wife would transfer the weed-filled contraceptive into the mouth of the male prisoner who would later sell the drugs for profit. Consequently, the prison cells stank not only of bodily substances but, also, of marijuana.

Apparently, prisoners would smuggle not only drugs but, also, mobile phones, often inserted into the rectum, and sometimes these items would not be detected, even during one of the frequent strip searches.

At times, life inside would become incomparably terrifying, and the prisoners would have to deal with the suicide of fellow inmates, as well as death threats from other men in the prison, not to mention frequent acts of violence perpetrated by these convicted offenders or, even, by the "screws" themselves (i.e., the prison officers).

In a very short space of time, both Mike and Rob succeeded in portraying the lack of a sense of safety, both physically and psychologically, within British penal institutions.

Sadly, we learn from Mike and Rob that they received very little proper emotional comfort or practical assistance while locked away. Certainly, neither made any mention of the provision of physical healthcare or mental healthcare for themselves or for their fellow inmates. Indeed, we hear far more about the ways in which the prison system often prevents convicts from engaging in meaningful human contact; for instance, few men will be allowed to attend the funerals of their grandparents, although a prisoner could make a brief appearance at the burial of a mother, a father, or a sibling, albeit only for one hour, handcuffed to a guard. Inmates could also be transferred from one penal institution to another quite frequently, often with virtually no notice at all; thus, any precious interpersonal relationships which might have formed among prisoners would be ripped apart quite regularly with no opportunity for repair.

As the episodes of this remarkable podcast unfolded, I became increasingly attached to both Mike and Rob and, also, more and more impressed by their verbal capacities, their self-reflective abilities, their honesty, their thoughtfulness and, even, their playfulness. Each man spoke with great sensitivity and care, and each one listened to the other in similar fashion. Perhaps it came as little surprise when, during the tenth episode of the first series, Rob revealed that, upon his release, he spent two years undergoing psychotherapy at the cost of £50 per session. Undoubtedly, that experience might well have helped him to process the awful horror of his time inside.

Both Mike and Rob have since become great aids to their fellow prisoners, and each has reached out to former cellmates in various ways, knowing how important such basic human contact can be.

I strongly suspect that forensic mental health practitioners will appreciate this podcast series immensely. For those of us who lecture to students and trainees and supervisees about forensic issues, *Banged Up* could well become an indispensable resource. And for those of us who have worked in the field of forensic mental health for many years, these podcast episodes will serve as a very stark reminder of how much more labour we must undertake in order to humanise the penal system, namely, by underscoring the importance of preventative psychotherapy, by facilitating more psychotherapy within prisons, and by arranging for the provision of psychotherapy post-release.

Certainly, life within British prisons can be very grotesque at times. But it may well be the case that those imprisoned overseas in the United States of America might inhabit even filthier jails. As Ms. Alisa Roth (2018), an investigative reporter and sometime Soros Justice Fellow, has revealed in her horrifying study of American prisons, inmates would not only be confined to faecal-stained rooms but would also be deprived of virtually all human contact and would spend their days in handcuffs and leg shackles. Many of these already criminally-inclined men became even more vicious whilst in jail, and some, including one potentially H.I.V.-positive prisoner, would spit upon the security officers or would assault these guards with faeces. Based on her inspection of the Twin Towers Correctional Facility at the Los Angeles County Jail in California, Ms. Roth concluded,

> Jails and prisons are dehumanizing places: the uniforms that strip people of their individuality, the endless rules, the gruff way that many, though certainly not all, officers address prisoners. The sense of us and them, that divide between the prisoners and the officers or really the prisoners and the rest of us, is especially pronounced on mental health units like this one, where many people are either openly aggressive – growling, snarling, yelling, banging on doors – or completely unresponsive. Even the very legitimate caution with which the deputies approach the cells adds to the sense that these people are something other than human, creatures to be feared (Roth, 2018, p. 40).

In view of these devastating reports, it should hardly surprise us that, from time to time, prisoners will often jump out of windows – quite literally – no doubt keen to end such dreadful incarcerations (cf. Greenhalgh, 2021).

One might be justifiably horrified to discover that, nowadays, in the modern world, we treat our prisoners in such an arguably sadistic fashion. Fortunately, some of our forensic institutions, whether prisons or maximum-secure units, do relate to their guests with greater humanity, and a small number of staff members actually provide groundbreaking psychotherapy in an effort to heal these wounded offenders. But the vast majority of our contemporary institutions still treat their inhabitants in a much more neglectful manner.

Nonetheless, before we condemn the twenty-first century approach to criminality, let us remember that, however grotesque our modern prisons may be, by comparison with our ancestors of ancient times, we actually relate to our current incarcerated offenders in a far more kindly style. The further back in history one progresses, the more viciously human beings have treated those regarded as criminals.

Anyone who has ever worked in medium-security units, high-security hospitals, prisons, mental health clinics, or other forensic and penological institutions will certainly recognise the true ugliness described herein. When I encountered my first very own forensic patient, the aforementioned double-murderer Fred, I had to speak to this man in a grotesque physical setting, surrounded by floors stained with excrement. Mike and Rob, the two stars of *Banged Up*, have reported even more grotesque experiences. And Alisa Roth, the investigative journalist, has painted a truly shocking portrait of the disgusting, dehumanised atmosphere of some of the world's leading forensic institutions (Kahr, 2018f, 2018g).

Fortunately, the forensic psychotherapy community has, over recent decades, endeavoured to help encourage a more humane and kindly and psychologically intensive – and, hopefully, less ugly – approach to the care and treatment of such dangerous lunatics. But from whence did this relatively new branch of mental health care originate and how has our work in this new arena unfolded?

In the chapters which follow, I hope to provide a glimpse into the world of forensic psychoanalysis and forensic psychotherapy, exploring our historical origins, our hopes and dreams, and some sense of the theoretical and clinical conceptualisations of our often vicious patients who, in spite of their horrible acts of violence, or, indeed, because of such crimes, deserve our most compassionate, containing, protective, and vigilant clinical attention.

PART I

Forensic Psychotherapy as a Profession

"Let the great Axe fall"

From Ancient Babylonian Torture to Modern Forensic Psychotherapy

SECTION ONE: SADISM IN THE PRE-PSYCHOANALYTICAL ERA

The Treatment of Ancient Offenders

In previous centuries, any man, woman, or child regarded as a criminal perpetrator would, in all likelihood, be assaulted with tremendous physical cruelty, often of a lethal nature. According to Lewis Lyons (2003), an historian of punishment, those accused of offending could be subjected to any, or all, of the four primary treatments, namely (1) imprisonment; (2) corporal punishment; (3) torture; and, in many instances, (4) capital punishment as well.

Perhaps no one embodied this vicious approach to punishment as heartily as the Babylonian monarch Hammurabi who, during the eighteenth century B.C.E., authorised amputation and mutilation of body parts as an appropriate form of retaliation for anyone convicted of a crime. For instance, according to the code sanctioned by Hammurabi, perjurers would have their tongues eviscerated from their mouths; sons who struck their fathers would have their hands chopped off; rapists would be subjected to castration of the testicles; and burglars would be murdered at once before being gibbeted (Johns, 1914). Not only did Hammurabi authorise very cruel forms of violence, but he did so in a rather elitist manner, so that if a nobleman assaulted a fellow aristocrat, he would be punished severely, but if a wealthy man attacked a *servant*, then such an entitled person would receive absolutely *no* punishment at all. Hammurabi's code applied not only to men who committed offences but, also, to women who perpetrated acts of infidelity. Indeed, female infidels would be bound to their male lovers and would then be hurled into the Euphrates river, and would thus die from drowning (Harper, 1904).

Inspired by the Babylonians, the ancient Greeks eviscerated their criminals with comparable brutality. For instance, Draco, the noted Athenian lawmaker, who lived during the seventh century B.C.E., argued that perpetrators of many shapes and sizes, irrespective of the nature of their offence, should be sentenced to death; hence, the Athenians would often murder not only convicted killers but, also, those who stole fruit (Plvtarchi [Plutarch], n.d.). The Romans followed suit and would subject their criminals to such horrors as burning and crucifixion and, also, would

DOI: 10.4324/9781003546245-3

even hurl their offenders from cliff tops (Daube, 1947). Others would be thrown into public amphitheatres and ripped to shreds by wild animals – an act of retaliation and punishment known as "damnatio ad bestias" (Seneca, n.d. [c. 40s C.E.]).

Those accused of criminality by the Hebrews would either be stoned to death or, alternatively, hanged, strangulated, or slayed by a sword (Maimonides, c. 1170 – c. 1180; cf. Johns, 1914; Smith, 1931; Cohn, 1971). In similar vein, the ancient Chinese endorsed branding, castration, mutilation, and decapitation (Alabaster, 1899).

Across the ages, those responsible for the maintenance of law and order would subject those accused of criminality to such treatments as shaming, branding, flogging, beating, confinement in stocks and pillories, imprisonment, mutilation, amputation, the tearing of flesh with red-hot pincers, breaking on the wheel, as well as execution through hanging, stoning, burning, drowning, impalement, shooting, garrotting, drawing and quartering, poisoning, starvation, boiling, beheading, and, as time progressed, electrocution and the injection of lethal drugs (Cawthorne, 2006).

As the millennia unfolded, humanity made few, if any strides. We tend to idealise the so-called Elizabethan era as the very height of the English Renaissance – often known as the "Golden Age" – characterised by the works of art of Nicholas Hilliard and the dramas of William Shakespeare. But we must recall that, during the late sixteenth century, anyone accused of offending would still be subjected to the most evil of tortures. Consider, for instance, the case of Margaret Clitherow, a pregnant woman who had dared to harbour Catholic priests. In consequence, the authorities sentenced Clitherow to death in 1586, having stripped her of all of her clothing, and then having forced her to lie on the ground before placing a wooden door over her torso and stacking nearly 1,000 pounds of weights on top (Mush, 1849), thus breaking her ribs and, ultimately, crushing this young person to death (cf. Claridge, 1966; Lake and Questier, 2011).

Perhaps no one encapsulated the art of savagery as the treatment of choice for so-called criminality better than William Shakespeare himself. Indeed, in his iconic play, *The Tragedie of Hamlet, Prince of Denmarke*, written circa 1599–1602, a leading character, known as "Claudius King of Denmarke", pontificated about "turbulent and dangerous Lunacy" (First Folio, Act III, Scene i, line 4) and proclaimed, "And where th' offence is, let the great Axe fall" (First Folio, Act IV, Scene v, line 244). Thus, although twenty-first-century prisons and secure units evoke significant shame and concern, we must enjoy some relief knowing that, nowadays, we do not crush our pregnant patients to death by placing hundreds and hundreds of pounds of weight upon their nude bodies.

Psychiatry in the Pre-Psychoanalytical Era

But what about our ancestors in the so-called "caring" professions? Although Hammurabi and Elizabeth I may have supported torture and execution as standard treatments, how did physicians, especially psychiatrists, deal with offenders, particularly those whom we would now regard as suffering from one or other version of psychopathology?

Fortunately, most "mad doctors" or "alienists" – the predecessors of the professionals whom we would currently describe as psychiatrists or psychologists or psychotherapists – regarded criminals as victims of one or other form of brain degeneration. During the early nineteenth century, Dr. James Cowles Prichard (1835, p. 6), a Senior Physician at the Bristol Infirmary in England, explained that dangerous patients suffered from "*Moral Insanity*", and that they would be inclined to commit "every species of mischief" (Prichard, 1835, p. 22) as a result of their soiled minds. Prichard and his colleagues regarded such morally insane patients as neurologically damaged and made little reference to their early life experiences. In terms of treatment for those individuals whom we would now classify as "forensic patients", Dr. Prichard recommended bleeding, shaving of the head, ice-cold baths, and the administration of purgatives.

The nineteenth-century notion of brain degenerationism spread far and wide, and, in the United States of America, Professor Charles Coventry, a Professor of Medical Jurisprudence at the Medical Institution of Geneva College, in Geneva, New York, championed this increasingly popular concept. As he noted, "Probably no case of insanity occurs without more or less derangement of the general health" (Coventry, 1844, p. 143), and, moreover, that, "the functions of the brain remain impaired" (Coventry, 1844, p. 144). Professor Coventry's American contemporary, Dr. John Purdue Gray (1857, p. 141), a physician in Utica, New York, described perpetrators of homicide as suffering from "a marked hereditary predisposition". Dr. Gray (1857, p. 143) underscored that such patients suffered, in all likelihood, from a "*physical disease*", and he made no mention at all of the potential aetiological impact of truly traumatic infantile or childhood experiences.

Indeed, back in the nineteenth century, many esteemed medical practitioners argued that criminals could be defined simply on the basis of their physical appearance. Mr. Bruce Thomson (1870b, p. 332), a Resident Surgeon in Perth, argued that, "One of the most marked physical characteristics of female prisoners in the General Prison for Scotland is the luxuriant heads of hair which they have." At that time, physicians emphasised the importance of these inherited characteristics, including hairstyle, with such focus that most presumed that many individuals would become mad and criminal simply by virtue of their bodily characteristics. In consequence, Thomson (1870a, p. 488) regarded mental illness and criminality not only as inherited but, also, as "*incurable*". Few psychiatric researchers ever dared to consider whether early *childhood events* might have contributed to the development of either madness or violence at all.

In the nineteenth century, psychiatrists regarded lunatics, especially *dangerous* lunatics, not only as genetically predisposed to madness and to violence and, moreover, as incurable, but they offered virtually no treatment whatsoever, merely punishment. When, in 1872, Arthur O'Connor, a seventeen-year-old youngster, pointed a pistol at none other than the British monarch, Queen Victoria, the physicians diagnosed him as suffering from a hereditary taint; and one

Baron Anthony Cleasby, the presiding judge in this lad's trial, sentenced him to one year's imprisonment as well as twenty strokes from a birch, before committing him to an asylum (Geary, 1990). In point of fact, not only did physicians prioritise punishment over treatment, but, moreover, many leading psychiatrists at the time had virtually no hesitation about expressing their hatred in print towards forensic patients, including none other than the aforementioned Dr. John Gray, the editor of *The American Journal of Insanity*, who dismissed a certain forensic female, Mrs. Elizabeth Heggie, who had poisoned her two daughters, as little more than "cross, irritable, ugly, and repulsive" (Anonymous, 1868, p. 20). Mrs. Heggie would be sentenced to death and then executed for her crime, having received no treatment of any kind.

Some of the rare humane psychiatrists, such Dr. John Conolly (1856), Consulting Physician to the Middlesex Lunatic Asylum in Hanwell, in the western part of London, campaigned against chaining naked patients to their hospital beds – a common practice at that point in time. And Dr. Edgar Sheppard (1867), the Medical Superintendent of the Male Department at the Colney Hatch Asylum, in Friern Barnet, in North London, recommended that violent patients should receive warm baths, cold douches to the head, one and a half drachms of Battley's sedative (a mixture of opium, calcium hydrate, alcohol, sherry, and water) in a pint of beef-tea, and that they should also be placed in a padded room with only a shirt and a mattress. The vast majority of physicians in the mid-nineteenth century and the late nineteenth century dismissed these forensic lunatics as mere sufferers from brain degenerationism (e.g., Clouston, 1870; Anonymous, 1871), and, thus, unable to be improved in any way.

The advancement of the concept of brain degenerationism and the championship of biopathological factors as causes of madness and violence has persisted across the ages; and, even nowadays, many scientific researchers and biopsychiatrists continue to conceptualise criminality as, first and foremost, a medical illness. For instance, Professor Charles Golden, an American neuropsychologist, and his colleagues have argued that violence might well result from prefrontal brain damage and from temporal lobe dysfunction (e.g., Golden, Jackson, Peterson-Rohne, and Gontkovsky, 1996), while Professor James Fallon (2013, p. 74), an American neuroscientist, has hypothesised that criminals suffer from a so-called inherited "warrior gene." And, moreover, the influential Professor Adrian Raine, a British-born, American-based psychologist and neurocriminologist, has undertaken positron emission tomography scans and, also, magnetic resonance imaging scans of the brains of numerous murderers. His investigations have revealed a range of abnormalities, including a decreased glucose metabolism in the lateral prefrontal cortex and medial prefrontal cortex (Raine, et al., 1994), as well as asymmetries in the amygdala, thalamus, and medial temporal lobe (Raine, Buchsbaum, and LaCasse, 1997). Raine and colleagues also discovered that those men diagnosed as suffering from antisocial personality disorder would be much more likely to reveal a reduction in the volume of grey matter in the prefrontal cortex (Raine, et al., 2000), as well as a bilateral reduction in the volume of the amygdala (Yang, et al., 2009; cf.

Raine, 2013). The impressive work of Professor Raine fails, however, to offer sufficient consideration of the possibility that brain asymmetries might actually result from early-life trauma and might thus be *correlational* to acts of violence, rather than primarily *causal*.

In view of the lengthy history of punishing, imprisoning, torturing, and executing criminals (whether or not those individuals deserved to be described as such), and in view of the multiple centuries of biologising violent offences as a sign of brain degenerationism, it makes great sense that so many of our ancestors and, indeed, our contemporaries, should dismiss forensic men and forensic women as damaged and untreatable and, therefore, unworthy of any investment of thought or care. Consequently, it would hardly surprise us that the aforementioned modern British prisoners "Mike" and "Rob", the stars of the podcast *Banged Up* – to whom I have referred in the previous chapter – should have had to spend their days and nights locked in prison cells contaminated by faeces with no opportunity for psychological understanding.

Fortunately, however, a tiny côterie of bold and pioneering individuals have dared to challenge this long-standing narrative of criminality as little more than a punishment by God or as a sign of a damaged brain.

SECTION TWO: THE FREUDIAN ROOTS OF FORENSIC PSYCHOTHERAPY

Across the ages, a handful of highly visionary individuals have endeavoured to approach the subject of crime from a more humane perspective. For instance, back in the mid-eighteenth century, a Milanese aristocrat, Cesare Bonesana di Beccaria – the son of a *marchese* – argued passionately for the abolition of the common practices of torturing and executing offenders. Signor Beccaria (1764, p. 138), who had trained as a lawyer, actually urged, "È meglio prevenire i delitti, che punirli." ["It is better to prevent crimes than to punish them."].

Likewise, one of Beccaria's British contemporaries, the London-born John Howard, who became High Sheriff in the county of Bedfordshire, undertook many prison inspections. Horrified by the dreadful conditions therein, Howard – a true public servant – lobbied for the provision of healthier diets for the inmates and even testified before the House of Commons about the disgusting state of English prisons (Grünhut, 1941; cf. Howard, 1958; Southwood, 1958; Radzinowicz, 1978). His work ultimately inspired the creation of the Howard Association, which eventually became transformed into the impactful Howard League for Penal Reform – an organisation which continues to flourish to the present day.

Not only did Beccaria in Italy, and Howard in England, champion a kinder approach to the management of criminality, but so, too, did the esteemed British novelist Charles Dickens (1842, p. 238), who, in 1842, exposed the cruelty of American prisons, reporting, "The system here, is rigid, strict, and hopeless solitary confinement. I believe it, in its effects, to be cruel and wrong." After encountering one of the convicts in an American prison, Dickens (1842, p. 242) revealed, "He is a man buried alive; to be dug out in the slow round of years; and in the mean time dead to everything but torturing anxieties and horrible despair."

However, in spite of these crucial and transformative critiques and campaigns, few individuals, in my estimation, offered a greater gift to our understanding of the phenomenology of violence, its aetiology, and its treatment, not to mention its prevention, than the founder of psychoanalysis himself, Professor Sigmund Freud.

Although Freud's own career in the world of forensics began rather inauspiciously, having failed his university examination – the *Rigorosum* – in forensic medicine (Freud, 1900a; cf. Jones, 1953), he eventually undertook an internship in France and attended the autopsies at the Morgue de Paris (Freud, 1886), hosted by the esteemed French physician, Professeur Paul Camille Hippolyte Brouardel (1897), who wrote extensively about the victims of violence, including those who had succumbed to infanticide.

Fortified by his studies in Paris not only with Paul Brouardel but, most especially, with the influential neurologist, Professeur Jean-Martin Charcot (1887), who enlightened this young Austrian doctor about the potential reversibility of mental disorders through such techniques as hypnosis, Freud returned to Vienna and challenged the cruelty of late-nineteenth-century European psychiatry, which consisted predominantly of electrical stimulation of the muscles (e.g., Newth, 1884), hydrotherapy (e.g., Freud, 1886, 1925a; cf. Steward, 2012; Large, 2015), hypnotism (e.g., von Krafft-Ebing, 1895), and, even genital surgery (e.g., Church, 1893; Sims, 1893), by pioneering what came to be known as the "talking cure" (quoted in Breuer, 1895, p. 23). Throughout the 1880s and 1890s, Freud developed an increasing awareness that, by encouraging free association and catharsis, through the hosting of unrestricted and confidential conversations, his neurotic patients would begin to improve from their often dramatic hysterical and obsessional symptoms and could then embark upon more pleasurable lives. And in 1896, Freud (1896a, p. 166) first published the word "psycho-analyse", in a French neurological journal.

Across his long and unparalleled career, Sigmund Freud bequeathed to us a rich legacy of clinical insights and beautifully crafted publications which have helped to elucidate the nature and causes of criminality in its many forms. One might argue that Freud's early recognition of the toxic reality of sexual abuse – generally ignored by most, if not all, of his contemporaries – helped to shed great light on the ways in which such trauma would contribute hugely to the development of psychopathology in its many forms. For instance, it will not be widely appreciated or remembered that when Dr. Theodor Reik, a young Viennese psychoanalyst, consulted Freud about an adult patient who perpetrated sexual offences, Freud pontificated most succinctly, "He must have been seduced as a child" (quoted in Natterson, 1966, p. 256).

Indeed, in terms of our understanding of paedophilia and other acts of sexual violence, Freud hypothesised that such patients may themselves have suffered similar assaults during their own upbringing (cf. Freud, 1905a; Anonymous, 1995; Kahr, 2010), which would then be re-enacted in later years; but, moreover, he noted, with much sagacity, that sexual crimes can be perpetrated not only by adults but, also, by children themselves. And in his essay on the aetiology of the neuroses, Freud observed,

> In seven out of the thirteen cases the intercourse was between children on both sides – sexual relations between a little girl and a boy a little older (most often her brother) who had himself been the victim of an earlier seduction. These relations sometimes continued for years, until the little guilty parties reached puberty; the boy would repeat the same practices with the little girl over and over again and without alteration – practices to which he himself had been subjected by some female servant or governess and which on account of their origin were often of a disgusting sort. In a few cases there was a combination of an assault and relations between children or a repetition of a brutal abuse (Freud, 1896b, p. 152).[1]

Thus, by foregrounding the aetiological role of sexual trauma in the genesis of adult paedophilia, Freud challenged the prevalent narrative of brain degenerationism and helped us all to understand the role of real-life invasions as a cause of sexual criminality.

Over the course of a long and impressive psychological career, Freud offered many insights into a plethora of clinical manifestations of forensic enactments, ranging from sexual perversity to violence (e.g., Freud, 1916, 1919, 1924a, 1925b, 1927a, 1930a, 1931a). Alas, we cannot do full justice to the enormity of Sigmund Freud's contributions to the field of forensic psychoanalysis, not least, his creation of the possibility that one might offer treatment, simply by talking and listening, and that one could discover the roots of criminality by investigating the deeper, unconscious regions of the human mind. But, in this brief encapsulation of Freud's forensic insights, let us recall that, in addition to having invented the "talking cure" and, also, having recognised that violence could well result from trauma and abuse, Freud also communicated boldly about the need to treat offenders with greater humanity. As I have already mentioned in the "Series Editor's Foreword" to this collection of essays, as early as 6th February, 1907, Freud spoke to a group of colleagues in Vienna, Austria, expressing his consternation about the "unsinnige Behandlung dieser Leute (soweit sie Demenz zeigen) in Gefängnissen" (quoted in Rank, 1907a, p. 101), namely, the "nonsensical treatment of these people in prisons (in so far as they are demented)" (quoted in Rank, 1907b, p. 108).

Furthermore, and perhaps of greatest importance, Freud underscored that we simply cannot attribute human violence to merely a small handful of convicted offenders. On the contrary, according to Freud (1900a, p. 176), every single man, woman, and child possesses the psychological capability of harbouring a "Todeswunsch", namely, a "death wish", and that although most of us will, thankfully, develop a sufficiently sturdy ego structure which will reduce the likelihood of enacting these unconscious death wishes, each person still possesses the capacity for murderousness. Moreover, Freud noted, those of us whom we might describe as honourable, law-abiding citizens will often derive much pleasure from treating our criminal neighbours with great hostility as an unconscious means of projecting our own sadism into others. In 1931, Freud lamented to Professor Georg Fuchs, a German political dissident,

> I could not subscribe to the assertion that the treatment of convicted prisoners is a disgrace to our civilization. On the contrary, a voice would tell me, it is in perfect harmony with our civilization, a necessary expression of the brutality and lack of understanding which dominate the civilized humanity of the present time (Freud, 1931c, p. 252).[2]

Freud certainly came to appreciate that murderousness lurks in the heart and soul of every human being, but that by articulating these ugly, painful feelings, one might be less inclined to enact them. For that very reason, he underscored to his American analysand, the psychiatrist Dr. Joseph Wortis (1940), that when a patient enters treatment, he or she must reveal everything to the psychoanalyst, including theft, treachery and, even, murder.

From an organisational perspective, Freud undertook unique work by rallying and cultivating a group of colleagues and by creating both a local Wiener Psychoanalytische Vereinigung [Vienna Psycho-Analytical Society], founded in 1908, and an Internationale Psychoanalytische Vereinigung [International Psycho-Analytical Association], established in 1910, as well as innumerable journals. In doing so, he engineered an entirely new profession of psychotherapy and psychoanalysis, and, ultimately, sponsored formalised training programmes based on in-depth, multi-frequency personal analysis, clinical seminars, and supervision. Freud focused his energies on every single aspect of human psychology; and, in view of these extensive, unparalleled tasks and undertakings, he devoted little time, alas, to the specific enhancement of a psychodynamically informed *forensic* mental health community. He did, however, write at length about the subject, and he did foster relationships with those who specialised in forensic medicine. For instance, in 1930, the father of psychoanalysis hosted visits at his home with Professor Nerio Rojas, from Buenos Aires, in Argentina (Freud, 1930b), and with Professor Gregorio Berman from Córdoba in Spain (Freud, 1930c). Likewise, he engaged in a correspondence with the English physician, Dr. Grace Pailthorpe (Freud, 1933), who had recently produced a report on behalf of the Medical Research Council, arguing instead for the use of Freudian psychoanalysis in the treatment of criminals (Pailthorpe, 1932). And, moreover, he exchanged missives with Señor Raúl Carrancá y Trujillo, a Mexican judge who attempted to psychoanalyse offenders, investigating their dreams, their slips of the tongue, and their sexual fantasies (Gallo, 2012). In this regard, Freud not only helped to establish the profession of psychoanalysis but, also, he devoted true energy to the facilitation of an informal cluster of forensic colleagues.

Regrettably, due to his metastasising maxillofacial cancer, first diagnosed in 1923, and to his hatred of the United States of America, Freud (1924b, 1924c) turned down a unique opportunity to travel to Chicago, Illinois, to serve as an expert witness in the trial of two teenage offenders, Nathan Leopold, Jr. and Richard Loeb, who had kidnapped and then murdered a fourteen-year-old boy, Bobby Franks, by having bashed his skull brutally with a chisel (e.g., Baatz, 2008). Had Freud accepted this lucrative offer (Seldes, 1953), he might well have advanced the burgeoning field of forensic psychoanalysis more efficaciously, as that trial would attract immense press attention. However, Sigmund Freud could not be omnipotent, and we simply cannot expect this overburdened man to have advanced every single sub-field of human psychology to its maximum potentiality during his own lifetime.

Needless to say, not all members of the mental health community have embraced the work of Sigmund Freud. For instance, Professor David Canter (1994, p. 21), widely regarded by many as the most distinguished forensic psychologist in the United Kingdom, dismissed the creator of psychoanalysis as little more than "fanciful" and as someone who has burdened us with "ever more elaborate accounts of the underlying mechanisms" (Canter, 1994, p. 216) of human behaviour. But, many of us would disagree with Professor Canter's assessment, and, by contrast, we experience much gratitude toward Sigmund Freud not only for alerting us to the fact that criminals will have endured traumatic childhoods but, also, for advocating that psychoanalytical treatment might help to alleviate distress and, even, severe psychopathology.

Freud also taught us much about the necessity of compassion towards every single patient. In 1934, he explained to his American analysand, the aforementioned Joseph Wortis, "We are not here to judge, not even if you were a criminal" (quoted in Wortis, 1934a, p. 55).

Thus, Freud became, in my estimation, the veritable grandfather of the discipline that we would now describe as forensic psychotherapy.

SECTION THREE: TOWARDS A PROFESSION OF FORENSIC PSYCHOTHERAPY

Post-Freudian Colleagues

In addition to his many unique contributions to the development of depth psychology, Sigmund Freud became a source of great inspiration as a pedagogue who encouraged colleagues and students to expand his work in numerous ways. As early as 1907, Freud's young disciple, Dr. Fritz Wittels, presented a paper in Vienna about the underlying role of repressed sexuality in the case of Tatjana Leontieva, a Russian woman who had murdered a Tsarist official (Rank, 1907c). And, in 1912, another early Viennese comrade, Alfred Freiherr von Winterstein (1912), recommended that psychoanalytical practitioners should not confine their investigations to the consulting room but should, in fact, endeavour to apply Freud's insights to such diverse fields as art, linguistics, morality, mythology, pedagogy, religion, sociology, and, moreover, criminology.

Perhaps Herr August Aichhorn deserves our greatest appreciation as the first psychoanalyst since Freud to have made a truly immense contribution to the study of forensic mental health. Aichhorn devoted many years to the treatment of delinquent youngsters who perpetrated crimes, ranging from theft to sexual perversions, including male prostitution (Mohr, 1966). In his noted monograph about the psychology of delinquency, Aichhorn (1925) underscored the heart-breaking role of trauma in the genesis of acts of criminality. For instance, Aichhorn traced the delinquent behaviour of one of his patients to the very fact that this young vagrant lad had lost his father at the age of twelve years, and then, two years thereafter, his mother had died, whilst working in a factory, viciously mangled in a dangerous machine. Based on his copious clinical experience, Aichhorn reported that psychological traumata, such as gross bereavement, formed the very backbone of delinquent behaviour. Whereas most authorities at that time recommended that punishments such as enforced labour might well be the very best treatment for criminal youths, Aichhorn (1932) offered residential care and psychological interventions, inspired by the work of Freud himself.

Psychoanalytical insights into violence soon progressed from Vienna in Austria to Budapest in Hungary, and, in 1913, Dr. Sándor Ferenczi, one of Freud's closest comrades, campaigned for more humane treatment of prisoners and even dared to speak openly about abuses committed by the prison guards themselves. He strongly championed the application of psychoanalysis to the study of perpetrators (Ferenczi, 1919a, 1922), so much so that one of his Hungarian juniors, Dr. Franz Alexander, extended Ferenczi's approach and, together with the criminologist Dr. Hugo Staub, began to teach arguably the world's first formal course on forensic psychology, foregrounding the need for "einer psychoanalytischen Kriminologie" (Alexander and Staub, 1929, p. [5]) – "a psycho-analytical criminology" – critiquing the crude biologisation of offenders as mere degenerated souls and arguing for the dissemination of psychoanalytical forms of treatment. This work became impactful in Germany, and, by the early 1930s, the contributions of Alexander had actually helped to inaugurate a psychological presence in the courtroom (Zilboorg, 1931). As the decades unfolded, Franz Alexander continued to lobby for a more psychologically orientated approach to violent offenders. Indeed, as we have already noted, Alexander, in collaboration with the French princess and psychoanalyst, Marie Bonaparte, and with the Los Angeles-based psychiatrist and psychoanalyst, Dr. Isadore Ziferstein, petitioned Edmund Brown, the Governor of California, to release a convicted rapist and kidnapper, Caryl Chessman, from being executed, albeit, alas, without success (Bertin, 1982).

As a result of the work of these Viennese and Hungarian psychoanalysts, the Freudian approach to criminality began to spread far and wide. For instance, in 1925, the founder of the psychoanalytical movement in India, Dr. Girindrasekhar Bose, lectured to the parliament in Calcutta about the ways in which depth-psychological insights could enhance our understanding of violence (Anonymous, 1926). In due course, Bose began to teach a course on crime at a school for Indian detectives (Hartnack, 2001), arguing that early intervention might help to prevent future disasters (Bose, 1945). Likewise, Dr. Juan Ramón Beltrán pioneered the use of Freudian psychotherapy in a prison in Argentina (Abraham, 1924); whilst Dr. Clara Lazar-Geroe (1942) offered psychoanalytical instruction to the Children's Court Probation Officers in Melbourne, Australia.

Alas, we certainly cannot do full justice to the wide range of achievements in the burgeoning field of forensic psychoanalysis which began to emerge across the globe, particularly during the 1920s and 1930s, and which featured contributions from such pioneers as Dr. Maurice Hamblin Smith (1924), an early Associate Member of the British Psycho-Analytical Society who worked at His Majesty's Prison Winson Green in Birmingham, as well as Dr. John Holland Cassity (1927), a psychoanalyst who treated patients in the criminal department at St. Elizabeths Hospital[3] in Washington, D.C., and who traced acts of paedophilic violence to early infantile trauma. And we must, of course, recall the remarkable efforts of Dr. Edward Glover, a Scottish-born, German-trained pioneer of psychoanalysis, who helped to launch The Association for the Scientific Treatment of Delinquency and Crime, an organisation which would eventually be rebranded as The Institute for the Scientific Treatment of Delinquency and, ultimately, as the Institute for the Study and Treatment of Delinquency (Rumney, 1992), which offered psychotherapy to those who perpetrated acts of criminality. Glover not only enlisted the cooperation of colleagues from the British Psycho-Analytical Society to participate in the running of this new psycho-criminological institution (*Institute Board Meetings: 16.1.1925 to 30.4.1945*, 1925–1945) but, also, he helped to develop the psychologically orientated periodical, *The British Journal of Delinquency*.

The growth of forensic psychoanalysis continued intergenerationally. Two of Glover's most esteemed trainees at London's Institute of Psycho-Analysis, namely, Dr. John Bowlby and Dr. Donald Winnicott, followed in the footsteps of their teacher, and each made even more iconic contributions to the field. Bowlby (1944a, 1944b, 1945–1946, 1946) did so by having undertaken systematic clinical research which demonstrated the role of early childhood loss in the genesis of juvenile delinquency. As Bowlby (1944b, p. 126) urged, "Well-trained play-analysts must be provided to give treatment. Medicine must step in and cure these cases long before they are even eligible to come before a Court of Law."

Winnicott undertook constant work with evacuated children during the Second World War and documented the ways in which parental separation contributed to the surge of juvenile violence (Winnicott and Britton, 1947; cf. Winnicott, 1943, 1945; Winnicott and Britton, 1944). After the war, Winnicott (1949c) urged British government ministers to recognise criminality as a form of psychological illness. And boldly, Winnicott, along with several of his colleagues at the Institute of Psycho-Analysis, argued for the abolition of the death penalty in Great Britain and actually wrote to the Royal Commission on Capital Punishment, critiquing this approach and underscoring that the threat of being executed by the state might even entice some people to commit murder (*Memorandum Submitted by the Institute of Psycho-Analysis to the Royal Commission on Capital Punishment*, 1950).

Indeed, Winnicott championed psychoanalytical insights as a means of providing a better understanding of destructive behaviours. In a letter to the editor of *The Times* newspaper, Winnicott (1949b, p. 15), reflecting upon the "knotty problem of crime and insanity" among juveniles, underscored,

> It is very seldom that the comments of a psycho-analyst are asked for or printed; instead it is assumed that the psychologist has an attitude, probably a sentimental one. The idea that psycho-analysis has no attitude, but that it can enlighten, seldom percolates (Winnicott, 1949b, p. 15).

Donald Winnicott (1956, p. 306) might best be remembered for his encapsulation of what he came to refer to as "the antisocial tendency", explaining that juvenile criminality derives from early experiences of deprivation. In his exploration of the case of a little boy called "John", Winnicott investigated the childhood origins of John's episodes of theft and, moreover, he hypothesised that stealing might well represent not only an aggressive act but, also, most surprisingly perhaps, an expression of *hope* – an indication that a youngster recognises theft as a means of communicating early deprivation as well as a desire to restore one's lost psychic nutrients. Indeed, in his stand-out essay on "The Antisocial Tendency", Winnicott described how he had consulted to John's mother in order to help her better understand the roots of her young son's offending behaviour. As Winnicott (1956, p. 307) explained to John's mother, "'Why not tell him that you know that when he steals he is not wanting the things that he steals but he is looking for something that he has a right to: that he is making a claim on his mother and father because he feels deprived of their love.' I told her to use language which he could understand." John's mother absorbed Winnicott's thinking on this matter, and she began to discuss the problem with her son. She wrote to Winnicott sometime later that, "I told him that what he really wanted when he stole money and food and things was his mum; and I must say I didn't really expect him to understand, but he did seem to. I asked him if he thought we didn't love him because he was so naughty sometimes, and he said right out that he didn't think we did, much. Poor little scrap! I felt so awful, I can't tell you." (quoted in Winnicott, 1956, p. 307).

Thus, following in Freud's footsteps, Winnicott endeavoured to facilitate the "talking cure" with his delinquent child patients and, moreover, with their parents as well, in an effort to offer greater insight and containment. Indeed, in 1962, he spoke about crime to the National Association of Probation Officers and produced several short publications about psychoanalysis and delinquency (Winnicott, 1962a, 1962b, 1962–1963, cf. Winnicott, 1966). And then, in 1967, he delivered an address to the Borstal Assistant Governors' Conference at King Alfred's College in Winchester, in the English county of Hampshire, on "Delinquency as a Sign of Hope" – a stellar paper which would eventually appear in the *Prison Service Journal*, and would thus be read by many probation officers (Winnicott, 1968).

Certainly, Donald Winnicott drew upon his own clinical experiences as a wartime child psychiatrist; but, moreover, he had already incorporated the pioneering forensic contributions of Sigmund Freud, who had long ago come to recognise the importance of early childhood experiences in the development of violent fantasies. In his essay on "Psycho-Analysis and the Sense of Guilt", delivered in honour of Freud's centenary, Winnicott (1958, pp. 31–32) argued that, "More than anyone else it was Freud who paved the way for the understanding of antisocial behaviour and of crime as a *sequel* to an unconscious criminal intention, and a symptom of a failure in child-care." This crisp summary aptly highlights the major ideas espoused by Freud, namely, that crime and perversion originate in the nursery. Indeed, Winnicott always encouraged violent children to transform their unprocessed emotions into language, just as Freud had done. In fact, when, in 1969, a colleague wrote to Winnicott, asking for advice on how to handle children who might use foul language, the great child psychoanalyst replied, "How much nicer is hate than murder and how silly we are if we mind when children scream out 'fuck' and other obscenities" (Winnicott, 1969b; cf. Kahr, 1998b).

John Bowlby and Donald Winnicott did not collaborate extensively, in spite of the tremendous similarity in their work. They did, however, co-publish a brief letter in the *British Medical Journal*, shortly after the onset of the Second World War in 1939, in collaboration with a fellow child psychiatrist, Dr. Emanuel Miller. Collectively, these three psychologically astute physicians expressed tremendous concern about the plans to evacuate British children to the countryside, in order to avoid bombings. Although such separation from mothers and fathers might be wise at one level, these men worried about the impact of painful, broken attachments, which, they knew only too well, would place evacuated children at greater risk of developing juvenile delinquent behaviours, which often form the basis of criminality in adult life. As they underscored,

> If these opinions are correct it follows that evacuation of small children without their mothers can lead to very serious and widespread psychological disorder. For instance, it can lead to a big increase in juvenile delinquency in the next decade (Bowlby, Miller, and Winnicott, 1939, p. 1203).

Although the contributions of such impactful figures as Bowlby and Winnicott remain seminal in contemporary mental health practice (e.g., Kahr, 2001c, 2015b, 2019c, 2019d, 2022c, 2024a), the work of many other originators during the first half of the twentieth century has become completely repressed... and lamentably so. For instance, in 1933, Dr. Vernon Branham, a disciple of the early American psychoanalyst Dr. William Alanson White, helped to create the Section of Psychiatry of the American Psychiatric Association, which boasted a psychoanalytical lens; and, some six years later, in 1939, Branham became the founding editor of the *Journal of Criminal Psychopathology* (Overholser, 1952) – the first exclusively forensic psychoanalytical periodical – which, regrettably, ceased publication after a short period of time. In similar vein, a much-overlooked British physician,

Dr. John Charsley Mackwood (1949, 1954), became one of the very first practitioners to offer not only individual psychodynamic psychotherapy but, also, group psychotherapy in prison settings.

The Welldonian Era

It saddens me that, due to restrictions of space, we cannot provide a more detailed analysis of all of the many great disciples of Sigmund Freud who contributed to the foundations of forensic psychotherapy in such creative ways, whether Mrs. Melanie Klein (1932a), who argued that early intervention through child psychoanalytical treatment can reduce the likelihood of criminality in later life, to Dr. Ismond Rosen (1964a), who published one of the first forensic textbooks on the psychodynamics of sexual deviation, to Dr. Murray Cox (1992a, 1992b, 2001) and Dr. Leslie Sohn, both of whom pioneered the practice of psychotherapy in a maximum-secure unit setting. We warmly await fuller histories of our field (e.g., Kahr, 2018c, 2020b, 2022d).

But since the death of Sigmund Freud, no one will have enriched this body of knowledge as much as the esteemed Argentinian-born, British-based psychiatrist, psychotherapist, and group analyst, Profesora Estela Welldon, who, inspired by her mentor, Professor Karl Menninger (1968) – noted for his description of punishment as a crime in and of itself – became the veritable founder of the more formalised profession of forensic psychotherapy. Over more than *seven* decades, Welldon has made innumerable contributions to the expansion of forensic psychotherapeutic theory and practice and to the growth of our community of colleagues.

It will, of course, be widely known that Welldon challenged certain orthodoxies within the forensic psychoanalytical team at the Portman Clinic in London, where she worked as a National Health Service Consultant for many years, including the notion that only men could perpetrate sexual perversions. Welldon (1988, 1991, 1996, 2001, 2011, 2012) broke new ground by helping us to appreciate that mothers can assault their babies and young children, just as readily as fathers do, and that women will also be at high risk of attacking their own bodies in a violent manner through endangerment, self-mutilation, and a host of other self-inflicted atrocities. In this respect, Welldon reconfigured the traditional conceptualisation of the criminal as a violent man. Moreover, Welldon (n.d. [1985], 1993, 2001) questioned not only the genderisation of forensic psychology but, also, its treatment, and helped to pioneer both the use of traditional, classical, one-to-one psychoanalytical psychotherapy and, most helpfully, the deployment of group psychotherapy.

Over the decades, this remarkable woman has shared her knowledge with great generosity, not only through her copious teaching and lecturing but, also, in many publications, including her now classic tome, *Mother, Madonna, Whore: The Idealization and Denigration of Motherhood* (Welldon, 1988). Other memorable Welldonian titles include such masterpieces as *Sadomasochism* (Welldon, 2002); *Playing with Dynamite: A Personal Approach to the Psychoanalytic Understanding of Perversions, Violence, and Criminality* (Welldon, 2011); *Sadomasochism in Art and Politics* (Welldon, 2016), not to mention the playful and blunt *Sex Now Talk Later* (Welldon, 2017), and, furthermore, her wonderful collection of essays, *A Practical Guide to Forensic Psychotherapy*, co-edited by Dr. Cleo Van Velsen (Welldon and Van Velsen, 1997).

But Estela Welldon has illuminated the field of forensic mental health not only through her clinical and scholarly contributions but, moreover, by having created, *inter alia*, the very first formalised training programmes in forensic psychotherapy. During her tenure at the Portman Clinic in London, Welldon launched a specialist certificate course as well as a diploma course in forensic psychotherapy, which, thanks to her collaboration with the distinguished director of the British Postgraduate Medical Federation, Professor Sir Michael Peckham, eventually received validation by the Faculty of Clinical Science at University College London in the University of London (Kahr, 2021e). Furthermore, she inaugurated the International Association for Forensic Psychotherapy – an organisation now more than thirty years of age – as well as our increasingly influential publication, *The International Journal of Forensic Psychotherapy*, for which she serves as Founding Editor.

By having undertaken such important institutional achievements, in addition to her many clinical discoveries, Welldon has very much followed in the footsteps of none other than Freud, who, alongside his own creation of the theory of the unconscious mind and the invention of psychoanalytical treatment, also crafted organisational structures and training programmes, without which, none of our "talking cure" professions would exist to this very day. Clearly, Estela Welldon deserves our appreciation as the veritable Sigmund Freud of forensic mental health.

It will be of no surprise that, in recognition of these remarkable achievements, the American Psychoanalytic Association elected her as an honorary member, the British Psychoanalytic Council presented her with a lifetime achievement award (Kahr, 2019f, 2019g, 2020d) and, moreover, Oxford Brookes University bequeathed upon her an honorary doctoral degree, presented by none other than Sir Louis Blom-Cooper, Q.C., the distinguished lawyer and judge (Kahr, 2000a).

Thanks to the inspiration of Profesora Welldon, many of her former students – now quite experienced practitioners – have undertaken similar groundbreaking work, helping to create or lead various professional organisations, such as the Forensic Psychotherapy Society in the United Kingdom (Kirtchuk, Gordon, Doctor, and Ingram, 2016), or book series, such as the "Forensic Psychotherapy Monograph Series" (originally produced by Karnac Books of London and subsequently published by Routledge / Taylor and Francis Group of London and of Abingdon in Oxfordshire). Moreover, through the role-modelling provided so generously by Estela Welldon, the Royal College of Psychiatrists launched a Forensic Psychotherapy Special Interest Group. Additionally, the British Psychoanalytic Council validated the professional title of "Forensic Psychodynamic Psychotherapist", which has become recognised by the Professional Standards Authority for Health and Social Care. And, in 2016, the University of London awarded a special post, namely that of Professor of Forensic Psychotherapy and Medical Education, to

Dr. Gill McGauley, one of Welldon's most esteemed students, who, alas, passed away, shortly after having assumed that vital new role (Adshead, 2016).

Perhaps of greatest importance, Estela Welldon's daring work as a clinician and as a teacher in the field of forensic psychotherapy has encouraged her many one-time students and trainees and mentees to publish clinical works of their own, helping us to appreciate more fully the psychodynamics of murder, of paedophilia, of rape, of arson, of infanticide, and of criminality in all its many forms (e.g., Kahr, 2001b, 2001c, 2018d, 2019e, 2021c, 2021d; Minne, 2008, 2009; Motz, 2008, 2009, 2014; Curen, 2009, 2018; Corbett, 2014; Collier, 2015, 2019; Stewart, 2016a, 2016b, 2019; Adshead, 2018; Doctor, 2018; Adshead and Horne, 2021). And some have even inaugurated special new projects, designed to introduce greater humanity into the care of imprisoned, incarcerated offender patients (Minne and Kassman, 2018). Those of us who had the privilege to study with Welldon directly will have gained an immense amount of bravery and potency, owing to the fact that this blue-sky woman helped us all to speak more fully and more directly about this important work, devoted to the humanisation of the dehumanised (Kahr, 2018b).

Through the encouragement of Welldon, various sub-fields within forensic psychotherapy have emerged, not least what I have come to refer to as *"forensic disability psychotherapy"* (Kahr, 2014a, p. xix), namely, the championship of the talking therapies in the treatment of those offenders who have long struggled with handicaps and intellectual disabilities and, also, brain damage (e.g., Kahr, 2004a, 2019e, 2020a, 2021c; Curen, 2009, 2018; Sinason, 2012). Indeed, the late Dr. Alan Corbett (2014) even managed to write a whole book about forensic disability psychotherapy, prior to his own untimely death, entitled *Disabling Perversions: Forensic Psychotherapy with People with Intellectual Disabilities*, which, happily, appeared in the "Forensic Psychotherapy Monograph Series".

Not long ago, I had the privilege of communicating with Profesora Estela Welldon about *how* and *why* she devoted so much of her creative energy to the inauguration of a new branch of mental health care. Welldon (2021) spoke with great passion and underscored how, back in the 1960s, both the British criminal justice system and the psychiatric community restricted themselves to the task of *judging* and *dismissing* forensic patients. Tragically, no one ever dared to *understand* the patients. By having launched the field of forensic psychotherapy, Estela Welldon has helped us to transform our profession from groups of workers who had once marginalised these troubled people, to those who, at long last, endeavour to comprehend such struggling individuals in a truly profound and compassionate manner.

SECTION FOUR: CONCLUSION

Since the preliminary forays of Sigmund Freud, and in the wake of the researches of such pioneers as Franz Alexander, Edward Glover, Estela Welldon, and others, numerous visionary colleagues have made remarkable contributions to the study of forensic psychotherapy. Alas, we cannot pay tribute to all of the amazing work which has ensued, and it will be my hope that many more histories of this discipline will be written in years to come, documenting these amazing achievements (Kahr, 2018c, 2020b).

To quote but one example of visionary work, which unfolded at the Tavistock Clinic in North-West London, only feet away from Estela Welldon's long-standing headquarters at the Portman Clinic, the esteemed Dr. Eileen Vizard, a British forensic child psychiatrist and psychoanalyst, established the Young Abusers Project in 1992, in collaboration with the National Children's Home, the National Society for the Prevention of Cruelty to Children and, also, the United Kingdom's Department of Health, arranging for psychotherapeutic assessment and treatment of both child and adolescent sexual perpetrators. Vizard, with whom I had the privilege of working, endeavoured to engage in prevention, by identifying those youngsters at highest risk of offending, and then providing in-depth psychoanalytical psychotherapy as a means of reducing the likelihood of future assaults (e.g., Mezey, Vizard, Hawkes, and Austin, 1991; Vizard, Monck, and Misch, 1995; Vizard, et al., 1996; Vizard, 1997; Woods, 1997; Kahr, 2004a, 2020a). The Young Abusers Project offered interventions to large numbers of young criminals with great success, forestalling many potential violent attacks. In recognition of her leadership of this pioneering project, Vizard became a Commander of the Most Excellent Order of the British Empire.

Needless to say, we must find more ways to acknowledge the extraordinary work of a whole range of other individuals from multiple disciplines who have toiled with such brilliance, and who have thus contributed to our field, whether the late Professor Flora Rheta Schreiber (1983), who authored the most detailed psychoanalytical study of the early traumatic childhood of a multiple murderer; whether the late Mr. Lloyd deMause (1973, 1974, 1982, 1984, 1991, 2002a, 2002b, 2006, 2012a, 2012b), who pioneered the field of psychohistory and the application of psychoanalysis to the study of global warfare; whether the late Professor Rudolph Binion (1975, 1976), who produced riveting studies of Adolf Hitler's early years – one of many such vital volumes (e.g., Langer, 1972; Bromberg and Small, 1983); or whether such impressive contemporary colleagues as Professor James Gilligan (1996, 2001, 2016), whose extraordinary work on the role of shame in the aetiology of violence deserves widespread dissemination (cf. Iremonger, 1970, 1984; Abse, 1973, 1989, 1994, 1996; Coleman, 1985; Miller, 1988, 1998).

For those of us devoted to the emerging disciplines of forensic psychotherapy and forensic psychoanalysis, we should derive great comfort that we now boast not only national and international membership organisations, a book series, a journal, and several training courses worldwide, but, also, of greatest importance, a creative consortium of clinical colleagues who have implemented remarkably forward-thinking treatments and interventions of many shapes and sizes.

Thankfully, due to the humanity which accompanies depth psychology, we no longer inhabit a world in which the punishment and torture and execution of ancient and medieval times have remained the gold standard.

Let us recall that, nearly a millennium ago, back in thirteenth-century Staffordshire, in the West Midlands region of England, a man called Hugo committed an act of theft and, in consequence, the authorities arranged for him to have his head cut off as an appropriate punishment. Unsurprisingly, Hugo's wife, Matilda, no doubt consumed with rage and fear, responded to her husband's execution by then murdering her three children not long thereafter (JUST 1/802 (Staffs. 1272), m. 46 dorse, n.d.). Sadly, we know, only too well, that violence breeds violence.

Happily, the narrative of the forensic psychotherapy movement has endeavoured to reverse the notion of punishment as the best form of treatment. Nowadays, if a man such as Hugo engaged in an act of theft, we would hope to offer him psychotherapy in a prison setting or, better yet, to identify Hugo, whilst still a school child, as a youngster at risk who might benefit from some variety of psychological assistance.

Regrettably, in spite of the growing availability of forensic psychotherapy, not all institutions provide much-needed talking cures. As we know, a very large percentage of psychiatric hospitals and prison services ply their inmates with heavy dosages of medication, such as antipsychotic agents, antidepressants, mood stabilisers, benzodiazepines, adrenergic blockers, stimulants, and opiate antagonists (Stahl and Morrissette, 2014), or will respond, predominantly, with neglect. And many of those incarcerated still endure rape and other sexual assaults by fellow inmates, whilst under lock and key (Starchild, 1990), or will continue to perpetrate acts of violence upon fellow residents (Walker and Seifert, 1994) or, indeed, upon staff members themselves (van Leeuwen and Harte, 2017). No wonder the aforementioned Alisa Roth (2018, p. 11), who undertook an extensive survey of the American prison system, lamented, "we continue to treat people with mental illness almost exactly as we did before electricity was invented, before women had the right to vote, and before the abolition of slavery."

As colleagues will know only too well, if we do not offer modern psychotherapeutic treatments to forensic patients, both during incarceration and, also, *beforehand*, through early intervention, we will never witness a decrease in global violence during our lifetime. Indeed, as we appreciate, if we avoid psychological work and continue to neglect our forensic patients and forensic prisoners, we will all endure the horrific fall-out of recidivism (Seruca and Silva, 2015), which, according to a report from the Bureau of Justice Statistics of the United States Department of Justice, estimated that some eighty-three per cent of prisoners released from their cells will be rearrested and reincarcerated on at least one occasion, if not more, over the next nine years (Alper, Durose, and Markman, 2018; cf. Yukhnenko, Sridhar, and Fazel, 2019).

In spite of the long and ugly history of human violence, and of the management of cruelty through the perpetration of even *more* violence, we now possess a special vaccination to prevent its further spread, namely, psychotherapy and psychoanalysis, in many shapes and forms. As colleagues will appreciate, the Freudian method of the "talking cure" has aroused much suspicion over the decades, especially in the forensic world. Back in 1936, the esteemed psychiatrist Dr. William Norwood East (1936, p. 320), then His Majesty's Commissioner of Prisoners and Director of Convict Prisons in Great Britain, as well as Lecturer on Crime and Insanity at the Maudsley Hospital, part of the University of London, vocalised his concerns that forensic patients might be subjected to "hours of compulsory association with a Freudian investigator." Three years later, Dr. Eric Strauss (1939, p. 167), a Physician for Psychological Medicine and a Lecturer in Psychological Medicine at St. Bartholomew's Hospital in London, campaigned against the emergence of so-called "Over-enthusiastic psychotherapists".

Had Estela Welldon endeavoured to launch the International Association for Forensic Psychotherapy at St. Bartholomew's Hospital back in 1939, I suspect that the inaugural conference might never have materialised, owing to the incomparable hatred towards psychoanalysis at that period of time. Thankfully, in 1992, due to Welldon's young colleague, Dr. Timothy Scannell, a psychoanalytically sympathetic Consultant Psychiatrist who worked at St. Bartholomew's Hospital, this vital organisation came to life in the most encouraging of manners (Kahr, 2011b) and has continued to expand over more than thirty years.

Forensic psychotherapy might well be the best "*psychological vaccine*" (Kahr, 2021a, p. 128) against lethal global violence and, thankfully, we know that it works extremely well. Now all we have to do is administer the jabs.

Notes

1 The original French passage reads: "Sept fois sur treize il s'agissait d'une liaison infantile des deux côtés, de rapports sexuels entre une petite fille et un garçon un peu plus âgé, le plus souvent son frère, et lui-même victime d'une séduction antérieure. Ces liaisons s'étaient continuées quelquefois pendant des années jusqu'à la puberté des petits coupables, le garçon répétant toujours et sans innovation sur la petite fille les mêmes pratiques, qu'il avait subi lui-même de la part d'une servante ou gouvernante, et qui pour cause de cette origine étaient souvent de nature dégoutante. Dans quelques cas il y avait concurrence d'attentat et de liaison infantile, ou abus brutal réitéré" (Freud, 1896a, p. 167).

2 The original German sentence reads: "Ich könnte zum Beispiel den Satz nicht unterschreiben, daß die Behandlung der Strafgefangenen eine Schande für unsere Kultur ist. Im Gegenteil, würde mir eine Stimme sagen: sie ist ganz in Einklang mit unserer Kultur, notwendige Äußerung der Brutalität und des Unverstandes, die die gegenwärtige Kulturmenschheit beherrschen" (Freud, 1931b, p. x).

3 The title of this institution, St. Elizabeths Hospital, does not contain an apostrophe in the word "Elizabeths"; hence, we have rendered the spelling correctly from an historical perspective.

2

Explosive Patients

Surviving Petrifying Psychotherapeutic Experiences

BOMBS IN THE HISTORY OF PSYCHOANALYSIS

Throughout the twentieth century, psychoanalysts had to negotiate bombs on far too many occasions across two world wars.

During the *Weltkrieg* of 1914 to 1918, many practitioners of psychoanalysis had to treat the survivors of horrific bombings. For instance, Dr. Karl Abraham, the leader of the German psychoanalytical community, wrote very chillingly about his work with those soldiers who suffered from shell explosions. In his essay on the war neuroses, Abraham (1919) described a soldier who, in 1914, endured multiple attacks and who had even lapsed into unconsciousness for two days after a bombing, which he survived. Other soldiers with whom Abraham consulted succumbed to organic injuries due to severe bodily attacks, including one man who, in consequence, could no longer retain either urine or faeces. Heartbreakingly, Abraham also consulted to young children, such as a twelve-year-old boy who developed a severe phobic reaction to daily air raids.

Decades later, the Second World War provided clinical practitioners of psychoanalysis with far more direct experience of bombings.

In September, 1939, shortly after the declaration of war in Europe, the eighty-three-year-old Professor Sigmund Freud, then battling carcinoma, had to be moved to a special "'safe' zone" (Schur, 1972, p. 527) in his home at 20, Maresfield Gardens, in North-West London, away from the windows (Young-Bruehl, 1988), in order to protect him from air raids. Certainly, as someone who had survived the first *Weltkrieg* – namely, the Great War of 1914 to 1918 – he understood only too well the potential of being bombed on British soil; but he died on 23rd September, 1939, long before the full horror of the Nazi *Blitzkrieg* (Woon, 1941; Stansky, 2007; Grayzel, 2012; Ward, 2015).

Miss Anna Freud, the youngest child of the father of psychoanalysis, had to navigate a much more prolonged relationship with bombs. During the Second World War, she and her intimate friend and colleague, Mrs. Dorothy Burlingham, created a nursery to care for children who had lost their homes and, sometimes, their families during the frequent attacks by the German *Luftwaffe*. Anna Freud shepherded many of those young people into specially constructed underground

DOI: 10.4324/9781003546245-4

air raid shelters, and within such protected confines the children slept not in beds but, rather, on the floor, covered by special rope netting, woven by Miss Freud and her staff team, to prevent the little boys and girls from rolling around when nearby bombings would shake the very foundations of the house (Young-Bruehl, 1988). Quite understandably, many of the children developed severe air raid anxieties (Freud and Burlingham, 1941; Burlingham and Freud, 1942).

Although Miss Freud endured a considerable number of nearby bombings, she maintained her characteristically optimistic and hopeful state of mind and observed that, during air raids, children would not become particularly frightened if they could enjoy the protection of a responsible grown-up. As the father of one of the six-year-old youngsters in Miss Freud's care explained, "You would have to drop a bomb down her back before she would take notice!" (quoted in Freud and Burlingham, 1941, p. 8). Some years later, Anna Freud (1973, p. 412) summarised the experience of having navigated the wartime bombings thus: "We are in trouble in various ways, with heat, light, strikes, bombs and similar matters. Sometimes I think it is only the experience of the two world wars that I have behind me which makes me look at such occurrences as if they were an ordinary part of life."

Dr. Donald Winnicott, perhaps Great Britain's most famous home-grown psychoanalyst, worked as an air raid patrol warden during the Second World War. Winnicott had to survive not only the bombs which dropped close to his marital home in London but, also, those which fell on his one-time childhood home in Plymouth, in the county of Devon. In 1943, the *Luftwaffe* bombed Plymouth viciously and nearly destroyed the house in which Winnicott had grown up as a youth (cf. Goodman, n.d.). His father, Sir Frederick Winnicott, still lived there with his spinster daughters Miss Violet Winnicott and Miss Kathleen Winnicott. Chillingly, all three of them nearly died in one particularly vicious assault (Winnicott, 1943). The following year, in 1944, Donald Winnicott's long-standing spouse, Mrs. Alice Winnicott, sustained some sort of facial laceration, and nearly lost her eyesight (Brennan, 1944), during a London bombing (cf. Kahr, 2025b).

According to Miss Una Cormack, a British social worker who practised during the Second World War, bomb victims would often present to the local Citizens Advice Bureaux. She described them thus: "Their minds are dazed, their spirits apathetic; their symbols of security have been swept away in a night and they are left part of a wave of helpless humanity eddying to and fro in a sea of misfortune" (Cormack, 1942, pp. 178–179). Many Britons suffered from significant sleep disruption as a result of the noise and the threat of the bombs (Mackintosh, 1944).

Not only did inhabitants of Great Britain experience devastating consequences from the physical bombings of the Second World War but so, too, did institutions. The Tavistock Clinic, London's largest psychotherapeutic organisation, had to move from its premises in Malet Place in Central London to Hampstead, in North-West London, outside the very heart of the country's capital. Not long thereafter, the Nazis, alas, bombed the Tavistock Clinic's premises in Malet Place (Dicks, 1970).

The "Blitz" proved deeply terrifying, not only to Britons but, also, to the Swiss. In 1941, Dr. Carl Gustav Jung (1941), often thought to be a Nazi sympathiser, wrote to his American colleague and sometime patient, Mrs. Mary Mellon, that he found the bombings of London extremely painful, and that this devastation hurt him as much as if someone had bombed his own country.

Although Jung expressed a great sense of sadness at the horror of the bombings, other clinicians reacted in very different ways. Some of the British psychoanalysts had become so numb that, in true Churchillian fashion, they soldiered on. Famously, during an evening meeting of the British Psycho-Analytical Society, held in Gloucester Place, in Central London, an air raid siren began to blare during Dr. Elizabeth Rosenberg's (1943) presentation on the war neuroses. Apparently, in spite of the loud warning noises, the analysts sat silently and continued to listen to Rosenberg's talk until Dr. Donald Winnicott – ever aware of external realities – stood up and cried, "I should like to point out that there is an air-raid going on" (quoted in Little, 1985, p. 19). According to the testimony of Dr. Margaret Little, none of the members of the psychoanalytical group took much notice of Winnicott's warning, and they remained in their seats and simply continued to engage, perhaps defensively, with Dr. Rosenberg's talk.

No one encapsulated the experience of the bombing of Great Britain during the Second World War as economically as Mrs. Enid Eichholz – later known as the psychoanalyst Mrs. Enid Balint – who had volunteered to serve as an untrained social worker, in order to help families devastated by the Blitz. As Mrs. Eichholz (1944, p. 92) observed, "When the flying bombs first began to fall most of us disliked them considerably." Whether this attitude represents true courage or, perhaps, the use of minimisation as a form of denial, one cannot know with full certainty. But whatever the emotional state of the psychoanalysts during that time, most of them soldiered through with considerable fortitude.

In more recent times, psychoanalysts have endured horrors from on high in different parts of the world. For instance, Dr. Hadnan Houbbalah, also known as Adnan Hobballah – a student of Dr. Jacques Lacan, based in Beirut, Lebanon – continued to practise psychoanalysis in spite of the seemingly endless air raids and bombs which had ravaged the Middle East (Millot, 2016).

Of course, one need not be assaulted by an actual mechanical bomb, with a fuse and a trigger and a timer, in order to experience what I have come to refer to as "bombs in the consulting room" (Kahr, 2020a, p. 4). Sometimes, one can be threatened, assaulted, or shot. To cite but three heart-pounding examples, let us recall the following horrific moments from the history of psychoanalysis and psychotherapy.

Not long after the Nazi rise to power, the noted German-Jewish psychoanalyst, Dr. Ernst Simmel, one of the pioneers of the Freudian movement in Berlin, received an alarming telephone call while mid-session with a patient, fellow physician Dr. Martin Grotjahn. The caller, who worked in the police department on Berlin's Alexanderplatz, warned Simmel that Nazi officers would soon be arriving at his home to arrest him. In view of the gravity of the situation, Dr. Simmel explained the nature of this telephone call to his patient, instructing him, "Please get up, we have to run" (quoted in Farber and Green, n.d., p. 25).

Recalling this chilling episode many decades later, Dr. Grotjahn (1987, p. 34) reminisced, "I sat up and reached for one of his cigarettes, an unheard of liberty. Since he assumed that his house was under surveillance, we escaped through the back window from the staircase and climbed down into the backyard, over a fence and into an alley." Fortunately, both Ernst Simmel and his patient, Martin Grotjahn – a Gentile, married to a Jew – managed to avoid capture, just in the nick of time.

Also, in 1934, in Vienna, Austria, Dr. Ruth Mack Brunswick, one of Sigmund Freud's most loyal acolytes, had to curtail a session abruptly, in mid-stream, with her patient, fellow physician Dr. Muriel Gardiner, because dangerous rioting had begun in the streets between the Austrian fascists and the social democrats, in what eventually became known as the *Österreichischer Bürgerkrieg*, namely, the Austrian Civil War. As Gardiner (1983, p. 1) recalled, she and her psychoanalyst could readily hear "the tat-tat-tat of the machine guns"[1] nearby. As Dr. Brunswick did not wish for her analysand to walk through the streets of Vienna, she instructed her personal chauffeur to drive the patient from the consulting room on the Hasenauer-strasse, in the eighteenth district, back to Gardiner's own residence, an experience which Muriel Gardiner (1983, p. 2) would still recall, years thereafter, as both "ominous"[2] and, also, "heart-sinking" (Gardiner, 1983, p. 2).[3]

Contemporaneously, in 1937, the Viennese physician Dr. Viktor Frankl, an early advocate of both Freudian psychoanalysis and Adlerian psychotherapy, opened a private practice for psychiatric and neurological patients. On one occasion, Frankl welcomed a large, athletic, male schizophrenic patient into his fourth-floor consulting room. The weather proved sufficiently clement on that occasion for Dr. Frankl to have kept the windows open. But suddenly, the patient hurled a "bomb" at Frankl by threatening to throw him out of the window. As Frankl (1997, p. 75) reported, "I was not nearly strong enough to resist him. But I didn't beg for my life, or for anything. Rather, I pretended to be deeply offended. 'Look here,' I said, 'that really hurts me to the core. Here I make every effort to help you, and what do I get? You break up our friendship, and I did not expect that from you. It really hurts.'"[4] Frankl's verbal intervention proved successful and, mercifully, the patient did not push him onto the street below.

Neither Ruth Mack Brunswick nor Muriel Gardiner grew up in Jewish homes, but, nevertheless, they had to endure life in Vienna surrounded by violent eruptions and bombs. Extraordinarily, both Ernst Simmel and Viktor Frankl – each of Jewish origin – survived the potential bombs of being arrested by Nazis or murdered by a Viennese schizophrenic. Dr. Simmel eventually escaped to the United States of America where he became one of the progenitors of psychoanalysis in California. And although Dr. Frankl managed to avoid being thrown out of a window by a patient, he did end up incarcerated in several concentration camps, but, mercifully, he lived to tell the tale.

Other psychoanalysts have endured near-fatal attacks, not by bombs *per se* but, rather, by guns. On 26th October, 1951, Dr. Ishak Ramzy, an Egyptian-born psychoanalyst, suffered a gunshot wound from a distressed patient during a consultation

(Ramzy, 1953; King, 2002; Kahr, 2004b). Thankfully, Ramzy survived and ultimately enjoyed a lengthy and successful clinical career. He even became the editor of Dr. Donald Winnicott's (1977) memorable book on "The Piggle" (cf. Ramzy, 1977; Kahr, 2021b, 2024a).

Tragically, another psychoanalyst – a contemporary of ours – would not be so fortunate and died at the hands of an awful "bomb" in the form of an actual terrorist shooting.

On 7th January, 2015, in the heart of Paris, two men, Saïd Kouachi and his younger brother, Chérif Kouachi – both members of the Al-Qaeda terrorist group – burst into the headquarters of the French satirical weekly magazine *Charlie Hebdo* and shot and killed not only seven journalists and a building maintenance worker but, also, a visitor, as well as a security guard and a police officer, who had attempted to contain this murderous incident. Additionally, the terrorists assassinated a female member of the staff, none other than the psychiatrist and psychoanalyst Dr. Elsa Cayat, who supplied the magazine's biweekly column "Charlie Divan" ["Charlie on the Couch"]. Tragically, bombs such as those which nearly killed Donald Winnicott's wife can fall from the skies during a world war or, more shockingly still, they can occur even in times of peace and can deprive working mental health professionals of our lives.

EXPLOSIVES ON HAMPSTEAD HIGH STREET

The Case of "Verna"

One must be very cautious when describing complex, painful episodes in the psychotherapeutic consulting room as "bombs" because, as we know, many of our colleagues, past and present, had endured far more deadly explosions, which often claimed their lives, whether perpetrated by Nazi soldiers who had raided psychoanalytical offices, or by members of the *Luftwaffe* who had dropped bombs on the homes of psychoanalysts, or by the Al-Qaeda terrorists who had opened fire with real guns and murdered Dr. Elsa Cayat at the office of *Charlie Hebdo*. Fortunately, most of us will not ever experience such horrors and, happily, most of our patients do not carry actual weapons into the consulting room (cf. Doctor, 2018).

But, as we know from the case of the Viennese schizophrenic man who threatened to eject Viktor Frankl from a window, we all find ourselves at risk when highly troubled patients, often those who might qualify as forensic patients, or those with forensic potentialities, enter our lives (Kahr, 2018d). Thus, although I appreciate the enormity of the distinction between bombs with triggers which can blow up cities versus bombs as psychological metaphors, I shall retain the use of that term because, from time to time, even those of us who work in cosy offices in leafy parts of town can be barraged by *emotional* bombs, some of which can cause great distress to the clinician and can, nevertheless, threaten our mortality.

More than thirty years ago, an exceptionally beautiful and sexy, twenty-two-year-old blond woman called "Verna" entered my consulting room in Hampstead, in North-West London, where I practised for many years, in order to undergo a first assessment session. She wore an incredibly short white skirt, which barely covered her thighs, as well as a low-cut blouse, which barely hid her breasts. On her feet, she sported pointy stilettos. Verna looked like a cross between Marilyn Monroe and Brigitte Bardot, but, in spite of her evident eroticism, she conveyed, however, a rather more sinister quality. I invited her to sit in the chair opposite mine; but, privately, I gawped with amazement, never having seen such a scantily clad woman in my office before.

Within moments of meeting me, Verna told me that she feared for *my* life: not *her* life but, rather, *my* life. I stared at this person in utter bewilderment, desperately hoping that I might have misheard her opening statement. Soon, my heart began to race faster than ever before, and I became quite queasy and started to experience a series of wretched knots in my stomach.

This prospective patient, who, it seemed, comported herself like a very special kind of bomb, namely, a "sex bomb", explained that she had suffered greatly at the hands of her boyfriend, whom she described as a man riddled by pathological jealousy. Verna then explained that this person – a high-ranking member of a dangerous underground organisation – would become extremely wary whenever she would so much as look at, let alone speak to, another male. I soon learned that, on various occasions, this very jealous boyfriend had actually beaten several potential rivals to a pulp.

Somehow, I managed to maintain a certain degree of composure as I listened quietly and carefully to this extraordinary recitation, but throughout our initial consultation, I kept glancing at the door to my office, lest the boyfriend should suddenly barge in unexpectedly and attack me physically. I also kept staring at the open window, fearful that this Mafioso man might even climb up a ladder, enter my consulting room, and murder me, simply for having dared to talk to his girlfriend, in a professional context, without his knowledge.

With my anxiety escalating and with my pulse racing at well over 100 beats per minute, I knew that I had to find a way to extricate myself from this terrifying situation, as it became increasingly clear that it would be potentially dangerous to work with Verna ongoingly. And yet, I also felt acutely aware of my responsibility as a clinician to a patient who had attended for a consultation seeking help. I simply could not throw her out of the room, even though I strongly wished to do so.

Uncertain how best to proceed, and desperately struggling between my wish to assist the patient and my need to protect myself, I explained to Verna that, having now listened to her story for nearly an hour, it might be of help for us to reflect upon the best course of action. I told her that, in my estimation, psychological treatment could well be of value, but I raised the possibility that one of my colleagues might be better suited to offer assistance. Verna looked completely unfazed by my remark. I then mentioned that I would think carefully about our meeting over the next twenty-four hours and that I would telephone her with a treatment recommendation.

Verna left the room and, after she had done so, I then breathed an immense sigh of relief. I locked the door to my consulting room, waited until I heard Verna leave the building, and then I reached for my coat and quickly bolted onto Hampstead High Street and proceeded to run at rapid speed down Fitzjohns Avenue towards the Portman Clinic. Ordinarily, this journey would have taken me approximately fifteen minutes, but I ran so quickly on this occasion that I arrived there in less than eight minutes! Having once trained at the Portman Clinic as a student, the receptionist knew me extremely well and responded in a helpful fashion when I told her that I desperately needed to see my old mentor, Dr. Estela Welldon, the clinic's longest-serving Consultant Psychiatrist, for an immediate conversation. Fortunately, Estela had just finished work for the day, and she kindly invited me upstairs into her office.

Dr. Welldon could readily detect my acute distress, and as soon as she asked me why I looked so unusually nervous, I did what any self-respecting psychotherapist would do, and I burst into tears, and then managed to convey something of the terror of my recent consultation with Verna.

With characteristic bluntness, Estela scolded me, "You would have to be a bloody idiot to take on this case. You must refer her to a psychiatrist in a *hospital* setting. It would be physically unsafe to see her in your own private office. This woman and her boyfriend could be in collusion and could be very dangerous."

Happily, Estela Welldon, the founder of modern forensic psychotherapy, helped me to defuse this explosion in just a very short while. The following day, I telephoned Verna, as I had promised, and I spoke to her directly, explaining that, in view of the seriousness of her concerns, she needed a physically safe environment in which to speak – a protected hospital with security at the gate – in which she could undertake psychotherapeutic sessions with a Consultant Forensic Psychiatrist, supported by a full nursing and social work team. I then referred her to a senior colleague who had treated so many multiple murderers that he found the case of Verna to be rather "light-weight" by comparison.

I had no difficulty overcoming my guilt at not having provided treatment for this woman who, clearly, required help. Although working with Verna would have proved to be an interesting experience, I could not guarantee that I would have lived through the treatment if the dangerous boyfriend decided to do away with me before my time.

In retrospect, I realise that my consultation with Verna, though memorable, proved so anxiety-provoking and so potentially endangering that I found it difficult to think or to ask myself some compelling clinical questions. If I had begun to work with Verna in ongoing, long-term psychotherapy, would that actually have endangered my life? Perhaps she really did have a deadly boyfriend who would have beaten me up or might even have murdered me in a paranoid, jealous rage? But, only later did it occur to me that the most truly dangerous person could well have been Verna herself. Perhaps she derived much unconscious pleasure from projecting her own fears and anxieties onto or into another person.

Only after I completed my further training in couple psychotherapy and couple psychoanalysis did I begin to revisit the case in my mind and reconsider that most unusual, indeed rather frightening, consultation in even greater detail. If Verna really *did* have a Mafioso lover, what unconscious factors had propelled her into such a relationship, and what had prompted her to dress in such a provocative manner? Furthermore, to what extent did that woman evoke terror in her psychotherapist as a means of recapitulating some early abandonment experience, knowing, unconsciously, that I would be forced to send her away?

Regrettably, or relievedly, I met Verna only once; hence, I had little opportunity to learn anything more about the complexities of her history. Perhaps if we had continued to work further, we might have unearthed some important details about her own early traumatic history, which had become sexualised, and perhaps I might have helped her. But, fortified by the encouragement of my esteemed teacher, Dr. Welldon, I permitted myself to make a referral to an institutional-based colleague, and hence, I lived to tell the tale. Fortunately, so did *he*!

The Case of "Albertina"

As a very young practitioner working in the field of intellectual disability, then known as "mental handicap", I had the opportunity to embark upon a very lengthy psychotherapeutic experience with a highly damaged individual, whom I shall call "Albertina", a woman in her sixties who, at birth, had suffered from perinatal anoxia and had sustained some brain damage in consequence, and, subsequently, developed a schizophrenic psychosis and thus had to spend her entire life in an institutional setting.

Though well maintained within a specialist facility, Albertina, alas, had never received any formal psychological treatment as such. Regrettably, she had few opportunities to discharge her rage at being so disabled and at being so deprived of a more normal, ordinary, fulfilling life; thus, she had, over recent years, begun to spit compulsively. Indeed, Albertina often spat upon the walls and the floor and on the furniture; and, moreover, she even spat upon her own body. Furthermore, she salivated upon the fellow residents at her in-patient clinic; and she even expectorated upon the members of the staff. Albertina's treatment team attempted to forestall this increasingly explosive symptom by isolating her, by punishing her, and by ignoring her. But, over time, the spitting became more and more intense – upwards of *1,000* spits per day.

In desperation, Albertina's family, in conjunction with the doctors and nurses at the in-patient clinic, sought specialist psychotherapeutic treatment from the Mental Handicap Team at the Tavistock Clinic in London, where I worked for many years. When, during a staff meeting, Dr. Sheila Bichard, the chief educational psychologist, read out the referral letter, everyone squirmed uncomfortably, in spite of the fact that, as disability specialists, each of us had treated patients who screamed, shouted, urinated, vomited, or defaecated in sessions, rather like uncontained babies in desperate need of maternal cleansing. When Dr. Bichard asked who, among us, would be willing to arrange a consultation with Albertina, each of my colleagues either looked sheepishly at the ground or curled their faces in disgust. But as the youngest and, undoubtedly, the most naïve member of the team, I offered to provide an initial assessment. My colleagues began to giggle and told me that I should rush to the shops and purchase plastic sheeting to cover the furniture in my office and that I should also arrange to receive a hepatitis injection!

Prior to my first appointment with Albertina, I facilitated a preliminary meeting with her younger sister, who functioned as legal guardian and who wished to provide some important family background information. To my surprise, the sister – a thoughtful and honourable woman – arrived at my office, several minutes late, carrying no fewer than six extremely heavy bags of shopping, with which she struggled. The sister sat down, breathed an intensely audible sigh and then apologised for her slight tardiness, explaining, "I searched in vain for a car to bring me here, but I couldn't find one, and so I had to lug all of this shopping by hand."

Although one must formulate psychoanalytical transference interpretations very judiciously, especially during a first consultation with a family member, the material in front of me screamed out for some basic understanding, and so, after the sister relaxed into the chair, I commented, "I wonder whether the six heavy bags that you have brought with you might, in some way, represent the huge burden with which you and your family have struggled, caring for Albertina over these many years, and that you have also been searching for a "car" to help you carry those burdensome bags. Perhaps you hope that coming to see a man called Brett *Kahr* might offer some assistance."

The sister responded enthusiastically to my interpretative comment, and she then proceeded to describe her exhaustion at having spent a lifetime caring for such a disabled, damaged, and psychotic sibling who brought untold sadness and shame and fury to the family. As this consultation ended, the sister and I agreed that I would meet with Albertina on one occasion, in the first instance, to see whether psychotherapy might even be possible.

The following week, Albertina arrived at my consulting room, escorted by a care worker whom her sister had selected. Short in stature and slender in frame, with wild, scraggly white hair, and with a look of terror in her eyes, Albertina resembled a hunted rabbit. I introduced myself to both Albertina and to the care worker, and I then invited Albertina into my office. Little did I know that our association would last for as many as eight years.

Albertina never spoke in words, although the staff members sensed that she *did* possess some rudimentary language skills. For the most part, however, she remained completely silent. But, nevertheless, this woman certainly did have the capacity to hurl bombs in the consulting room.

After she seated herself in a chair, I explained to Albertina that, as she might know, I had already met with her sister, who believed that a conversation with a man such as myself could be of some potential use. Albertina stared blankly. I continued to talk, noting that she and I now had an opportunity to learn more about her.

Within moments, Albertina began to churn her mouth in a circular fashion, and she then launched her first attack of spittle onto the carpet of my consulting room. Only seconds later, she spat once again, with a trail of saliva dripping across her lower lip and then onto her chin. During the first few minutes of our meeting, Albertina spat at least twenty times. She then lifted herself from the chair and began to walk around the consulting room, expectorating on different parts of the floor.

I must confess that I felt rather nauseated, never having endured a spittle attack before. I desperately wished that I had refused to see this woman, and I feared that I would be of little use to someone so incredibly mad and uncontained.

As that first consultation continued to unfold, Albertina dashed round the room, rather like a wild animal marking her territory, and she expectorated more and more. At one point, I felt as though I might vomit – an undoubtedly profound countertransferential reaction to such an outrageous form of behaviour within a psychotherapeutic consulting room. I believe that, at the time, I thought to myself, "Thank goodness I have been sufficiently well-analysed and that I have not collapsed, because this is truly awful."

In an attempt to be of some use, I rendered several verbal observations to Albertina which, I hoped, might have some small impact. I suspect that I did no better than eke out a few platitudinous comments in an effort to be of assistance. Although I cannot recall my precise words, I suspect that I might have uttered something simple, such as, "You're really working very hard to show me how frightened and distressed you must be." My words fell upon deaf ears. Albertina did not even glance in my direction. She simply persevered with her increasingly violent spitting ritual, hurling bomb after bomb after bomb.

Throughout these spittle explosions, I kept myself mentally purified from all of this overt dirtiness by fantasising about where the cleaner in the office building kept her mop, knowing that, afterwards, I would have to scrub the floor of my room for some considerable time. Confident that, at the end of the hour, I could run in search of a cloth and some cleaning spray made me very happy indeed.

At one point, Albertina started to march in my direction, towards the leather chair on which I sat. My heart began to race as I became terrified that she might spit upon me directly and I simply did not know quite how I would manage such an attack. Instead, Albertina stopped in front of the tiny table perched next to my chair, upon which I kept my red leather appointment diary. Although merely an administrative object, I do regard my diary as an extension of my body, as it contains every single detail of my working life, and I felt extremely protective of this small book, and thus, as Albertina began to fill up her mouth with saliva, I quickly grasped the diary and pulled it to my chest, away from the table. Fortunately, the patient took the hint, and she ran to the other side of the room, towards the door. I breathed a small sigh of relief that both my own body and, also, my diary, a symbol thereof, had escaped this liquid assault.

At that point, Albertina then picked up the white plastic entryphone, attached to the wall, near the door to the office. She stared into the receiver and then dribbled a long chain of saliva from her mouth into the speaking end. I became instantly terrified that the introduction of bodily fluids into this electrical object might cause a fire of some sort, no doubt a partly appropriate fear but, also, perhaps, an unconscious countertransferential reaction spurred by the dread of some further explosion from Albertina.

Fortunately, my capacity for symbolic thinking and psychoanalytical conceptualisation returned at this point, and I formulated my first truly helpful interpretation. In soft tones, I pontificated, "As I have said, I know that you must be scared. You do not know whether I am a safe person or whether I will harm you in some way. And you are here in an unfamiliar room that you have never visited before, and you might be wondering why you have been brought here. I think that you are covering the entire room with spit to make it your own, so that it becomes a safe place. And I think that by spitting into the telephone, as you are doing now, you are trying to find a way to talk to me. I know that it is difficult for you to speak in words, as I am doing, so you are using your spit as a way of communicating with me." To my delight and amazement, Albertina did, indeed, listen to my words, and, in spite of her brain damage and her psychosis, she actually seemed to understand something of what I had just communicated.

The patient then sat down quietly in the centre of the consulting room, crossed her legs, and began to weep slightly. Suddenly, the tears had replaced the spittle as a more touching and less aggressive form of bodily discharge. Although my work with Albertina had only just begun, and although I knew that we still had many struggles ahead, I felt a tremendous sense of relief that this traumatised, violent, and hated patient could demonstrate her wish to communicate by spitting into the receiver of an entryphone and, moreover, that she could appreciate the efforts of a listener, desperate to find some way of understanding and of making some small amount of contact.

Towards the end of our first consultation, I explained to Albertina that we would need to pause in a short while, but that if she wished to return the following week for a further meeting, I would be very pleased to see her again. Albertina made no reply; she simply sat silently on the floor with a pensive face. But she did not spit at that moment, which I interpreted as both a sign of her wish to refrain from attacking and, also, her desire to reach out to me in some way, as she had done with the entryphone. I explained that I would speak to the escort and that I would confirm our next appointment. I then opened the door to my office, whereupon the very composed and calming escort greeted us. In Albertina's presence, I told the escort that we had agreed to have a further consultation the following week at the very same time. This woman nodded and understood, and I then bid Albertina farewell.

I regret that in the context of such a brief communication, I cannot provide a more detailed examination of the myriad ways in which my work with Albertina unfolded (cf. Kahr, 2017, 2020a, 2022a, 2022b), but I can report that the patient did attend on a weekly basis thereafter, and that she continued to do so for a full eight years, during which time her spitting began to decrease in intensity by gradual steps. Throughout our second consultation, Albertina spat only half as much as she had done during the first session; and with each successive appointment, her "acting-out" behaviour diminished more and more, until, at long last, she stopped spitting entirely and turned, instead, to a pad of paper and to a box of crayons, transforming her angry feelings from spittle into scribbled pictures. Although Albertina used very little verbal language, she communicated more and more through artwork and through an increasingly contained style of comportment. Over time, I developed a way of speaking to Albertina, informed by classical psychoanalysis and by infant observation, commenting upon her movements, upon her behaviours, and upon her facial expressions.

Eventually, the bomb-like explosions of the early sessions turned into rather more calm and much more depressive encounters in which Albertina ceased to spit as a manic defence and as a form of self-protection, and she then began to reveal, instead, the deep sadness which lurked beneath – a sense of sorrow derived from the loss of her brain, the loss of her freedom as an in-patient, and so much more.

Although the spitting decreased markedly with each passing month, Albertina did, however, find other ways of dropping bombs in the consulting room. On one unforgettable occasion, she entered the room on a cold wintry day without any overcoat. Instead, she wore merely a long, flowing caftan. This unusual form of dress struck me immediately and I found myself wondering why on earth the staff at her institution had allowed her to arrive at my office in Hampstead, in North-West London, in this manner. I sat down in my chair, and, within seconds, Albertina tugged at the caftan and, in one fell swoop, she ripped this piece of clothing off her body and stood before me completely naked, with no undergarments whatsoever!

Years previously, as a very young psychologist, I had worked on the back wards of a regional psychiatric hospital with long-stay schizophrenic patients, many of whom would strip off their clothing from time to time before sprinting up and down the corridors. These brief displays of patient nudity always occurred in full view of the entire staff team and the other patients, and no one seemed to bat an eyelid. However, I had never before found myself alone in a room with a nude patient and I became extremely worried on many levels, wondering whether this sudden behaviour had a particular meaning for Albertina. I endeavoured desperately to figure out how best to respond, highly fearful lest someone should walk in and accuse me of unethical behaviour or sexual impropriety in a professional context.

In retrospect, I realise that my own sense of bewilderment and my own fleeting, transferentially-provoked fear of being caught red-handed for a sexual crime might well have mirrored an early experience of sexual abuse in the patient's own history. During my initial consultation with Albertina's sister, I learned that, in early childhood, a part-time male employee who worked for the family had actually molested Albertina. But no one in the family knew any of the specific details, and Albertina herself simply could not speak about the matter to anybody.

Drawing upon all of my knowledge about psychoanalysis and all of my experience with survivors of abuse and trauma, I offered an observation to my temporarily naked patient. I knew that it would be imperative for Albertina to put her clothing back on immediately, but I also appreciated that both she and I needed to understand something of this complex, bomb-like situation. And so, I interpreted: "I think that you are showing me that your body has never been private. Your body has never been your own. And you want me to know this. I think it will be important for us to speak about this, but first I think it will be important for you to put your clothing back on." Without a moment's hesitation, Albertina absorbed my words and she reached for her caftan and redressed herself in a calm and quiet manner.

Throughout this process, I struggled, not knowing where to place my line of vision. It felt invasive to stare at the patient directly in her nude state; and yet, I thought that it might be quite shaming to Albertina if I turned away, as if in shock or disgust. Consequently, during this bomb-like interchange, I found a way to tilt my head sideways, so that I maintained the most minimal amount of eye contact possible.

Although Albertina could not speak in words, she then proceeded to spit upon her finger and to ram it penetratively in and out of her ear, as though simulating the motions of sexual intercourse. I commented that, perhaps, by having removed her clothing, and by having inserted a moistened, saliva-streaked finger into her ear, she wished me to know that, at one point, many years previously, someone might have removed her clothing and might have stuck something long and hard and wet into her. My interpretation seemed to defuse the bomb, and, once again, Albertina stopped harming herself and simply sat down on the consulting room floor, with tears streaming down her cheek.

Over eight long, exhausting, and challenging years, Albertina and I continued to work together on a regular basis, fully supported by the steadiness of the remarkable escort, without whom the treatment would have failed utterly. Happily, as psychotherapy progressed, Albertina became increasingly less provocative and destructive and endangering, both in our private sessions and, also, at her long-standing psychiatric in-patient facility. Gradually, her barrage of spitting behaviour ceased entirely, and she eventually stopped attacking members of the staff team and, also, her fellow patients.

In our very last session, I bid Albertina farewell and told her how much I had appreciated the privilege of working with her over such a long period of time. As she took her escort's hand and began to march down the corridor, she turned her head in my direction and uttered, "Bye Bweh … Bye Bweh", which I translated as "Bye Brett … Bye Brett".

The Case of "Alfonso"

During my tenure as Staff Psychotherapist for the Young Abusers Project, a visionary clinical programme co-sponsored by the Tavistock Clinic and the Department of Health of the United Kingdom, in association with the National Society for the Prevention of Cruelty to Children and the National Children's Home, I had the privilege and, also, the challenge of working with young sex offenders. Dr. Eileen Vizard, the noted forensic child psychiatrist and psychoanalyst who founded this project, hoped that, by intervening with juvenile perpetrators during their adolescence, shortly after having committed their very first sexual crimes, we might be able to stave off a lifetime of subsequent sexual offences during their impending adulthood.

Through the Young Abusers Project, I had the opportunity to work with a rather terrifying sixteen-year-old called "Alfonso" – a very tall, young, black male, more than six feet and six inches in height, and approximately 250 pounds in weight. The sheer heft of Alfonso's physicality frightened me from the outset; and I felt very small by comparison. No doubt, I had already begun to identity with some of the three young children whom he had abducted from a school playground and whom he then raped quite savagely.

I shall not attempt to provide a more detailed overview of the case at this point, having already done so in print on two previous occasions (Kahr, 2004a, 2020a), but I will share a very frightening moment, which occurred quite early on in our weekly psychotherapeutic work in my private consulting room.

Rather like Albertina, this adolescent paedophile also arrived by escort from his remand home, as neither the police nor social services trusted Alfonso to roam the streets of London on his own, lest he should perpetrate more sexual offences. Thus, knowing that a burly escort sat in the adjacent waiting room gave me huge comfort indeed.

Nevertheless, Alfonso could be quite menacing in sessions. Over the course of many weeks he struggled to speak about having raped those three little girls. Instead, he explained to me that, in his spare time, he worked as head of security for the noted pop star Michael Jackson. Needless to say, I very much doubted the veracity of this claim, knowing that Alfonso actually spent his days under lock and key. But he remained firm in his conviction that he served as a special security officer for this internationally renowned singer and recording artist. As one might imagine, I interpreted that, perhaps, as a little boy, Alfonso wished that he might have had his own head of security to keep him safe and protected. But this sixteen-year-old patient merely laughed contemptuously at my ostensibly ridiculous comment.

As the weeks and months unfolded, Alfonso spoke more and more about his fabricated duties as chief security officer for Mr. Jackson. He explained that, owing to Michael Jackson's celebrity status, he and the other guards had to keep any interlopers away, especially white men who might wish to harm Mr. Jackson. Indeed, he told me that, only recently, a certain white man who wore glasses (as I do) had attempted to attack the famous pop star, and thus, in order to protect his boss, Alfonso and his men had kidnapped this person and then tortured him with knives before slicing his body into many little pieces and then disposing the severed parts into the River Thames. Alfonso related this story in such a convincing and sinister manner that, although I knew it to be an elaborate fabrication, I also had to entertain the possibility that it might be true, or that, at the very least, he harboured such detailed murderous wishes towards white men with spectacles.

One day, Alfonso entered the consulting room for his weekly session and immediately perched himself on the chair. He then dropped a true bomb on me. With a deadpan face, he explained that he had recently acquired a shotgun and that neither his escort nor the staff in his facility knew anything about this. He explained to me that he had brought the gun with him to my consulting room. He then took his large hand and patted his huge thigh several times, as if to communicate, "Here it is, in my pocket." At that moment, my jaw froze, and a chill descended my spine. Alfonso then began to run his finger up and down his trouser leg in a seductive and menacing manner, telling me that he had spent quite a lot of time thinking about how easy it would be to shoot me dead.

Of all the bombs and explosives that I had ever experienced in my office over the years, this one seemed to be the most frightening of them all. My pulse raced, and I could feel pains deep in my ribs, wondering whether I should scream for help, whether I should render a brilliant Freudian interpretation, or whether I should simply sit in silence in the hope that, by doing so, I might somehow contain the situation. Certainly, I felt very, very scared indeed.

Over the next few minutes, Alfonso continued to touch his pocket and then threatened me further, snarling that if I displeased him in any way, then I, too, would end up like that other white man with glasses, sliced up into a million pieces.

Alfonso then stuck his large hand into his pocket, and, in a flash, removed it and thrust it out in front of him, shouting, "Pow", in a menacing voice, pretending to shoot me dead. I cannot remember the last time that I had felt so terrified in my life, and, although I could see no gun, for a brief moment I could not actually determine whether he had shot me in pretend fashion with his fingers or whether he had *truly* shot me with a gun. I looked down at my increasingly tachycardic chest and sighed with relief that I could see no signs of blood.

With a cruel sadism – the sort required to rape little children – Alfonso giggled, knowing that he had frightened me immensely, and then he boasted that, after the session, he would escape to the airport with his fellow security officers who, ostensibly, worked for Michael Jackson. Alfonso explained, "My men are gonna *beat* me at Heathrow Airport and drive me to Mr. Jackson's mansion." Of course, consciously, he had intended to say, "My men are gonna *meet* me at Heathrow Airport", but, he had, at that moment, made a slip of the tongue, and he used the word "beat" instead of "meet".

Suddenly, my terror began to abate, and, internally, I experienced great relief, having become aware that the patient had perpetrated an old-fashioned parapraxis (Freudian slip). I had now accumulated sufficient clinical data to craft an interpretation, and I pointed out Alfonso's slip of the tongue, reminding him that he had just told me that his men would "beat" him, rather than "meet" him. I wondered aloud whether he worried that some men, perhaps his escort and I, would want to beat *him* up for his violence and cruelty towards his young victims, and that, in order to avoid such a punishment, he would need to beat *us* up first or even pretend to shoot us and frighten us to death.

To my utter surprise, Alfonso did not respond verbally to my comment but, instead, he reached for the nearby box of tissues, unfolded a large Man-Size Kleenex, and placed the white piece of paper over his black face. I commented that perhaps he felt very ashamed for having tried to shoot me with his fingers and that he wished to cover his eyes and that, perhaps, a part of him also wished that he could have a white face, like me (or, indeed, like the increasingly light-skinned popstar, Michael Jackson), and not be such an angry young man, full of "black" feelings.

Alfonso became slightly teary-eyed for the very first time and, thereafter, he finally allowed me to see aspects of his quite considerable vulnerability in a more fulsome manner. In due course, he began to tell me much more about his early history. I knew already, from the psychiatric reports that I had received about this patient, prior to the onset of treatment, that, shortly after Alfonso's seventh birthday, his father had died from a heart attack. The reports offered no further information and I had simply assumed that the father must have suffered from long-standing cardiac disease which eventually claimed his life. But Alfonso told me that his father did *not* have heart disease as such; however, on the day of his death, the parents had begun to fight viciously, screaming loudly and throwing objects at one another. Alfonso sat in the room at that time and he had observed this entire ghastly parental interchange in which he felt extremely unsafe. At one point, the mother grabbed a large knife from the kitchen and began to thrash it about. She did not actually stab her husband – Alfonso's father – but she had certainly attempted to do so, whereupon the father immediately clutched his chest and then collapsed dead on the floor.

As soon as I heard this horrible and (literally) heart-breaking tale of violence and terror and loss, which Alfonso had never articulated previously, I realised that his subsequent paedophilic attacks on the little girls contained numerous elements of a re-enactment of this trauma, as he attempted to derive an angry pleasure from inserting his large kitchen knife-like penis into their fragile bodies, and that he endeavoured to recreate that very situation in the transference by attempting to shoot me with his long, penetrative fingers.

Our psychotherapeutic work continued for some time thereafter and Alfonso gradually became less violent as a personality; indeed, his long-standing depression and sadness soon emerged, and he then began to cry. Having previously feared that I would harm him, Alfonso ultimately grew increasingly attached to me, and, on one occasion, he even picked up a book from my shelf – a heavy clinical tome – and whispered, "With this book, I thee wed", thus indicating his growing fondness and gratitude that I had not retaliated by shooting him in return.

SURVIVING PSYCHOLOGICAL SHRAPNEL

Not long before the eruption of the coronavirus pandemic, I popped into my local post office to pick up a parcel and, on the counter, I spied an extraordinary notice, warning customers that we must not, under any circumstances, send any "Prohibited and Restricted items" through the mail. The prohibited substances highlighted on this warning sign included aerosols (not used for toiletry or medicinal purposes); alcohol (above seventy per cent A.B.V.); compressed gases; corrosives; fireworks and flares; flammable liquids and solids; lighters and refills containing flammable liquid or gas; lithium batteries; matches; oxidising agents and peroxides; pesticides and poisons; solvent-based paints and varnishes; toxic gases and liquids; weapons; wet spillable lead acid or lead alkaline batteries; and, of course, explosives and ammunitions.

As I glanced at this rather chilling poster, I experienced a tremendous sadness, realising that, nowadays, we inhabit a world in which certain individuals do actually use the postal service *not* for letters, as I do, but, rather, for sending corrosive and flammable substances and, even, explosives and ammunitions and bombs.

Certainly, I appreciate the very large difference between the explosives used by terrorists, which have claimed innumerable lives in the most violent of circumstances, and the more metaphorical explosions which we encounter in our work as psychotherapeutic practitioners. Nevertheless, being attacked by threats from the Mafia, by copious amounts of saliva, or by imaginary guns can still be extremely frightening.

As a supervisor of many thoughtful colleagues, I know that my clinical experiences will be regarded as by no means unique. Everyone who has ever worked in the mental health profession must navigate unpleasant, even petrifying, explosions from patients – these "bombs in the consulting room" – from time to time. Those who work more regularly with violent, forensic patients or with the profoundly disabled will have to endure such instances on an even more frequent basis, rather like the members of staff in a hospital department of accident and emergency.

And yet, in spite of the ubiquity of such consulting-room explosions, none of us has ever received any formal or detailed training in how we might defuse these "bombs" which appear all too frequently in the course of our ongoing clinical work with very troubled, very fragile, very damaged, and very angry men, women and, even, children.

Strikingly, psychoanalysts and psychotherapists have experienced bombs and explosions on a regular basis since the inception of the discipline. As early as 1910, Professor Sigmund Freud complained to his Hungarian colleague, Dr. Sándor Ferenczi, about a new patient, one Sergéi Konstantínovich Pankéev, who would later become known as "Der Wolfsmann" ["The Wolf Man"]. Freud (1910b, p. 138) explained that this patient referred to him as a "Jewish swindler",[5] and noted that, "he would like to use me from behind and shit on my head" (Freud, 1910b, p. 138).[6] Unsurprisingly, the father of psychoanalysis felt rather abused and denigrated (cf. Freud, 1918).

Dr. Donald Winnicott also experienced a bomb from one of the very first children with whom he worked psychoanalytically back in the 1930s. As Winnicott (1956, p. 306) reminisced subsequently, "For my first child analysis I chose a delinquent. This boy attended regularly for a year and the treatment stopped because of the disturbance that the boy caused in the clinic. I could say that the analysis was going well, and its cessation caused distress both to the boy and to myself in spite of the fact that on several occasions I got badly bitten on the buttocks. The boy got out on the roof and also he spilt so much water that the basement became flooded. He broke into my locked car and drove it away in bottom gear on the self-starter. The clinic ordered termination of the treatment for the sake of the other patients."

Across the decades, Winnicott endured "bombs" of a more physical nature. For instance, in the middle years of his career, he became the psychoanalyst to one of his colleagues, the aforementioned Dr. Margaret Little. In spite of the fact that this woman had already qualified as a psychoanalyst in her own right, she still suffered, nevertheless, from profound emotional problems. On one occasion, she even smashed a vase in Winnicott's consulting room. As Little (1985, p. 20) reminisced, quite some time later, "In one early session with D.W. I felt in utter despair of ever getting him to understand anything. I wandered round his room trying to find a way. I contemplated throwing myself out of the window, but felt that he would stop me. Then I thought of throwing out all his books, but finally I attacked and smashed a large vase filled with white lilac, and trampled on it. In a flash he was gone from the room, but he came back just before the end of the hour. Finding me clearing up the mess he said, 'I might have expected you to do that [clear up? or smash?], but later.'"

More perilously, Winnicott had to endure at least two assaults on his body. As a result of my long-standing archival and oral history research about the life and work of Winnicott, I discovered that, at some point, probably in 1963, one of his autistic child patients poked him in the eye (Kahr, 1997b); and, in consequence, Winnicott suffered considerable ocular pain for many years thereafter (cf. Kahr, 2021b, 2024a). Perhaps more shockingly still, another patient – an adult – also bashed him in the eye round about that same time[7] (Kahr, 2021b, 2024a). Thus, psychoanalytical practitioners must confront "bombs" in many, many forms.

Having to endure a patient's fantasies of defaecating upon us, or having to survive the patient flooding our consulting room and biting us on the buttocks, or even endangering our eyesight, might be understood, in many ways, as the very bread and butter of our psychoanalytical labours. Perhaps it might be of comfort to know that even Freud and Winnicott felt sufficiently vexed by their troublesome, explosive patients that they became compelled to record such disturbing vignettes in print. Indeed, Dr. Wilfred Bion once remarked that, when treating a very ill patient, we have only two alternatives: one must either terminate the work or else one must *write* about it (MacCarthy, 2002).

In other words, in order to survive bombs and explosives, we need to verbalise our hate in the countertransference (Winnicott, 1949a) – those awful feelings of being abused, attacked, denigrated, insulted, or injured in some way. By remaining silent, weighed down by the fear of ridicule or, indeed, by the shame of inadequacy, we will perhaps suffer unnecessarily from the burden of the powerful experiences which certain patients project onto us or into us and with which we might at times identify (Klein, 1946).

Verbalisation of our hatred in the countertransference – either in the form of spoken words or in the form of writing – will be of inestimable value in the management of these bombs which sometimes explode in our presence. But we may also be helped by a recognition of the fact that the bomb might well be a re-enactment of the patient's early traumatic experience. And though aimed in our direction, and rather unpleasant to boot, the explosion in the consulting room may actually represent a perverse form of hope, once we come to realise that the patient has entrusted us sufficiently to tolerate a repetition of an infantile or childhood experience. The patient yearns for us to know about this experience, often of a preverbal nature, and hence, will act it out in concrete form, rather than in words. Thus, the healthy clinician might benefit from conceptualising the bomb *not* as an attack but, rather, as an unusual, albeit challenging, sort of gift.

In my work with forensic patients and with disabled patients, I have, over the years, come to appreciate that such explosive events often unfold in four distinct phases or stages. In the first phase, the clinician will be forced to endure a profound sense of *stupefaction*, in which the bomb causes shock and fear and thus prevents the practitioner from thinking. The stupefaction must be felt and experienced so that its impact will register with profundity. In the second phase, which I have come to conceptualise as one of *toleration*, the psychotherapist will begin to enjoy the capacity to endure the explosive symptom in a more considered and familiar way. (For instance, after several sessions of Albertina's spitting, I no longer felt that initial sense of stupefaction and nausea; rather, I began to tolerate the messiness of the symptom in a relatively straightforward manner). And in the third phase, I will always rely upon the use of traditional psychoanalytical *interpretation* in order to unravel the unconscious meaning or meanings of the bomb-like symptom, before proceeding onto the fourth and final phase of the treatment process, namely, that of *resolution*, in which both parties, in traditional psychoanalytical style, will have experienced the bomb, will have understood its meaning, and will have mourned its loss (Kahr, 1995, 1997a, 2017, 2020a).

Thus, the clinician most likely to survive the bombs in the consulting room must be well-analysed, must have ample professional opportunities to process and digest his or her countertransferential hatred (whether in supervision, in collegial discussion, or through writing), and must, also, take great comfort in the ongoing availability of the psychoanalytical approach to the interpretation of patient communications which, when fully internalised, can actually save us in our work with the most difficult of patients. These ingredients serve, in many respects, as the very platform upon which we practise.

Often, if mental health clinicians cannot find a means of understanding or containing or defusing the bomb-like manifestations, we develop a greater risk of destroying the treatment, either covertly, by disappointing the patient through a lack of compassion and insight, or by terminating the work abruptly. Sometimes, psychoanalytical practitioners will even evict patients from the office. The esteemed American psychoanalyst, Professor Richard Chessick (2018, p. 79), an expert in the study of borderline personality disorder, revealed in his autobiography that, "I have consulted on several cases where the therapist became so enraged at a borderline patient that he literally chased him out of the office."

Back in London, during the 1940s, many Britons experienced immense distress in the wake of the Nazi bombings, but others soldiered through in a far more robust fashion. The noted songwriter, dramatist, and actor, Noël Coward (1941, p. 6), reminisced that, on Saturday, 19th April, 1941, he "Had a few drinks, then went to Savoy. Pretty bad blitz, but not so bad as Wednesday. A couple of bombs fell very near during dinner. Wall bulged a bit and door blew in. Orchestra went on playing, no one stopped eating or talking. Blitz continued."

Psychological bombs and emotional explosions strike, often quite unexpectedly, throughout the course of our clinical careers; and just as no two individuals will navigate a bomb from on high in quite the same manner, likewise, no two mental health practitioners will respond to an unexpected consulting room incident in similar fashion.

Moreover, each worker will have a different level of prior experience and a different capacity to navigate tricky encounters, so much so that a sturdy psychotherapist may not be fazed at all by a particular episode, whereas another colleague might regard that same episode as rather traumatising. For instance, Dr. Michele Gomes (2018a, 2018b), an American psychoanalyst, published a case history about a patient called "Ben" who terrified her when, on one occasion, he entered his session carrying a kitten which he dropped in her presence, forcing her to catch the animal. As Dr. Gomes (2018a, p. 250) remarked, "My heart continued to pound quickly". Although most patients do not deposit pets in the laps of their psychoanalysts or psychotherapists on a regular basis, one wonders whether this experience would really constitute a bomb as such. Having had patients who often fantasised about sending me to concentration camps and watching me and my family suffocate to death in gas chambers, the prospect of stroking a kitten in my consulting room seems, by contrast, an utter delight.

These psychological bombs often cannot be predicted or, indeed, prevented. They will unfold as an occasional component of the clinical process. But if the psychoanalytical practitioner continues to hold a professional setting in his or her mind at all times (Temperley, 1984), one will be far better prepared for the unexpected. For instance, when Alfonso, the juvenile paedophile, threatened to murder me with a gun, I took great comfort from his slip of the tongue, which I analysed incessantly, I believe, to great effect. I have absolutely no training in avoiding gunfire, but I do have a considerable amount of training and experience in the interpretation of parapraxes, and that gave me a great sense of comfort.

Throughout this chapter, I have focused exclusively on the bombs – whether concrete or metaphorical – endured by psychoanalytical clinicians across the twentieth century and beyond. Needless to say, not only do mental health professionals navigate bombs, but so, too, do our patients. Years ago, I treated an elderly German woman of Aryan background who had emigrated to Great Britain in the 1950s. Although by no means a victim of the Nazis – in fact, her father had worked for Adolf Hitler – she, nonetheless, had endured the Allied bombings throughout her childhood, and she suffered a lifelong depression which developed after her best friend died when the Americans dropped a bomb on my patient's schoolhouse.

Other patients have experienced long-term, intergenerational effects of real bombs. Some years ago, I worked with a marital couple. The husband, whom I shall call "Giuseppe", grew up in Italy, although his wife spent her childhood in Wales. Throughout the sessions, Giuseppe would yell at the wife, often unceasingly, so much so that the wife felt as though she became the regular recipient of bomb-like explosions. In attempting to understand the roots of this angry behaviour, Giuseppe explained that his mother had yelled at him extensively during childhood; and his grandmother had screamed at the mother even more extremely. In fact, the patient's grandmother seemed to be so full of rage that she would often take a bin of rubbish onto the roof of the house and then drop it onto the ground below as a means of discharging her rage.

One day, while reminiscing about his family history, Giuseppe told me that, during the Second World War, his grandmother – then a young woman – had to witness several bombs exploding nearby her house. Although she survived, three of her siblings died in the process, resulting in a long-standing grief and depression. Suddenly, with this new information to hand, we began to hypothesise that the grandmother may, perhaps, have thrown rubbish from the rooftop as a symbolic means of mastering the trauma of the dropping of Allied bombs. Similarly, Giuseppe's verbal rage might well have resulted, at least in part, from the tremendous fear of the bombs which this Italian family had to endure decades previously. The revelation of this awful piece of biography certainly helped us to understand the contemporary marital aggression much more fully.

Throughout the Second World War, physicians in the Royal Air Force worked hard to care for British pilots fighting overseas. For example, an air physician, Squadron Leader Samuel Cuthbert Rexford-Welch (1958, p. 276), and his colleagues documented that, among flyers in Malta, "After prolonged bombing, concentration on work was diminished and the amount as well as the quality of muscular and mental activity was reduced." Rexford-Welch's men also noted that pilots involved in such bombings suffered from "waves of depression" (1958, p. 276). We know that "real" bombs exert quite a devastating impact. But so, too, do the emotional bombs of the consulting room, and the psychological shrapnel which ensues, which I have chosen to underscore throughout this brief contribution.

I shall conclude my remarks with one more story.

Some thirty years ago, a female patient developed a very profound erotic transference towards me and, to my utter shock and horror, had discovered the location of my private residence. One morning, she greeted me outside my home and offered to drive me to my consulting room. I found this a rather scary experience. Needless to say, I refused the invitation but agreed to meet the patient at the office for our regular appointment later in the day so that we could discuss this episode of gross acting-out. As the patient's erotic transference grew in intensity, one of my teachers at the Portman Clinic suggested that I might benefit from a supervisory consultation with the venerable, elderly psychoanalyst Dr. Arthur Hyatt Williams,[8] a noted mental health expert who had worked extensively in prisons and who had accumulated a great deal of experience with both erotic and violent stalkers and other types of forensic patients (e.g., Williams, 1964; Hyatt-Williams, 1998). Though very frail by that point, Dr. Williams kindly granted me a one-off appointment, nevertheless. In due course, I sat down in his office, fully prepared to summarise the case, but, before I could speak, Williams immediately began to tell me about one of *his* stalker patients who threatened to kill him, and then reminisced about another stalker patient, and then he elaborated upon his experiences with yet *another*. Before long, the fifty-minute supervision came to an end, and I had still not had a single second of space in which to convey to Dr. Williams anything about *my* stalker. Being young and naïve and rather softly spoken at the time, I simply stood up at the end of the hour, thanked Dr. Williams profusely, and then departed, never having had a chance to receive direct help. But, in retrospect, I realise that Arthur Hyatt Williams had given me a great gift. Though he did not learn *anything* about my patient *at all*, he demonstrated to me that *he* had survived his own bomb-throwing, forensic, stalking patients, and that he went on to live a very long and full and productive life.

I found my consultation with Dr. Arthur Hyatt Williams deeply reassuring and I took great comfort from the fact that, although bomb-throwing, explosion-inducing patients might frighten us profusely, the sturdy clinician, well supported by a collegial team and by an internal psychoanalytical framework, can, indeed, survive the bombs in the consulting room very well and can live to tell the tale, passing on some hopeful reassurance to a new generation of brave and bold colleagues who have dared to undertake this challenging and often life-changing work to which we have all devoted ourselves.

Notes

1 In the original German version of this text, Dr. Muriel Gardiner (1978, p. 31) reported on "das Knattern von Maschinengewehren vernahmen".
2 In the original German version of this text, Dr. Muriel Gardiner (1978, p. 32) deployed the word "ominöse".
3 In the original German version of this text, Dr. Muriel Gardiner (1978, p. 32) described this painful situation as "beklemmende", which might be translated more accurately as "nightmarish", "oppressive", or "disturbing".
4 The original German passage reads: 'Ich wäre ihm kräftenmäßig nicht gewachsen gewesen. Ich bat ihn aber nicht um mein Leben, ich bettelte überhaupt nicht um irgend etwas, sondern ich tat nur tief gekränkt: "Sehen Sie", sagte ich, "das kränkt mich jetzt wirklich: da setze ich alles daran, um Ihnen zu helfen, und was ist der Dank? Sie kündigen mir Ihre Freundschaft auf. Das hätte ich von Ihnen wirklich nicht erwartet. Jetzt kränke ich mich wirklich."' (Frankl, 1995, p. 54).
5 The original German phrase reads: "Jüdischer Schwindler" (Freud, 1910a, p. 214).
6 The original German passage reads: "er möchte mich von hinten gebrauchen und mir auf den Kopf scheißen" (Freud, 1910a, p. 214).
7 Although I always endeavour to provide highly detailed referencing to every single historical fact, I have elected to refrain from furnishing a precise bibliographical citation for this clinical anecdote, which I found in one Dr. Donald Winnicott's unpublished typescripts. Had I elected to do so, I would thereby have revealed the location, and,

potentially, the identity of this particular patient. In this instance, I have decided to prioritise my commitment to clinical confidentiality above my passion for scholarly meticulousness.

8 The noted British psychoanalyst Dr. Arthur Hyatt Williams would sometimes be referred to as "Dr. Arthur Williams" and sometimes as "Dr. Arthur Hyatt-Williams" or as "Dr. Arthur Hyatt Williams", with or without a hyphen. I have referred to him predominantly as "Dr. Arthur Hyatt Williams" – the more commonly used form of address – but I have retained the original version of his surname in one of his publications (Hyatt-Williams, 1998) for the sake of bibliographical accuracy.

PART II

Sexual Forensics

Genital Exhibitionism and Paedophilia

Why Do Men Expose Their Genitals?

The Unconscious Origins of Exhibitionism

SECTION ONE: THE PSYCHOPATHOLOGY OF FLASHING

Troubled men and women have engaged in exhibitionistic activity throughout the course of human history. For instance, in the fourteenth century, Geoffrey Chaucer wrote about a frisky gentleman, known as "Nicholas the Gallant", in a story entitled "The Miller's Tale", part of *The Canterbury Tales*, in which this character went "up the wyndowe dide he hastily, / And out his ers he putteth pryvely / Over the buttok, to the haunche bon" (lines 693–695). And sometime later, in the sixteenth century, the Chinese novel, 金瓶梅 [*Jin Ping Mei*], known in English as *The Plum in the Golden Vase*, conveyed the tale of a young man who had displeased a certain lady, and, not long thereafter, this aggrieved woman's serving maids then attacked that man with a variety of long and short cudgels. In a desperate effort to free himself, he removed his trousers, and the sight of his genitalia caused the maids to disperse.

As long ago as 1550, a Venetian commission against blasphemy prosecuted an Italian man called Domenego for having exposed his penis to various ladies during a mass in several local churches. According to the report, Domenego "harboured such extreme temerity and impudence that he has again and again dared display his pudendal member" (quoted in Rooth, 1970, p. 139). Marco Antonio Bragadin, Francesco Longo, and Marc'Antonio Trevisan, the three commissioners responsible for eradicating blasphemy in Renaissance Venice, sentenced Domenego to six months of imprisonment, as a punishment for his ostensible wickedness, followed by ten years of banishment from Venice and its nearby territories. The commissioners stipulated that should Domenego dare to escape, he would have to be captured; and they offered a reward of 400 piccoli.

More than 100 years later, in 1663, an English baronet, the Honourable Sir Charles Sedley, became drunk at the Cock Tavern on Bow Street, in the Covent Garden region of London, in the presence of several comrades, including Charles Sackville, Lord Buckhurst (the future 6th earl of Dorset) and Sir Thomas Ogle; and these revellers then proceeded to expose themselves from the balcony of the tavern to the passers-by below. Sir Charles, in particular, undressed himself completely, and he "harangued the populace in such profane language that the public

DOI: 10.4324/9781003546245-6

indignation was wakened" (quoted in Rooth, 1970, p. 136). The records of his indictment ("Le Roy versus Sir Charles Sedley") charged the inebriate gentleman with "several misdemeanours against the King's Peace, which were to the great scandal of Christianity" (quoted in Rooth, 1970, p. 139). Owing to Sedley's status as a gentleman from an ancient family, The Lord Chief Justice, Sir Robert Foster, imprisoned him for only one week and fined him 2,000 marks. Sir Charles re-offended some five years later, in 1668, during yet another escapade with his companion Lord Buckhurst; and, on that occasion, the monarch, Charles II, had to intercede on Sedley's behalf.

In reviewing these two prominent cases of exhibitionism from the sixteenth and seventeenth centuries, one cannot help but notice the lack of psychological insight into either the causes of, or the precipitating factors for, these acts of genital exposure in an Italian church and in an English tavern. Our forefathers regarded indecent behaviour of this variety merely as a form of sin or lewdness, rather than as an expression of psychological turmoil, or as an attempt to communicate some internal distress. Nevertheless, the sense of effrontery remains apparent, and there can be little doubt that Domenego's church women and, also, Sedley's Covent Garden strollers became offended by these episodes of flashing.

But if one does not subscribe to a religious theory of aetiology, we must then wonder why men engage in such an act of sexual exposure, which often brings much fear and terror to the victims of these episodes of genital exhibitionism.

Forensic enactments of this variety can be very damning indeed. As we know from important psychopathological research, many men who do perpetrate such sexual crimes will also be much more likely to engage in other forms of even more dangerous sexual perversions, ranging from frotteurism to rape to paedophilia (Abel and Osborn, 1992).

Dr. Philip Sugarman and his colleagues at the Reaside Clinic in Birmingham studied a sample of indecent exposers referred to the West Midlands Forensic Psychiatry Service between 1967 and 1984, inclusive; and they conducted an investigation of the criminal careers of these men up until 1992 through the Criminal Record Office. Sugarman and his colleagues noted that in their group of 210 cases, whom they examined in depth, some thirty-two per cent received a conviction for a more serious sexual offence, such as attempted buggery, attempted rape, actual buggery, and actual rape (Sugarman, et al., 1994). Some sixty-three per cent of these serious sexual offences occurred *after* the episode of indecent exposure, suggesting that many perpetrators do become more overtly dangerous with the passing of time, and that as many as seventy-five per cent had committed other offences apart from indecent exposure, totalling more than 2,000 separate convictions including arson, attempted murder, breach of the peace, criminal damage, major assault, minor assault, property offences, and robbery. Helpfully, Sugarman and colleagues reported that those flashers who had exposed themselves solely on one occasion proved less likely to re-offend in more serious ways, whereas those flashers who had either touched their victims, spoken to their victims, pursued their victims, or masturbated whilst exposing themselves would be at higher risk for committing serious crimes at a later point in time. This research data will offer much helpful insight to psychiatrists and psychologists and to the courts in terms of assessing the potential risks of re-offending and, moreover, to psychotherapists and psychoanalysts who embark upon the treatment of such offenders.

The case of the infamous cannibalistic, necrophilic serial murderer Jeffrey Dahmer certainly underscores the potential sadism inherent in the act of penile exposure; for little do we realise that long before Dahmer killed his young male victims, he had actually begun his criminal career by having engaged in acts of genital exhibitionism. On 7th August, 1982, Dahmer committed an act of Disorderly Conduct at the Wisconsin State Fair Park, in West Allis – a suburb of Milwaukee, Wisconsin – by having urinated in public with his penis exposed in front of twenty-five women and children. As the years unfolded, his behaviour escalated in even more gruesome ways. According to Brian Masters (1993, p. 70), author of the principal biography of Jeffrey Dahmer, "Exhibitionism was, for him at least, a fruitless and arid kind of being with somebody at a safe remove" (cf. Kahr, 2019e, 2020b, 2023b).

Fortunately, most exhibitionists do not progress to such extremes of murderousness. Nevertheless, cases of this nature certainly underscore the vital need to understand the origins of this form of forensic enactment.

SECTION TWO: THE PSYCHODYNAMICS OF EXHIBITIONISM

Although many behavioural psychologists and biologically orientated psychiatrists have undertaken a massive amount of illuminating research into the psychopathology of exhibitionism, very few of them have actually understood the more private internal world of the exhibitionist sufficiently; and although traditional psychiatrists can tell us the time of day at which a flasher will most likely expose himself, these colleagues have offered very little clarification about the patient's deeper, unconscious motivations. In fact, most mental health researchers have hypothesised that exhibitionists suffer from neurological defects (e.g., Flor-Henry and Lang, 1988; cf. Jones and Frei, 1979; Flor-Henry, 1987), thus marginalising, if not dismissing, the need for fuller psychological investigation.

Fortunately, the discipline of psychoanalysis has, as ever, provided us with a far more profound understanding of the nature of this presenting symptom.

In his magnum opus, *Die Traumdeutung* (Freud, 1900a), better known in English as *The Interpretation of Dreams* (Freud, 1900b, 1900c), the father of psychoanalysis, Dr. Sigmund Freud, wrote at some length about the very widespread occurrence of exhibitionist dreams containing nudity and genital exposure. Five years later, in his seminal monograph, *Drei Abhandlungen zur Sexualtheorie* (Freud, 1905a), translated into English as the *Three Essays on the Theory of Sexuality* (Freud, 1905b), he observed that, as young children, many of us will have displayed parts of our bodies naked, before we would have become subjected to the maturational processes of socialisation and acculturation which permit us to control our infantile exhibitionistic urges. Freud noted however that, in some individuals – those whom one might describe as sexually perverse – the infantile tendency to exhibit will persist, and that individual will develop into a clinical genital exhibitionist. Freud conceptualised this act as a deviation in respect of the sexual aim. In other words, in the more usual scenario, one's sexual urges will be directed at genital intercourse, but, in the case of the exhibitionist, the goal will be display, rather than copulation. Freud recognised that sexually perverse people, including exhibitionists, will enact their libidinal desires overtly, while the more repressed neurotics will merely fantasise about perverse desires and refrain from any gross forms of acting-out.

Freud seems to have had little clinical experience of treating overtly exhibitionistic patients, but he certainly knew about these individuals. For example, as early as 1895, he wrote to his colleague Dr. Wilhelm Fliess, describing a young woman who, whilst tidying up the room of a stranger, suddenly found that the man had exposed his penis, and had then placed it in her hand. This experience of exhibitionistic molestation, involving contact, became one of the triggers which eventually contributed to this woman's subsequent paranoid, persecutory state (Freud, 1895).

Without doubt, Freud's greatest contribution to the study of exhibitionistic behaviour must be his insistence that each one of us will have begun our lives as an exhibitionistic infant; and although most of us will come to contain the urge to display ourselves unduly, the clinical pervert will continue to do so in a very baby-like manner. Thus, by insisting that every grown-up man and woman has not only engaged in infantile genital exposure, but has also derived pleasure therefrom, Freud has certainly helped to *humanise* the condition, and, in doing so, he has, I trust, assisted us in our campaign to approach the clinical offender with greater compassion and empathy.

Several of Freud's early disciples offered useful insights about the nature of genital exhibitionism. The Hungarian clinician, Dr. Sándor Ferenczi, wrote about exhibitionism in a number of prescient, pioneering contributions to the psychoanalytical literature. Ferenczi realised that the urge to exhibit one's powerful penis, which might be alluring, will have become so deeply repressed, that it could readily be transformed into its very opposite, namely, a fear of looking at oneself, thus representing a defence against showing off. Ferenczi (1915) published a very short contribution on "Spektrophobie" – the German term for *spectrophobia* – which might be defined as the fear of looking into mirrors, which he conceptualised, rather creatively, as a flight from the potential pleasure of exhibitionism. In his subsequent article on nakedness, Ferenczi (1919b) reported the case of an hysterical woman who dreamed of undressing in front of her son and washing her naked body with a sponge. He theorised that, in such a circumstance, nudity and exhibitionism might serve as a means of instilling fear. Ferenczi also described the case of a little boy who had difficulty sleeping. In order to frighten the child away, his mother would remove all of her own clothing in the boy's presence. Ferenczi's work has helped us to appreciate that acts of exhibitionistic undressing, whether in dreams or in waking life, can be perpetrated by women as well as by men, and can serve the function of inducing terror.

Many, many other early psychoanalysts published important insights about the problem of exhibitionism. For instance, Dr. Jenö Hárnik (1923), a much-neglected figure in the history of this profession, wrote one of the very first papers which dealt with this subject. Based in part on some clinical observations from Dr. Hanns Sachs, the early Berlin psychoanalyst, Hárnik reasoned that, in men, exhibitionism serves an important function, namely, a defence against castration anxiety. In view of the actual vulnerability of the genitalia, especially so during the earliest, long-forgotten years of boyhood, adult men will become temporarily reassured by the act of exhibitionism which reinforces the idea that one still possesses an intact penis. Hárnik also helped to explain why cases of genital exhibitionism occur so infrequently in women. He suggested that because women experience a sense of shame at not having a penis, as Freud had theorised, they do not wish to reveal their genitalia, thus exposing the shameful absence. Additionally, Hárnik argued that although most women do not flash their genitals in the way that some perverse men often do, women will, nevertheless, exhibit the entirety of their bodies by dressing in certain types of clothing, so that they will often remain permanently on display (cf. Maeder, 1909; Flügel, 1932).

In similar vein, Dr. Sandor Lorand (1933) also recognised the importance of exhibitionism as a defence against castration anxiety in his infrequently cited contribution on "The Psychology of Nudism". Lorand, a Hungarian-born psychoanalyst who emigrated to New York City, New York, noted that exhibitionism reinforces one's belief in the potency and security of the penis, and that, by unveiling it to unsuspecting bystanders, the perpetrator can elicit a reaction in the victim, emphasising that the penis does still exist, and that it might be very powerful indeed. Also, Lorand argued that exhibitionism protects the male from his fear of the *vagina dentata* (the vagina lined with teeth) about which the patient might fantasise, and thus the exhibitionistic act of exposure still allows that individual some sexual proximity with women, nonetheless.

Clinicians have amassed much data from treatment experiences to support the castration anxiety hypothesis as one of the very cornerstones in the development of exhibitionism. Dr. Ismond Rosen, a South African-born, British-trained psychoanalyst, treated flashers in psychotherapeutic groups at the Portman Clinic in London. In his memorable chapter on "Exhibitionism, Scopophilia and Voyeurism", he described the case of a man called "Peter", who suffered from "constant recurring fantasies that his genitals would be bitten off by sharks in the swimming pool, bath water and bed" (Rosen, 1964b, p. 299). And Anna Freud (1974) reported the plight of a little boy who began to show off his penis to girls in the local neighbourhood, after he had undergone no fewer than three separate surgical procedures on three of his appendages, namely, one of his fingers, one of his toes, and, also, his penile foreskin. No doubt the boy's exposure of his genitalia will have served as an attempt to provide reassurance against fears of having his fingers, toes, or penis cut off by the doctors.

The little-known Swiss psychoanalyst, Dr. Hans Christoffel (1936, 1956), published two studies about his psychoanalytical work with exhibitionistic patients, noting that many would lead ostensibly heterosexual lives, but that they would often marry older women with whom they might not engage in coitus. Some of these men suffered from colpophobia – fear of the vagina – hence, they would develop a predilection for genital *exposure*, rather than genital *insertion*. For Dr. Otto Fenichel (1945), the great Austrian-born encyclopaedist of the psychoanalytical literature, exhibitionism could, potentially, serve several important functions. In agreement with Freud, Fenichel regarded indecent exposure as an *overcathexis* of a *partial instinct* or *component drive*, which represents a regression to a more infantile form of sexuality. He also confirmed Hárnik's observations about castration anxiety, suggesting that the act of exhibitionism would often dispel inner doubts about the durability of one's penis. Further, the act of exhibitionism would ensure that others become fearful; thus, in consequence, the exhibitionist could readily function as an aggressor, rather than as a victim, which he would fear even more. Finally, Fenichel speculated that exhibitionism serves as a defence against a powerful voyeuristic impulse, an idea to which Freud (1905a) had already alluded.

The British paediatrician and psychoanalyst, Dr. Donald Winnicott, reinforced Freud's earlier writings about the ubiquity and normality of phallic display in little boys. He actually referred to this period of oedipal development as "the phase of swank and swagger" (Winnicott, 1964, p. 186; cf. Winnicott, 1971). Other important British contributions include those of Dr. Mervin Glasser (1978), a one-time Director of the Portman Clinic, who wrote about deficits in the superego structure of exhibitionists, and, additionally, those of Dr. Christopher Lucas (1990), a psychoanalyst who also treated exhibitionists at the Portman Clinic. In Lucas's important essay on exhibitionism, he supported the castration anxiety hypothesis, and he noted that exhibitionism provides relief for the patient from internal turmoil. By evoking fear in the female victim, the exhibitionist will succeed in projecting his own distress into someone else. Lucas (1990, p. 23) described the very act of exposure as "both successful and unsuccessful", in that the revelation of the penis provides relief and sexual stimulation, but it also causes harm to the victim and, ultimately, to the exhibitionist and to his family as well.

In terms of early childhood events, it seems that future exhibitionists might not only experience deprivation of care in the mother-baby relationship, but, as the early years unfold, pre-exhibitionistic children will often become subjected to actual scenes of bodily exposure in the household. Dr. Sandor Lorand (1933) described the case of a sixteen-year-old girl who would undress completely at a party, in an effort to provide erotic flirtation and stimulation. On one occasion, she encouraged a twenty-year-old male to remove all of his clothing, eventually causing him to climax. In consequence, the girl's mother consulted with Dr. Lorand about her daughter's behaviour; and, before long, it soon emerged that during the sixteen-year-old's early childhood, this same mother used to walk around naked, as did the children. Therefore, we can surmise that infantile and childhood experiences of nudity and exposure will certainly contribute to a subsequent sense of familiarity with later acts of public undressing.

In similar vein, Dr. Frank Caprio (1948) described the early years of a male clinical exhibitionist whose mother used to enter the bathroom nude, ostensibly in order to comb her hair, whilst her son stood in the shower (cf. Caprio and Brenner, 1961). This patient, a nineteen-year-old who had begun exposing his penis as early as fourteen years of age, reminisced, "Sometimes when I was in a bathtub taking a bath, my mother would come in to get a towel. Once or twice when I was taking a shower she would come in to urinate. I could hear her urinating. My father would do the same thing. I could see my mother wipe herself with toilet paper. When I would be shaving, my mother would come in to urinate or defecate" (quoted in Caprio, 1948, p. 591).

One discovers these sorts of early experiences with widespread frequency in the families of many exhibitionists. For instance, Professor Robert Stoller (1979), the American psychoanalyst who had written so extensively about perversions, published the case of a woman called "Olympia", a centrefold in the pornographic magazine *Raunch*, who, as a child, used to frequent male toilets with her father, watching the grown men urinating. Olympia's mother also paraded nude around the house.

Christopher Lucas (1990) observed, quite tellingly, that several exhibitionists with whom he worked clinically would even become stutterers or stammerers. This observation prompted him to speculate that these men had grown up in homes with limited verbal communication, and thus, they came to develop a tendency to use *action*, rather than *verbalisation*, as a means of expressing internal conflicts. I have certainly worked with several mentally handicapped patients who had exhibited their genitalia publicly, and, in every case, those patients struggled to produce words with clarity, offering stuttering and stammering (cf. Christoffel, 1936; Fenichel, 1945).

Psychoanalytical workers have also made a number of astute observations about the immediate triggers of an exhibitionist episode, often linking the act to a recent trauma, abandonment, or humiliation (Stoller, 1975, 1985). Dr. Clifford Allen (1962) related the case of a man who exposed his penis after a woman rebuffed his marriage proposal. The aforementioned Dr. Christopher Lucas (1990) wrote about a man who displayed his genitals immediately after having argued with his wife. And Professor Wayne Myers (1991) noted that his photoexhibitionistic patient showed a picture of his erect penis to one of Myers's other patients in the waiting room, shortly after Myers had announced his own forthcoming holiday break (cf. Hirning, 1947).

Summarising the psychoanalytical contributions to the study of exhibitionism as a form of sexual perversion, we can enumerate the following observations:

1) Exhibitionism serves as a communication of internal distress, usually linked to early childhood traumata.
2) Exhibitionism functions as a defence against castration anxiety, and, also, as a means of reinforcing masculine potency.

3) Exhibitionism protects the patient from intercourse with women who may be conceived as dangerous or castrating.
4) Exhibitionism protects the patient against the fear of homosexuality.
5) Exhibitionism permits the patient to express sadism towards women, especially hatred toward the mother.
6) Exhibitionism operates as a narcissistic display.
7) Exhibitionism expresses the patient's masochistic tendencies and, moreover, his or her unconscious need to be captured by police and other authorities, thus gratifying the desire to be punished.
8) Exhibitionism serves as a means of restoring the patient's damaged self-esteem.
9) Exhibitionism permits the patient to transform aggressive affects into sexual activities.

Before we conclude our survey of psychoanalytical research on exhibitionism, let us examine in somewhat greater detail the problem of female exhibitionism. For many years, psychoanalysts did not believe that women ever exhibited themselves. Even the aforementioned Ismond Rosen (1964b, p. 293), an immensely erudite student of the world literature on the subject, stated quite categorically that, "The perversion of genital exhibitionism does not occur in women." However, as early as 1945, Otto Fenichel did describe the story of a woman who cut a piece of fabric out of her dress in order to expose her genitals and then facilitate cunnilingus. Some decades later, the Canadian-based psychoanalyst, Dr. George Zavitzianos (1971), published a study of a twenty-year-old psychopathic woman called "Lillian", who sat in her father's car, devoid of any clothing, exhibiting herself to passers-by. Unsurprisingly, as a little girl, Lillian used to walk around naked (cf. Hollender, Brown, and Roback, 1977; Zavitzianos, 1977; Grob, 1985).

Dr. Estela Welldon – later known as Profesora Welldon – the eminent forensic psychotherapist and psychiatrist, completely challenged early psychoanalytical ideas about the seeming absence of exhibitionistic perversions and other forms of sexual perversions in the female (cf. Welldon, 1996). In her landmark publication, *Mother, Madonna, Whore: The Idealization and Denigration of Motherhood*, the first book-length psychoanalytical study of female sexual perversions, Dr. Welldon (1988) described, among other cases, the tale of "Miss E", a thirty-four-year-old woman who began to expose her genitalia to female authority figures, in particular, since the age of seventeen years. In order to flash, Miss E wore a special overcoat, and she derived great pleasure from shocking her victims, including her doctors, whom she tracked to their private homes. Over the years, Miss E's exhibitionism resulted in expulsion from schools, jobs, training centres, and even counselling groups and mental hospitals. Sadly, Miss E could not control her urges at all, and, on a certain occasion, one of Miss E's victims slapped her.

Dr. Welldon noted that during the patient's developmental years, Miss E's mother would masturbate her, as well as the other siblings, as a means of pacifying the children. Miss E's mother actually confirmed this type of so-called child-rearing practice, confessing, "it was easier than to use a dummy" (quoted in

Welldon, 1988, p. 96). The mother, alas, had to endure beatings from her drunken husband; and, in consequence, the rhythmical masturbation of her children brought her some gratification.

In view of such an early experience, Miss E grew to depend upon sexualisation as a predominant mechanism of defence in her interactions, transforming complicated negotiations with authority figures into sexual encounters involving exhibitionism. Welldon also conceptualised Miss E's stripping as a form of manic enactment. Furthermore, Miss E had identified with the aggressor – her mother – by pestering others in an inappropriately sexual manner, just as her own incestuous mother had done to her. Shrewdly, Welldon observed that, by choosing powerful women as her victims, Miss E had secretly wished that her doctors and other such women would actually contain her, and thus become better mother-figures than her own biological mother had done. As Welldon (1988, p. 97) suggested, "Her hope for a shocked response in her victims had to do with a hopeful outcome in which women in authority – symbolic mothers – would not respond like her own mother, using and exploiting her as a part-object".

The work of Estela Welldon has confirmed once and for all that exhibitionism, though perhaps more widespread among male patients, can never be the exclusive domain of men, and that women will also display sexual perversions, including exhibitionistic perversions (cf. Holtzman and Kulish, 2012). Furthermore, Dr. Welldon's clinical researches demonstrate the widespread incidence of abuse and molestation in the backgrounds of so many perverse, forensic individuals.

In terms of treatment and rehabilitation, generations of psychotherapists and psychoanalysts have made great strides in providing psychologically orientated opportunities for exhibitionistic patients to receive help. Eschewing shaming programmes, hypnosis, pharmacotherapy, and incarceration as first lines of defence, the psychoanalytically-inclined psychotherapists have deployed traditional "talking therapy" with often good results. Sometimes we have even attempted to do so with zeal, as had occurred when Freud's disciple, Princesse Marie Bonaparte, one of the founders of psychoanalysis in France, encountered a flasher who had exposed himself to her while strolling through the Bois de Boulogne in Paris. According to members of her family, the Princesse remained unperturbed, and, rather than screaming or fainting – as many people might have done – she calmly handed her business card to the exhibitionist, offering him a free psychoanalytical consultation. As one might imagine, the chap in question bolted with all due haste (Bertin, 1982; Vickers, 2000).

Although sustained psychoanalytical treatment can operate very effectively with the exhibitionist, one must work through the strong defence mechanisms of splitting and denial utilised by the patient as a means of warding off discomfort and anxiety (Stoller, 1985; Pfäfflin, 1996). The defences can often be deeply entrenched, as we can detect in the case reported by the American psychologist Dr. David Shapiro (2000, p. 61), who wrote, "a middle-aged man with a long history of exposing himself briefly to young girls admits, indeed emphasizes, that he is a 'weak' person, a person lacking in self-control. He says (in his defense) that he does this only when drinking. However, he expresses no wish or intention to stop drinking." Other exhibitionists will deny the offence, often claiming to be urinating, for example, rather than exposing their genitals (Murphy, 1997).

Fortunately, if one can sustain the treatment relationship, then both the clinician and the patient will have the opportunity to proceed through three general phases: (1) the denial of the severity of the offence; (2) the recognition of the psychopathology of the exhibitionistic act; and (3) the working through of the symptomatology and broader character structure (cf. Warren, 2001). Although we do not have the space to discuss treatment issues in this context, psychoanalytical workers have reported some very impressive results in the rehabilitation of the exhibitionist (e.g., Rosen, 1964b; Socarides, 1988).

For example, Dr. Elif Gürisik's (1997) moving and convincing account of a flasher called "Peter", a thirty-four-year-old man who exposed and masturbated himself two or three times daily, provides a good indication of the potentialities of treatment. In spite of his compulsive masturbation, exhibitionism, and depression – all very understandable in terms of his history, which included a promiscuous mother who had sex with many men in front of Peter – the patient ultimately made a very good recovery in weekly psychoanalytically orientated group psychotherapy in a clinic setting. After five years, Peter ceased his flashing behaviours, although he remained in treatment for seven years in total, in order to consolidate his progress. Eventually, his impulsiveness of character became transformed into thoughtfulness, and he gradually developed into a more mature person, indulging in fewer sadomasochistic encounters with lovers and with family members. Eventually, he became a fervent skier, and, moreover, a competitive ballroom dancer, winning several medals. As Gürisik recognised, Peter's skiing and ballroom dancing served as a healthy and non-violent sublimation of his need to expose himself.

SECTION THREE: CONCLUSION

One need not search far before one will encounter evidence of exhibitionism in daily life. Virtually every museum and art gallery contains nude paintings and sculptures; practically every community boasts its own naturists or nudist beaches with genitalia on display; and every health club offers a profusion of saunas and steam rooms and showers, replete with naked bodies. Our cultural icons often practise versions of exhibitionism, ranging from the provocatively dressed actress and model Elizabeth Hurley – the former girlfriend of the actor Hugh Grant – and her famous 1994 "safety pin" dress, which left little to the imagination (e.g., Anonymous, 2024), to the legendary Hollywood actor Errol Flynn, who kept his friends entertained by exhibiting his full erection at parties (Gansberg, et al., 1981). Indeed, *The Full Monty*, a filmic festival of male genital exhibitionism, became one of the most celebrated motion pictures in the history of the British cinema, and it subsequently became a huge hit musical on Broadway.

Exhibitionism forms a very substantial part of adolescent subculture as well, evidenced by the penchant for "streaking" and "mooning" (in other words, displaying one's buttocks through a car window, for example), which one encounters frequently as part of football hooliganism. And adults continue to display themselves; indeed, anyone walking through London's West End on a Friday or Saturday night would have to be visually impaired not to notice the profusion of drunken men urinating against the sides of buildings.

Our relatives in the animal kingdom expose themselves with great regularity, as we know from observational studies of baboons, chimpanzees, gorillas, and orang-utans (Maletzky, 1997). And the male peacock will exhibit himself most of all with his resplendently phallic tail, designed to attract the female of the species.

As a number of psychiatric authors have suggested, exhibitionism may even form a part of our neurological hard-wiring (Jones and Frei, 1979).

And yet, as we have seen, this natural tendency to display can often become perverted and reach offensive, criminal proportions. Fortunately, more psychoanalytical theoreticians and clinicians have begun to derive an increasingly better understanding of the causes and consequences of clinical exhibitionism and, hence, have now developed more sophisticated ways of treating the exhibitionist in a psychotherapeutic situation.

Let us now examine a particular clinical case in great detail, which will, I trust, shed more light on the early origins of exhibitionist behaviour, and on the ways in which psychotherapeutic treatment might contribute to both the containment and, ultimately, to the eradication of this very common form of criminality.

From Penile Trauma to Flashing

A Case of Forensic Disability Psychotherapy

THE HANDICAPPED FILM STAR

The telephone in my consulting room rang.

"Hello, this is Brett Kahr speaking."

A polite and cultured gentleman with a very pronounced foreign accent replied, "Thank you, sir, for speaking to me. My family doctor has recommended that I should talk with you about my eighteen-year-old son."

I invited the caller to offer more information, whereupon he explained, "My beautiful boy, "Tobiasz", is such a sweet, young person. My wife and I love him very much. But the London police have just cautioned him for repeated acts of genital exhibitionism. He has been exposing himself in public."

The father, "Mr. X.", communicated this troubling and potentially shameful information in a very direct and straightforward manner, conveying a quality of deep concern for his son and, also, a sad recognition that his child had committed a series of crimes. I soon learned that the father, an émigré from Eastern Europe, held a demanding public role, which he executed with tremendous professionalism.

Mr. X. then elaborated, "I know that my son exhibited his private parts to various girls because he is mentally handicapped. He would not have done so had he not been handicapped. My wife and I think that he is very intelligent in many ways, but when you meet him, you will see that he suffers from some kind of disability and, at first glance, most people think that he is quite stupid."

I explained that I would be happy to meet with Tobiasz for a consultation, whereupon the father responded warmly, "Our son needs help, and if you agree to share your expertise with us, we would be extremely grateful. This is a top priority for us … *the* top priority … and we will bring Tobiasz to your office whenever it might suit. Just name the time and we will be there." The father also underscored that, in spite of Tobiasz's disability and, also, his Eastern European origins, he would be capable of speaking to me in perfect English.

I thanked the father for his clear and helpful summation, and then I offered an appointment for the following week.

Throughout this brief telephone conversation, I found myself deeply impressed by the courtesy, politeness, and seriousness of Mr. X. Unlike some patients (or

DOI: 10.4324/9781003546245-7

parents of patients) who convey immense resistance during the first telephone conversation, explaining – often rather grandiosely – that they can attend for a consultation *only* after 8.30 p.m. on a weekday or *only* on a Saturday or Sunday morning, and that they cannot afford more than fifteen pounds sterling per session, Mr. X. communicated with consideration and with gratitude, which made me hopeful that this family possessed a great deal of mental health and that, perhaps, the son, Tobiasz, might well be receptive to the psychotherapeutic encounter.

Those of us who work with patients diagnosed as intellectually disabled must devote considerable thought and care to the arrangement of the first consultation. In traditional psychotherapy with a *non*-disabled adult, one will speak to the patient directly and will not, under any circumstances, talk to other members of the family so that we may preserve confidentiality as fully as possible. With a child patient, by contrast, one *must* meet the parent or parents beforehand, or at least liaise with the caregivers on the telephone, in order to craft a plan. But how does one choreograph a first consultation with an eighteen-year-old person diagnosed as "mentally handicapped"?

Disability psychotherapists must consider whether an organically impaired or traumatised mentally handicapped patient (the phrase in standard use during the late 1980s when I first met Tobiasz) will require a formal escort (Kahr, 1998a, 2017, 2020a). Mr. X. explained that, although his child suffered from no physical disabilities whatsoever and could manage to travel to my office independently, Tobiasz might find a psychotherapy consultation frightening; therefore, the father and I agreed that he would accompany Tobiasz for the first session and would come into the office to meet me and to help the young man settle. Mr. X. explained that his wife – the mother of Tobiasz – had found the whole situation too disturbing and that she would not wish to attend. With some thoughtfulness, Mr. X. remarked, "In view of the fact that Tobiasz will no doubt wish to talk to you about private sexual matters, I think that it is best if we leave his mother out of this."

Once again, I regarded the sensitivity of Mr. X. as most sincere. Although he explained that he had no idea why his son had displayed his genitals to random females in a public setting – on a bus, in fact – he appreciated that a frank discussion of such behaviours would be required and that it might be quite shaming for his son to exhibit the contents of his mind – especially his *sexual* mind – in front of his own mother.

On the day of the initial appointment, the doorbell rang at the precise hour – neither a second early nor a second late. Mr. X., a well-dressed, distinguished looking man in his fifties, walked down the corridor with an equally well-groomed young man by his side. As father and son approached the threshold of my consulting room, I introduced myself and extended my hand, first to Tobiasz – the prospective patient – and then to Mr. X. – the father – and I invited them into the room, gesturing to the two empty chairs placed some six feet away from my own. After the three of us had taken our seats, I welcomed this son and father and then I turned towards Tobiasz and clarified that, as he may already know, his father and I had spoken briefly on the telephone during the previous week, but that I would be grateful to hear from him directly as to how I might be of assistance and, moreover, whether he would be happy for his father to sit in the room during the first part of our consultation.

Tobiasz, an extremely handsome young person with the classical looks of a film star, sported a highly exaggerated smile – often quite a characteristic defence against sadness and trauma (Sinason, 1986, 1988; cf. Sinason, 1999) – and he grinned at me quite broadly. He then turned to his father, as though seeking permission to speak. Mr. X. nodded at his son and encouraged him to communicate with me, whereupon Tobiasz opened his mouth for the first time. Within seconds, his handicap, by no means visible from his striking physical appearance, soon became quite apparent.

"I … uh … I … uh … uhhhh … uhhhh … uuuhhh …"

Tobiasz fumbled and stumbled, unable to articulate a coherent sentence.

I did not know to what extent his inability to speak with clarity stemmed from any baseline organic disability, or linguistic unfamiliarity, or, rather, from his anxiety about sitting across from a suited, bespectacled stranger in a potentially frightening context. Fortified by my prior teaching and supervision from Mrs. Valerie Sinason (1986, 1992) – later Dr. Sinason – one of the pioneers of disability psychotherapy, I knew that an exaggeration of the patient's handicap could often mask a fear of communication. Hopeful that Tobiasz might begin to speak more fully and clearly, I smiled benignly and nodded patiently as this young person struggled to find some simple words.

Mr. X., ever the helpful gentleman, gazed warmly at Tobiasz and intoned, "Brett Kahr is here to help our family. You can talk to him."

Tobiasz beamed, as though his father had suddenly and magically detoxified me. He then opened his mouth once again and attempted to speak.

"I … uh … uh … I … ahhh … uhhh … I …"

At this point, I made a comment that it might be quite frightening for Tobiasz to have come to meet me, especially after having already undergone an interview with a policeman, at the police station, some weeks previously. I underscored that Tobiasz might be worried that I, too, could become a psychological policeman of sorts who might send him to prison.

Apparently, the young man seemed relieved that I already knew something about his cautionary interview with the authorities, whereupon he replied in simple but, also, clear tones.

"Yes. The puuuh … leees. Puuuh … leees."

He struggled to vocalise the word "police", but in spite of his handicapped rendition, I could certainly understand these sounds.

Mr. X., recognising his son's long-standing difficulty at speaking in words, began, quite spontaneously and helpfully, to provide some further background information.

"As you can see, my son is a very handsome fellow. He has always been the most good-looking boy among his peers. All the girls want to marry him because he is so handsome. His mother and I have always thought that he should become a film star."

At this point, Tobiasz began to smile and to giggle and his face lit up with delight.

"Film star," he chirped, in completely audible tones. He had absolutely no difficulty articulating the phrase "Film star", and I sensed that he must have uttered those words many times previously.

Mr. X. then explained that, from the age of two years or thereabouts, Tobiasz had begun to display some sort of developmental delay of an indistinct nature. The doctors in their home country in Eastern Europe could not agree upon a diagnosis. One physician thought that he might be autistic; others suspected some sort of mental handicap. No one knew. But, clearly, Tobiasz demonstrated certain signs of difficulty with speech and concentration. As the parents boasted considerable financial resources, they had no difficulty employing a full-time nanny to support Mrs. X. as primary caregiver, while the father worked all day. Mr. X. insisted that, in spite of the disability struggles, Tobiasz had enjoyed a very loving childhood, full of comfort, luxury, and play.

"My son always had whatever toys and games he wished for. We deprived him of nothing. We think that he is a very lucky boy and he knows that he is our priority and that we love him very much."

Once again, Tobiasz smiled, pleased to hear such a good report about himself – a great contrast, no doubt, to the interview with the police, who berated him for having exposed his penis in public on multiple occasions.

At this point, I thanked Mr. X. for having introduced his son to me and for having provided me with such useful biographical background. I then turned to Tobiasz and asked whether he would be happy to speak to me privately so that the two of us could begin to talk about his situation in more detail.

With a huge grin on his face, he pointed his finger at his father and muttered, "You go away." Mr. X. sniggered affectionately, rose from his seat, shook my hand, and explained that he would meet Tobiasz after the end of the consultation and clarified that he would be waiting in his car, parked just outside of my office building.

Once Mr. X. had left the consulting room, Tobiasz looked at me with a wide-eyed expression which, I imagined, conveyed not only his anxiety about having to participate in a psychotherapy consultation but, also, perhaps, his relief that he could now enjoy some independence from his supremely articulate and competent father who suffered from no evident handicaps whatsoever.

Within seconds of Mr. X.'s departure, Tobiasz pounded his chest and boasted, "Film star. I be film star."

I looked at this strikingly handsome chap – a cross between Paul Newman and Robert Redford – and smiled softly as Tobiasz attempted to enhance his fragile ego structure by fantasising about himself as a movie icon. Although he had the looks to compete with Mr. Newman and Mr. Redford, he certainly lacked the verbal fluency and the mental acuity to become an actor.

With Mr. X. now safely out of earshot, I felt authorised to speak to Tobiasz in a more psychologically intimate manner and I risked a first interpretation.

"Your father has told us that both he and your mother are very proud of what a handsome young man you have always been and that you could be a film star. And *you* have just told me that *you* want to be a film star. But I think that a part of you must wonder whether this dream will ever come true. And in recent months, you have been showing off your penis to several young women. Perhaps you worry that, unless you display your body in that more striking way, no one will look at you or notice you. A young man exposing his private parts in public will attract a great deal of attention, just as film stars do."

At this point, Tobiasz's huge smile evaporated and he immediately began to appear more forlorn.

"I … very handsome."

I replied that as his parents, and many others besides, had often commented on his pleasant physicality, Tobiasz had certainly received a lot of confirmatory evidence about his good looks. But I wondered whether a part of him did not always feel quite so good looking.

"I … ugly too," he whispered, to which I replied, "Well, I would imagine that even though you look very handsome on the outside and you receive a lot of lovely compliments, I suspect that, on the inside, you do, perhaps, feel ugly at times, and that you may become very upset when you think you might be different from other boys."

He wasted no time in explaining, "Other boys … girlfriends. I … no."

I attempted to flesh out his cryptic statement: "You are letting me know how sad it is that other boys have pretty girlfriends but that you do not have a girlfriend. And that is very disappointing for you … even *angry*-making, especially when you have been told every day that you are so handsome."

He responded with sadness, "No girlfriend … no girlfriend."

I wondered aloud whether Tobiasz might also feel rather lonely, in spite of the fact that his parents have always doted upon him.

My comment seemed to touch a chord, and I derived some hope knowing that, in a more private conversation, Tobiasz could not only understand my speech, but, moreover, that *his* speech had become increasingly clear. Having begun the consultation uttering little more than occasional para-minimal encouragers (sounds such as "uhhh" and "ahhh"), he could now utilise longer words such as "girlfriend" and "handsome", which he could articulate with evident clarity.

I underscored that, although Tobiasz and I had only just met for the first time, and although I did not know a great deal about him as yet, I did have a sense that, in spite of being very handsome, and in spite of having very attentive and generous parents who love him greatly, he could be very sad and very angry at times that he might be different from the other boys. By wishing to be a film star he might hope that everything will turn out magically well. And by having displayed his private parts in public, he had found a way to be looked at, although this had placed him in a potentially very dangerous and destructive situation.

At this point, Tobiasz stopped grinning and he stared at me with a very sad expression. To my surprise and relief, he intoned, "I … uhhh … I … uhhh … not good what I did. Not good."

As our first encounter began to draw to a close, I explained that, as he knew, the family doctor had recommended that it might be useful for Tobiasz to talk to me about his situation. I underscored that although he and I had not yet discussed his genital displays in full, he might be willing to tell me more about what had happened and about his feelings, and that he and I could meet together, in private, on a weekly basis, to think about his life and to see whether such conversations could be helpful.

"Helpful," murmured Tobiasz. "Helpful."

He then smiled effusively and confirmed that he would be happy to talk with me again.

We arranged to have a second consultation the following week at the very same time, and I asked this young man whether he felt able to communicate this information to his father or whether he might wish for me to telephone his father to confirm the next appointment. Tobiasz seemed keen to keep his father out of the consulting room, and I had a sense that he wished to communicate only with me. He thus replied, "I tell him. Next week. Same time."

I repeated the day and time of our forthcoming appointment, stood up from my seat, and explained to Tobiasz that I very much looked forward to our next conversation and that I would do my best to be of assistance to him. A true gentleman, like his father, this young, handicapped man rose from his chair, extended his hand to me like an accomplished diplomat, and bowed his head in appreciation. As he began to walk down the corridor, he turned and waved, shouting, "Next week. Same time."

UNZIPPING THE TROUSERS

As our second appointment approached, I did worry that Tobiasz might not have understood the practical arrangements fully, but happily, one week later, the doorbell rang at precisely the correct moment, and Tobiasz and his father entered the building. Mr. X., with typical sensitivity, shook my hand, and noted that he had understood that Tobiasz and I had agreed to have a regular weekly session at the very same hour. I confirmed that Tobiasz and I thought this plan could be very useful. Mr. X. declared, "This is very good news. My wife and I are very pleased. I shall ensure that Tobiasz comes to you each week at this time." He then gave his son an affectionate hug and departed.

Tobiasz took his seat and we embarked upon our second session. The patient remained silent and, after a short interval, I asked him how he had experienced our first meeting during the previous week, and what thoughts, if any, had stayed in his mind.

"You nice man. Nice man."

I replied that if he considered me to be a "nice man", he might feel a bit more comfortable to talk to me about his life and his world in greater detail … especially about some of the more difficult experiences and feelings.

"Like my penis."

Previously, Tobiasz had not articulated the word "penis". Clearly, he possessed a more considerable capacity for verbal communication than he had revealed during the opening moments of our first consultation.

I then invited him to tell me about the times when he had displayed his penis.

Without hesitation, he explained that, one day, some three months earlier, he found himself seated in the back row of the upper deck of a bus, and, while looking at a very pretty girl across the aisle, he became "hard". He told me, in a very unhandicapped manner, that he wanted the girl to touch his penis, and so he unzipped his trousers and exposed himself, thinking that she would find his genitals attractive. The girl – some seventeen or eighteen years of age – rose instantly from her seat and disappeared from view, with a look of horror on her face. Tobiasz explained that he felt very saddened by this rejection and could not understand why she would not play with his penis.

"So pretty," he whimpered.

I commented that, although he had difficulty understanding why the beautiful girl did not touch his private parts, as he had wished, perhaps he also struggled to understand that the young woman could well have a mind of her own, and that, however handsome Tobiasz might be, he had probably scared this person by having exposed himself so abruptly.

He stuttered, "Me not dane ... dane ... dane ..."

"Dangerous?" I intoned.

"Me not dangerous," Tobiasz underscored.

I explained that while he did not consider himself to be dangerous at all, it might be challenging to imagine that he could well have had quite a frightening impact upon someone else.

"Me not dangerous," he repeated.

He then revealed that, over the course of several weeks, he had "unzipped" himself on four or five further occasions, always in the back row of the bus, and always in the presence of a pretty girl.

Although most of the young women to whom he exposed himself had walked away briskly in an act of self-protection, one of them ran to the driver, who stopped the bus and telephoned the police. Eventually, two officers escorted Tobiasz off the bus and then interrogated him.

He told me that he did not realise that the police would be so angry at him. Apparently, one of the policemen who removed Tobiasz from the bus pushed him rather aggressively and this frightened him considerably. The young man could not understand why the officer had to be so "mean".

As I listened to Tobiasz, I became increasingly impressed that, in spite of his handicap and his tendency to struggle verbally, he did manage to express himself with clarity and he could, albeit with some difficulty, narrate moments from his life history. This made me quite hopeful that we might eventually be able to learn something about his deeper motivations for these acts of genital exhibitionism.

Throughout this conversation, I became curious as to *when*, precisely, Tobiasz started to unzip his trousers. Had he done so for many years or had these illegal activities begun only quite recently?

Tobiasz responded to my query in a very straightforward manner and he told me that he had never taken his penis out of his trousers until just a few months earlier, not long after his eighteenth birthday. I attempted to discover why he had begun to exhibit himself at that particular point, rather than one or two or three years previously. Having worked with other male genital exhibitionists in my practice, I knew that the act of exposure often emerged in response to specific traumata, and I wished to discover whether some ugly event or fantasy had triggered Tobiasz's actions. Although I invited him to free-associate about what might have happened round about the time of his first offence, Tobiasz looked quite blank and did not seem to comprehend the meaning of my interest.

I thanked this young man for having begun to speak to me about a very important and very scary set of experiences which had resulted in a caution by the local police, and I underscored that, as our sessions progressed over the coming weeks, we would have an opportunity to think in more detail about these and many other biographical experiences so that we could both acquire a better understanding of the workings of his mind. Tobiasz smiled, then he rose from his chair and, once again, in rote-like fashion, repeated his exit line from the previous session, "Next week. Same time."

As the months unfolded, Tobiasz and I continued our regular psychotherapeutic work. His father, a remarkably loyal and reliable man, never failed to bring Tobiasz to my office, and the young eighteen-year-old always rang the bell at the correct time. Once each month, I handed Tobiasz an invoice to present to his parents and, the following day, I would always receive a cheque in the post. I certainly appreciated the seriousness with which the entire family attended to the formalities of Tobiasz's psychotherapy, which reflected their solidity and sanity, and this certainly enhanced my sense of hope. Many disabled patients, by contrast, have no supportive family members at all or, indeed, access to residency in an institutional setting which might prioritise talking therapies. But, in spite of his sexual offences of genital exhibitionism, Tobiasz lived in a world of considerable sturdiness and thoughtfulness.

Over time, I came to learn a great deal more about Tobiasz's early childhood. He began to reminisce, free-associatively, about his sixth birthday party, for which his mother baked a delicious chocolate cake with vanilla icing and his father took him riding on a pony. He recalled how, during his eighth year, he began to listen to pop music on the radio and he particularly enjoyed the songs of The Beatles, especially the classic "Yellow Submarine", which he began to hum for me. He talked of his grandmother, who doted upon him, and of his many aunts and uncles and cousins, all of whom treated him "nice". Unlike my other disabled patients, many of whom suffered horrific traumata at the hands of parents or institutional staff members, Tobiasz seemed to have had an idyllic childhood. And unlike my other exhibitionist patients, most of whom sat on the chair in my consulting room with their legs spread wide apart, as if to underscore how they frequently communicate with their genitals, Tobiasz seated himself in a modest and gentlemanly fashion, with his legs squeezed together. In many respects, he did not remind me of my other disabled patients or, indeed, of my other forensic patients.

And yet, he *had* displayed his private parts in public, causing great distress to several young females, and he did evoke the serious concern of the police. What on earth propelled a boy from such a seemingly loving and sturdy family to behave in such a manner?

EXPOSING THE TRAUMA

After several months of work, Tobiasz had painted an increasingly detailed and verbally rich portrait of his early childhood. But, thus far, we had devoted very little time to his schooling. I learned that, for the first ten years of his life, Tobiasz did not attend either a nursery or a primary school in his country of origin; instead, his wealthy parents paid for a tutor to educate him in the family residence owing to the fact that the local physicians explained that retarded children should be home-schooled. Tobiasz recalled a succession of very warm-hearted private instructors. Naturally, I had to entertain the possibility that one of these teachers might have harmed him in some way, but Tobiasz described each tutor in turn as a friendly and kindly person who taught him about letters and numbers and, moreover, about history. The teachers also watched movies with Tobiasz as special treats, and he particularly enjoyed reminiscing about how, on "nice days", he and one of his favourite instructors would watch cartoons together on television.

During one of our sessions, I expressed a curiosity to this young patient as to whether he felt disappointed that he had not attended a traditional school like all the other boys and girls in his home town. To my surprise, he told me that he did, in fact, become a "boarder" at the age of ten, although he quickly clarified that he had done so, "only for a bit … only for a bit." Over the course of several further psychotherapy sessions, Tobiasz shared some fairly anodyne memories of his time at boarding school, recalling, for instance, that he possessed a nice set of pencils and pens and, also, some lovely crayons. When I enquired about the teachers, he spoke of them in flattering terms. But he never mentioned the other boys at this single-sex school, nor did he speak of any sadness at having had to leave his family.

Eventually, after months of regular, sustained psychotherapeutic work, Tobiasz entrusted me with a vital memory and shared a very "big secret" that he had never revealed to anyone else before. I remained silent with a look of concern on my face, and, with a gentle nod of the head, I encouraged him to begin speaking, whereupon I learned that, not long after his arrival at the boarding school, the other ten-year-old boys began to tease him for being a "retard" and for speaking in a slow and indistinct manner.

One night, after the teacher had turned off the lights in the large dormitory, the other boys – about six or seven of them – attacked Tobiasz. In an effort to shame him, they pinned him to the floor so that he could not move, and then they stuffed a sock in his mouth so that he could not scream, ultimately stripping him of all of his clothing. The tormentors proceeded to make fun of Tobiasz for having a "little penis", and one of the more outspoken schoolmates humiliated him further by declaiming, "Look, even his dick is retarded." Most shocking of all, this gang decided that they would "torture" Tobiasz by "ripping off" his penis from his body, whereupon several of these abusive lads then began to pull on his genitals, tugging quite viciously, for several minutes, so much so that Tobiasz actually thought that they would succeed in detaching his penis completely.

This dreadful assault became an almost nightly ritual until, one day, Tobiasz received permission to telephone his parents, whereupon he demanded that he be removed from the school immediately. Sensing their son's unhappiness, the parents responded to his request and they returned him to the family home. But Tobiasz, full of shame at this castrating attack on his body and on his sense of self, had kept these episodes a complete secret, and neither his teachers nor his parents ever discovered quite what had happened to him.

Tobiasz became teary-eyed as he struggled to relate this traumatic episode to me. But to his credit, he did so in clear words, with much detail. At times, the tears simply streamed down his cheeks. Strikingly, he never reached for a tissue, readily available on a nearby shelf, and I commented that perhaps he had waited eight years for these tears to emerge and that by crying and by having shared this experience with me he might, at long last, begin to feel some relief.

Although it would be far too simplistic to conceptualise psychoanalytical work as the simple revelation of a trauma, leading to an immediate recovery, Tobiasz's narration of the attack on his penis as a ten-year-old boy certainly produced a tremendous sense of catharsis. Subsequently, he spoke with even greater verbal fluidity, as though he had finally begun to find his voice.

In subsequent sessions, Tobiasz and I reflected at great length about the impact of these episodes. We discussed his sense of shame at feeling "like a girl", unable to fight back "like a boy". We explored his fear that the other lads hated him for being a "retard" and, also, for having a rich and famous father. He also dared to suggest that, because he looked far more handsome than the other boys, they might have resented his appearance. Without having mentioned the word "envy", Tobiasz certainly theorised with the clinical intelligence of a seasoned mental health practitioner.

I admired this young man's ability to share his memories of these cruel episodes from his short time at boarding school. In view of the profundity of the attack on his body and on his growing sense of masculine potency, such an experience would certainly have provoked his castration anxieties and would have induced a sense of deep shame and insufficiency, in spite of his many capacities. Tobiasz and I also talked about the fact that these penile attacks occurred during his first prolonged separation from his very loving and attentive parents, and that he might have experienced some angry feelings towards both his mother and his father for having sent him away to such a dangerous school.

Eventually, after Tobiasz spoke at length about these traumata, we then began to consider the potential impact of such an emotionally shocking and physically painful experience – the near loss of his penis – upon his subsequent acts of genital exhibitionism eight years later. Once we had established a connection between his boarding school abuse and his eventual exhibitionism, Tobiasz could at last begin to appreciate that he might have needed to display his penis in front of those "pretty girls", as he actually believed that these young females would truly admire his genitals, thus helping him to repair the pain of having exposed his private parts in front of those violent "ugly boys". During this more prolonged period of "working through", he and I reflected not only about the potential causes of his criminal acts but, also, we began to imagine what impact his exposure might have had upon the "pretty girls" whom he imagined would simply stare in admiration and treat his penis as a film star in its own right.

As we began to understand more and more about the deeply painful and profoundly shaming experiences that Tobiasz had endured as a boarder at school, he became increasingly able to discuss private matters with me in a more straightforward way. Eventually, we devoted greater consideration to an exploration of why his genital exhibitionism had emerged in his eighteenth year, rather than at some other time.

Although there may be many factors which contributed to this young man's exhibitionist activities at that particular moment, we did come to discover that, shortly before his first public exposure of his genitals, Tobiasz had experienced an emotionally castrating attack from a stranger. With tears in his eyes and rage in his voice, Tobiasz told me that, one day, while out for a stroll, a boy no more than fourteen or fifteen years old, passed him on the pavement. Sensing that Tobiasz might have a learning difficulty of some sort, this young person began insulting him: "You're a fucking faggot. You're a fucking retard." Tobiasz did not retaliate; he simply continued on his walk. But he felt absolutely wretched. And only three or four days later, quite eviscerated and demasculinised, he displayed his penis on a bus for the very first time. Tobiasz enjoyed making connections of this sort and, gradually, he began to develop an infinitely richer understanding of his behaviours and his emotions.

After fourteen months of sustained psychotherapy, I received a telephone call from the father, Mr. X., informing me that a high-ranking official in his country of origin had invited him to return home to assume a new appointment and that, in consequence, he and his family would have to move back to Eastern Europe in two months' time. I must confess that this sudden announcement saddened me, as I had become very fond of Tobiasz and, also, quite impressed by his capacity for emotional growth. We had reached a point where he had become much more verbally fluent, much more insightful, and much more empathic, even expressing shame and regret that some of the girls might have found his penis scary. Fortunately, we had eight more sessions in which to prepare for an ending and to say goodbye.

In our final meeting, Tobiasz told me, quite touchingly, that he would miss me. I replied that I had very much appreciated the serious way in which he had committed himself to the psychotherapeutic process and that I would think about him afterwards and that I hoped that he would be well. Tobiasz parted with a warm handshake and with a look of deep kindness in his eyes.

Approximately six months after our psychotherapy ended, Tobiasz sent me a handwritten note, posted from his country of origin, in which he expressed his sincere thanks to me for our work together over the last year. To my relief and delight, he reassured me that, nowadays, while riding the bus, he behaves like "a very nice man." To the very best of my knowledge, Tobiasz engaged in no further acts of public genital exhibitionism in the years which followed.

CONCLUSION

Not all forensic patients must cope with intellectual disabilities and not all disabled patients will perpetrate crimes. But many of those men and women diagnosed as intellectually disabled will be at risk of committing offences, not least because of their struggles to transform their ordinary human sadistic affects into words. Consequently, over recent decades, with the growth of both forensic psychotherapy and disability psychotherapy as discrete professional specialities, a number of colleagues have begun to explore the intersection between these two fields with great success (e.g., Curen, 2009, 2018; Sinason, 2012; Hollins, 2019), so much so that Dr. Alan Corbett (2014) wrote an important textbook, *Disabling Perversions: Forensic Psychotherapy with People with Intellectual Disabilities*, about the new arena of *"forensic disability psychotherapy"* (Kahr, 2014a, p. xix; cf. Corbett, 2018).

As we know from the case of Tobiasz, described herein, penile trauma does, indeed, exist, and it certainly provokes profound, often forensic, consequences.

More than 250 years ago, the English novelist Laurence Sterne published *The Life and Opinions of Tristram Shandy, Gentleman*, in which the protagonist, as a little boy, could not find his chamber pot and, consequently, urinated out of a window, the frame of which fell, tragically, upon his penis. In order to dispel any rumours of having become completely castrated, the child's uncle recommended that he ought to exhibit his genitals in the public marketplace to offer reassurance. While this may have been a very sound treatment method for castration anxiety in the eighteenth century, we now have a much better remedy, namely, the capacity to offer our verbally compromised and bodily fearful patients a confidential psychotherapeutic space in which such traumata can be explored and, hopefully, healed.

5

Fragile Monster
How to Make a Paedophile Talk

I cannot do justice to the large and dangerous subject known as paedophilia in the space of a brief book chapter. In previous publications, I have endeavoured to encapsulate certain aspects of my psychotherapeutic work with young sexual offenders in the hope of understanding the origins of their symptomatology and, thus, helping them to improve and thereby become less likely to perpetrate more crimes in the future (Kahr, 2004a, 2020a). On this occasion, however, I wish simply to offer a brief glimpse into the moment-by-moment interaction with a juvenile paedophile in the psychoanalytical consulting room, so that colleagues and students might have an opportunity to learn how those of us who work in the field of forensic psychotherapy endeavour to listen to our patients and speak with them in more detail. In the interests of confidentiality, I have disguised not only the name of the patient in question, but, also, those of the professional colleagues who served as escorts, transporting this young man to my office.

***

At precisely 1.35 p.m., the doorbell rang.

This may seem an odd time for an appointment, but my psychotherapy sessions often begin, unusually, at twenty-five minutes before the hour, or ten minutes past the hour, so that when patients arrive at the office building, they will not bump into my colleagues' patients in the process. It would be rather crowded if everyone appeared at the stroke of twelve.

Complete privacy remains the absolute bedrock of psychotherapeutic work; hence, I make every effort to create as confidential an atmosphere as possible.

I picked up the entryphone.

"Hello."

"Professor Kahr, it's Giles Sweeney."

"Ah, please do come in. I'm on the second floor."

I then pressed the buzzer, and Mr. "Giles Sweeney" – a very experienced social worker – entered the building, accompanied by two other males. I already understood that my new patient would not be arriving on his own.

DOI: 10.4324/9781003546245-8

Ordinarily, patients travel to my consulting room all by themselves. But this patient had come under escort, having recently assaulted several little children of both genders.

"Brodie", a sixteen-year-old sexual offender, had forcibly stripped three youngsters of their clothing and had then fondled their genitals roughly, while masturbating himself to a climax.

This young person had committed a dreadful offence; and his progressive social worker, Mr. Sweeney, arranged for him to embark upon intensive psychotherapy, in the hope that a powerful treatment intervention might help to forestall the development of a full-fledged paedophilic personality.

My colleagues and I have discovered that if young sex offenders can receive psychotherapy while still in their teens, this often prevents them from becoming career paedophiles later in life. And as many invariant paedophiles target dozens – often hundreds – of youngsters, such work becomes imperative. Consequently, I agreed to the plan.

As Brodie now lived in a remand home for delinquent adolescents, Mr. Sweeney had to escort him to my office based, at that time, in Hampstead, in North-West London. The courts would not have trusted Brodie to travel alone, as he might conceivably have harmed some children along the way.

I perched myself at the entrance to my consulting room, at the very end of a long corridor, and I waited quietly.

Within seconds, I could hear a bevy of feet mounting the stairs, and then, two very large men appeared: Giles Sweeney, the social worker, and his colleague, "Jeffrey Lundgren", a probation officer, each dressed in smart, but casual, clothing.

Behind them trailed a much younger, much shorter person, perhaps no more than 5' 6" in height, wearing green denim jeans and a faded orange T-shirt, whom I knew must be Brodie.

Giles Sweeney, the taller of the two grown-ups, immediately took charge of the introductions.

"Professor Kahr, I'm Giles Sweeney. And this is my colleague from probation, Jeff Lundgren."

I nodded and shook each man's hand.

"And this is Brodie."

"Welcome," I replied, "I'm Brett Kahr."

I greeted Brodie, but I did not use his name. I knew only too well that while some patients enjoy being addressed by their first names straight off the bat, others experience this as far too intimate in the context of a psychotherapy session.

And although I had shaken Mr. Sweeney's hand and, also, that of Mr. Lundgren, I did not offer a hand to Brodie, as I would normally do with a new patient. I refrained from such a gesture as I could tell from Brodie's extremely downcast gaze and from his highly agitated appearance that he had no wish to engage in social niceties. I also knew that several police officers had recently manhandled him, following his detention and incarceration for the sexual offences against those three little children. Consequently, I refrained from any physical contact with this person.

Giles Sweeney, a diplomatic chap, appreciated Brodie's need for privacy, and he volunteered, "Well, Professor, we'll leave you to it. We'll come back in fifty minutes … at 2.25 p.m., if that's correct?"

I nodded to both the social worker and the probation officer, and then I invited Brodie to come into the office. After he crossed the threshold of my consulting room, I closed the door behind us.

I gestured to a large, comfortable chair, newly reupholstered in blue suede fabric, and then I sat in my own more weather-beaten, brown leather chair, positioned exactly six feet away.

I have always placed my consulting room chair at a distance of six feet from the patient … and *not* by accident.

Many years ago, as a young University Fellow at the Yale Psychological Services Clinic in New Haven, Connecticut, one of my teachers undertook a very clever investigation. He studied three groups of psychotherapy patients: those placed *three* feet away from their therapists, those placed *six* feet away, and those positioned at a distance of some *nine* feet. He then interviewed the patients afterwards. The men and women who sat quite close – three feet apart – and those, likewise, who sat quite far away – nine feet apart – all reported considerable discomfort. But six feet felt just right.

Consequently, I have always seated myself at this magical distance of six feet, as it seems neither too intrusive nor too abandoning.

With the social worker and the probation officer en route to the local Starbucks for a fifty-minute espresso or cappuccino, and with the door to my office now firmly closed and secured, the work of psychotherapy could finally begin in earnest …

… or so I had thought.

During the early years of my career, I often inaugurated my sessions in utter silence, so as not to interrupt the patient's free flow of associations. I had studied under many ancient Freudian teachers who advised that clinicians must *never* begin the session with even so much as a "hello", as that could intrude upon the patient.

But as the years unfolded, I found such advice really rather unhelpful. One of my old teachers once reminisced that one of *his* old teachers, the great British psychoanalyst Dr. John Klauber – a warm-hearted man of Hungarian extraction – would often counsel that we must never forget how much courage the patient will have required in order to mobilise himself or herself to attend that first clinical appointment. Appearing at the consulting room demands a great deal of psychological bravery. Practitioners must, therefore, make our patients feel welcome.

Bearing all that in mind, once I have sat down in my chair, I would always begin the first session with each new patient by asking how I might be of help.

I believe that I inaugurated the initial session with Brodie thus:

"Hello … as you know, I'm Brett Kahr, and as you *also* know, your social worker, Mr. Sweeney, has recommended that it might be useful for you to come to see me. Please tell me how I may be of assistance."

Brodie sat in the chair with his neck arched downwards, staring into his lap. My words of greeting seemed to fall upon deaf ears, because he made no response to my invitation to begin speaking.

Silence from a psychotherapy patient neither surprises me nor troubles me during introductory consultations. Encountering a psychotherapist for the very first time can be scary, and patients often fear that we will make some horrible pronouncement about their personalities, rather like an oncologist breaking the bad news that the cancer has metastasised.

In spite of the anxiety of being in the presence of a mental health professional, most of my more psychologically robust patients collect their thoughts and begin speaking in due course, with very little prompting. In fact, the vast majority of these men and women have *so* many anxieties on the tips of their tongues that they cannot wait to blurt out their stories, often before they have even removed their overcoats.

Brodie, however, wallowed in utter silence.

I used the quiet as an opportunity to study this young teenager more closely.

Most people imagine perpetrators of sexual crimes to be rather grizzled, ugly brutes, in dirty clothes. During my working lifetime I have, in fact, met many paedophiles who do, indeed, look deeply unattractive, with steely eyes and deadly expressions.

But Brodie had the face of an angel.

His rosy cheeks bore no trace of stubble, and his enviable mop of blond hair flopped across his brow. He certainly did not strike me as old enough to have reached the age of sixteen years. Had I not already known his date of birth, I might have guessed him to be a mere thirteen or fourteen.

In spite of his cherubic complexion, he looked desperately emaciated, and I wondered when he had last eaten a meal.

I had expected to meet an evil-looking adolescent sex offender who had perpetrated acts of immense cruelty upon not one, not two, but *three* small boys and girls; yet, by contrast, I found myself seated across the room from a simple-looking and deprived young lad – little more than a boy himself – who might easily have come straight from the pages of *Oliver Twist* or *Les Misérables*.

My own private free association to the novels of Charles Dickens and Victor Hugo hardly astonished me. I knew already from Giles Sweeney's extremely lengthy and detailed case reports – sent to me prior to this first appointment – that Brodie's father had disappeared soon after his birth, and that the mother had died in a car crash shortly after the boy's first birthday. This undernourished lad had already endured fifteen years as an orphan, reared in one foster home after another.

Brodie had still not spoken, and thus I tried, once again, to inaugurate a conversation.

"I know that this is your first time in a psychotherapist's office. Perhaps it feels a little nerve-wracking."

I waited … and waited … and waited for Brodie to speak … but he failed to do so. The silence grew: ten seconds … twenty seconds … then thirty – an eternity in the intense context of a psychotherapeutic consultation. But this teenage sex of-fender had still not uttered a single syllable.

After nearly a minute of increasingly stiff silence, I intervened once again, in my most calming and measured psychotherapeutic voice: "I know that you've never met a psychotherapist before and that you might be reluctant to talk. But please, do tell me how you've been and how you feel about having been asked to see me today."

Once again, Brodie made no reply.

This waif-like sixteen-year-old still wallowed in silence, looking rather fright-ened. His head continued to lurch in what seemed a most uncomfortable down-ward position. Perhaps Brodie had already begun to convey to me – albeit quite unconsciously – how heavy his head must feel: full of thoughts of sexual confu-sion, of guilt, of terror about his future, and goodness knows what else.

I must confess that having now extended several invitations to Brodie to begin speaking, and having received absolutely no verbal acknowledgement, my own level of anxiety began to rise.

But of course, as someone who has worked in the mental health field for a very long time, I had to remember that Brodie's lack of response actually provided me with much important information.

I thought once again about the lengthy documents that I had received from Giles Sweeney, which contained a chilling description of how Brodie, while baby-sitting for some neighbourhood children, had bound their wrists with bathrobe cords, and then, one by one, stripped them of their pyjama bottoms, and then rubbed their immature genitalia quite roughly with his left hand while masturbating himself to orgasm with his right hand.

Each of these three youngsters – a six-year-old brother, and his two sisters, aged four and three respectively – wailed and howled during this attack, unable to make any sense of why Brodie, the sweet-faced child-minder, would want to touch their private parts in this way. In all likelihood, none of the little ones had ever seen an erect penis before, and one can only imagine their terror as this familiar baby-sitter had suddenly turned into an unfamiliar hyperventilating monster.

As I sat quietly in my office chair, *still* waiting for Brodie to talk, I realised that this boy – like all paedophiles – communicates not with his mouth but, rather, with his sexual organ.

Nevertheless, I knew that, somehow, I would have to initiate a proper verbal conversation if I wished to make any psychotherapeutic progress with this very troubled young person, and so I persisted in my efforts to inaugurate some sort of dialogue.

"You know, I wonder whether you might be quite angry at Mr. Sweeney for having brought you here. And perhaps you might be quite angry with *me* as well. I suspect that you may not want to be here at all."

Once again, my comments evoked no reaction whatsoever.

I bore the silence, as a psychotherapist must do, and I continued to wait. But as I did so, the silence became increasingly noisy.

Although silence can be extremely frustrating, it also provides a space in which the psychotherapist might be able to think more fully and more broadly: studying the patient, searching for clues, and exploring hypotheses.

As I looked at this teenage sex offender, stationed some six feet away from me, I noticed something quite unusual about the way in which he had positioned his body in the chair.

Most patients will perch themselves in the blue suede chair in a rather straightforward manner. Women will often cross their legs demurely. Men will either fold one leg over the opposite knee, or they will sit with both feet securely planted on the ground, but with each leg pressed closely together.

Brodie, however, had splayed his legs quite widely: a true rarity among psychotherapy patients.

Over many decades of practising clinically, I have encountered only three groups of people who regularly spread their legs in such a bold fashion, namely, prostitutes, pornographers, and paedophiles.

Most of the people who have consulted me over the last four decades will have led very decent, very honourable lives, working as lawyers, doctors, accountants, businesswomen, and househusbands. Mercifully, fewer than one-tenth of one per cent of patients will have abused young children or will have contributed to the pornography industry.

But, in the course of my professional life, I have treated a fair few paedophiles, prostitutes, and pornographers – all of whom spread their legs while seated in the chair! This cannot be entirely accidental. I have come to regard this very unconscious but, nevertheless, very ritualised leg-splaying among such patients as a means of conveying how these people communicate with their genitals and how their private sexual organs become such visible public property.

I did entertain the idea that I might make an observation to Brodie about the position of his legs, but I rejected this notion as I suspected that he would experience this as a potentially shaming comment which might close down any hope of communication. And so I maintained my silence instead, just as he maintained his.

It occurred to me that Brodie could not bring himself to speak to me because he might have felt very ashamed of his vicious attack on those painfully young children.

Once again, I risked a comment.

"You are being extremely quiet. Perhaps you might be worried that if you start to speak about what has happened to you in recent weeks ... about what you have done to those children ... that I might condemn you or reject you. Perhaps you feel more protected saying nothing at all."

Brodie did not move a muscle. His mouth still remained tightly shut. I had no idea whether he even took in my words at all.

At this point, perhaps five or six minutes into our monastic silence, he surprised me by lifting his head from his chest and by glancing up into the extreme right-hand corner of the ceiling. He then craned his neck in the opposite direction, staring into the far left-hand corner.

Brodie repeated these very pointed neck movements five or six times in succession.

If a sixty-year-old patient twisted his neck from side to side in this fashion, gazing upwards and sideways, I might imagine that he would already have consulted with an osteopath or with a physiotherapist who would have suggested such stretching as a means of exercising a degenerative cervical spine.

But the sixteen-year-old Brodie had no need for such orthopaedic posturings.

I made a rather anodyne comment about his head movements, expressing curiosity; but once again, Brodie refrained from replying or, indeed, from offering any acknowledgement, and he then returned his head to a downward stare.

After several failed attempts to engage this young person in conversation, I became increasingly dejected and felt that I might be making no progress at all, in spite of my many, many years of clinical experience.

It occurred to me at this point that my feeling of helplessness could well have mirrored Brodie's own deep-seated sense of helplessness.

In psychoanalysis, we refer to this phenomenon by the somewhat clunky phrase *projective identification* – a term which describes how the patient creates an atmosphere in which he or she evacuates horrid, unwanted thoughts and emotions into the mind of the psychoanalyst or psychotherapist, who then experiences these feelings all too viscerally (e.g., Klein, 1946; cf. Ogden, 1982; Joseph, 1987). In other words, the clinician identifies with the patient's projections.

For instance, if a psychotherapist should suddenly become sleepy in the session, in spite of having had a good night's rest, it may be that he or she has begun to pick up – quite unconsciously – the patient's own weariness and fatigue. Should the psychotherapist start to feel angry without good reason, this could well be a sign of some repressed anger in the patient, bristling beneath the surface.

In other words, we become exceptionally sensitised conduits, identifying what the patient can neither tolerate nor verbalise.

Projective identification can be a nuisance but it also provides a great deal of important data.

Collecting my thoughts, I risked an interpretation.

"I mentioned a short while ago that you might be very angry, having been brought here against your will. I have also been wondering whether there may be times when you feel quite helpless … as though you have little control over your own life."

Once again, Brodie uttered not a peep, and he resumed his head-turning ritual, staring again and again at the corners of the consulting room ceiling.

With most of my more "normal" or "neurotic" psychotherapy patients, I know very little about them prior to the first meeting. Only the tiniest number of patients will arrive under escort by social workers and probation officers, preceded by a bundle of court documents.

But with Brodie – a forensic patient who had committed an extremely serious sexual assault on several rather small children – I had already learned a very great deal about him from Mr. Sweeney's summaries and from Brodie's prior psychiatric assessments and psychological test results. I discovered, for instance, that he had only recently undergone a series of interviews at a police station, after the parents of the children for whom he baby-sat had reported him for molestation.

"You know … I am so struck by the fact that you keep looking up at the corners of the ceiling, as though you expect to find something there …"

Brodie held his guard. In fact, I could see that my persistent attempts to engage him in verbal conversation had now begun to annoy him. He stopped looking upwards, and he began to stare at his shoes instead, avoiding any eye contact with me whatsoever.

Undaunted, I persevered.

"I know from Mr. Sweeney's report, which I *have* read, and from the police report, which I have *also* read, that you recently had to undergo an interrogation at the police station. I would imagine that must have been quite a scary experience."

Untouched by my remark, or so it seemed, Brodie kept his head bowed and his jaw locked.

"I'm so struck by the fact that you keep staring at the ceiling, and it occurred to me that there might well have been overhead video cameras in the interview room at the police station, recording the entire proceedings. That might have felt very frightening. And perhaps you're checking the corners of *my* office to see whether there might be cameras here … even *hidden* cameras … monitoring every movement, and listening to every word. If that is true, it makes great sense that you're not speaking to me."

I took an invisible breath, hoping that this interpretation might have registered. It certainly made great sense to me that his compulsive ceiling stares could well be indicative of a very reasonable examination of the physicality of the room. After all, when cats or dogs enter a new location for the first time, they sniff around compulsively to ensure that they will encounter no vicious beasts lurking beneath the settee. Brodie, likewise, would be well within his rights to scrutinise my office, lest I had a team of police officers hidden behind the bookcases, ready to pounce and take him to prison.

Alas, my remark, which I considered reasonably thoughtful, failed to elicit any overt response from this increasingly vexing young lad.

By this point, at least twenty-five, possibly thirty, minutes had elapsed, and I knew that Mr. Sweeney, the social worker, and Mr. Lundgren, the probation officer, would soon ring the bell again, thus signalling the end of the session. Although the specific contents of the session would remain confidential, I knew that I would have to speak to Giles Sweeney and confirm whether or not he would need to bring Brodie back for a follow-up appointment.

I felt under increasing pressure, and I began to squirm.

Over the years, I have met many, many patients who start the session in total silence. But after a while, most of them begin talking after two or three or four minutes.

I could not recall the last time someone had kept me waiting for nearly half an hour.

Desperate to hear this boy speak, I tried every trick in the book.

I hypothesised that Brodie might have a fear that, if he spoke to me about his crimes, I might turn him over to the police for further questioning, and I interpreted his anxiety that I might reveal to his social worker and his probation officer all of the details of our conversation, violating his right to confidentiality. I also pontificated about his terror that I might find his story to be so unbearably revolting that I would have no alternative but to throw him out of the office as a punishment for having harmed those children.

Brodie's eyes still looked glassy and vacant, and he continued to maintain his stony, almost catatonic, expression.

A sudden free association then popped quietly into my mind. I imagined myself working at a hospital, in a busy accident and emergency department, desperately trying to revive a patient whose heart had stopped beating. I fantasised about using some high-voltage electric paddles to shock the patient back to life.

But I had no paddles in my consulting room, and all of my efforts to bring this emotionally dead person into the land of the living kept failing miserably.

I experienced the unresponsive and emotionally flatline Brodie as dying before my very eyes. I even imagined having to confess to Giles Sweeney: "Time of death: 2.25 p.m."

Then it occurred to me that Brodie *did*, indeed, have a very broken heart … not in the *cardiological* sense, but in the *psychological* sense. After all, his father had walked out on him during early infancy, and then, little more than one year later, his mother had died in that awful hit-and-run.

Perhaps, at that very moment, Brodie did develop "heart disease" of some sort.

How, though, could I become his *psycho*-cardiologist? Would I need to shock him back to life with a defibrillator, or could I find a more gentle, less frightening way of getting his blood to pump?

And then, at that point, decades of training and experience finally "kicked in", and my clinical intelligence began to return.

I saw before me a young person whom many would regard as a brutal paedophile-in-training. I suspected that the parents of Brodie's three little victims might well wish him dead … and one could hardly blame them. After all, this sexually violent teenager had assaulted all three of their children, and it would not be unreasonable to suspect that each of those tiny survivors might require years of psychotherapy at some point in the very near future.

Of course I could see the monstrous side of Brodie, but I could also appreciate the Dickensian orphan boy who had never really had a daddy or a mummy or anything that might represent a safe, protected childhood. Between the ages of two and fifteen, he had lived in as many as five foster homes. No wonder he wished to destroy the childhood of three kids for whom he baby-sat, each of whom, quite enviably, *did* have a loving, dependable, reliable mother and father.

I took a deep gulp of breath … and then I spoke.

"You and I have been sitting here for more than thirty minutes... almost forty minutes now... and although I've offered you many opportunities to speak, you've kept really, really silent."

I paused again for another brief breath, and then I continued.

"I know you're frightened, as you've never met me before. Brett Kahr is a total stranger to you. And you've had so many interviews with the police and the social workers and the psychiatrists. You must be sick of all of these grown-ups talking to you … interrogating you. It makes perfect sense that you are keeping quiet."

Brodie's lips refused to budge.

I continued.

"You know that I've read the reports that Mr. Sweeney sent me, and therefore, I'm very aware that you have had a really, *really* difficult life, and that you've endured some truly painful experiences. I know your father disappeared. And I know your mother died, which is extremely sad. You've never really had a mummy all your own."

I had a sense that Brodie could hear me, but he still remained icy.

"Mr. Sweeney told you that he had arranged for you to see a man called Brett Kahr. As you know, that is my name. My surname is an unusual one, spelled K-A-H-R. But it's pronounced exactly like a car on the road: C-A-R. And it occurs to me that this could well be a very *provocative* name for you. Perhaps you might have wished that Mr. Sweeney had brought you to see a Dr. Brett *Smith* or a Dr. Brett *Jones*. But Brett *Kahr* is tricky name for you, because your mummy was run over and killed by a *car* – a C-A-R – and perhaps you might worry that I am going to be a very deadly car and that I might run you over in some way."

After I finished speaking, I gulped … privately … desperate for some sort of richer response from this fragile boy.

To my shock and, also, to my delight, Brodie lifted his head and, for the first time in forty-five minutes, he looked at me directly, across the six-foot divide, and then, within seconds, this hitherto statue-like lad suddenly burst into floods of tears.

At first, the teardrops began to stream down his cheeks in silence, but as he saw his very deep pain reflected in my facial muscles, which had, by this point, become furrowed with compassion, Brodie released several audible wails and, at long last, this troubled boy really let go, sobbing profusely.

Suddenly the monster could finally begin to reveal the fragility and the suffering that he had carried within both his body and his mind for at least the last fifteen years.

I let Brodie cry, and I certainly did not interrupt him, but I held his gaze with a look of deep concern.

Strands of mucous began to trickle from his nostrils, and he then reached into the pockets of his jeans in search of a tissue, but he had none; and so, at that point, I gestured to the box of Kleenex perched on the bottom shelf of the bookcase next to his chair.

He reached into the cardboard box, grabbed a clump of tissues, and then wept some more … and then some more.

After a minute or two of uninterrupted crying, I intervened in a very soft and gentle voice.

"I think that my remarks have touched a chord. I think you've been really frightened that, just as you did something awful to those little children, *I* might do something awful to *you*. Perhaps you fear that I would harm your body in some way, or run you over like a very dangerous car. Like the car – the C-A-R – that killed your mummy. No wonder you have been reluctant to look at me. No wonder you have struggled to talk to me, fearful that I might be a dangerous K-A-H-R."

Brodie nodded his head in agreement – the first time that he had deployed his neck muscles to convey affirmation rather than paranoid suspiciousness.

Using his right hand to daub his eyes, and his left hand to wipe his nose, this adolescent sexual offender finally uttered his very first recognisable words.

"You're right," he whispered.

"Am I?"

"Yeah, I've never had a family, not really."

And then he burst into another round of tears.

I asked him when he had last cried in this unrestricted way.

"Never."

I replied, "I rather suspected as much. Perhaps it feels a huge relief to be able to let someone know how very unhappy you've been … all this time."

"Yeah," he croaked. "Yeah."

I nodded silently in an attempt to convey that I understood.

After a few more moments, Brodie's tears began to subside. He reached for another wadge of tissues, and then he took an enormous breath and exhaled a great sigh of relief.

With our fifty-minute session fast approaching its conclusion, I knew only too well that the reliable Giles Sweeney would ring the doorbell in a very brief while, and I realised that Brodie and I had to formulate a plan.

"We have been together now for almost fifty minutes, and, as you know, your social worker and your probation officer will return in just a little while to take you back to the remand home. So we need to think about the next steps."

Brodie looked at me and nodded, as though the idea of some "next steps" might be most welcome.

"Psychotherapy is an ongoing process … a chance for us to really *talk* about your life … to *think* about your life … and although this might be a bit scary, I suspect that it could be quite useful for you. The fact that you've been able to cry so deeply in this way gives us both a real sense that you *do* wish to communicate all your pain and sadness and anger. So I'm wondering whether you might wish to see me again at this very same time next Tuesday, at 1.35 p.m."

Brodie nodded in silent approbation of the plan.

And then he chimed, "Yeah … that'd be good. 1.35 p.m., you said?"

"Yes, 1.35 p.m. I know that may seem a very idiosyncratic time, but my colleagues and I, who work in this building, always space our appointments accordingly, so that when you arrive you can do so quite privately."

"Yeah, I'd like to come back next week."

"Well, I very much look forward to seeing you again so that we can have another conversation and then we can both decide how best to progress from there."

"Do you think you can help me?"

"Yes. I think that psychotherapy could be very helpful for you, and it would be my privilege to assist you as much as I can."

"How long will it take to make me better?" he wondered.

Virtually every patient who attends for psychotherapy poses this question during the first consultation, and one can never provide a definitive answer, because some people require a shorter period of treatment, whereas others will need an infinitely longer stretch of time.

In many respects, the psychotherapist finds himself or herself in the same state of uncertainty as the oncologist whose patients invariably ask, "How long do I have to live?"

However, by contrast, our patients want to know, "How long will it be before I can *start* to live?"

I responded to Brodie frankly and I told him that as our work progressed we would both come to acquire a clearer idea.

"Thank you, Professor."

I realised that by having called me "Professor", Brodie no longer considered me to be only a deadly Kahr, but that he could also recognise me as a professional, keen to help.

At that moment, the bell rang, and I rose from my seat, walked over to the entry-phone, and buzzed in Messrs. Sweeney and Lundgren, fresh from having refuelled themselves at Starbucks. Brodie rose from his seat.

I opened the door to the consulting room just as the two escorts appeared in view. Briefly, I explained that Brodie and I had a very productive meeting and that we agreed that it would be useful to have another such consultation the following week, at 1.35 p.m.

True gentlemen, neither Giles Sweeney nor Jeffrey Lundgren asked any awkward or intrusive questions. They, too, wished to respect Brodie's privacy and dignity. Sweeney simply smiled, "Oh, that's great. That's *really* great. We'll come back at this same time next week. 1.35 p.m. Consider it done."

So, we confirmed that we would have a second meeting, after which time we could then decide whether it would be in Brodie's best interests to fix regular weekly meetings for the foreseeable future.

In view of Brodie's presenting symptoms – his cruel engagement in acts of sexual violence – I knew that we might need a longer, rather than a shorter, period of treatment.

We would have much work to undertake in order to make sense of his madness.

Everyone nodded and bid one another farewell, and then Brodie exited the consulting room. With his escorts in tow, he walked down the corridor, and just before he began to descend the staircase, he turned round and smiled at me bashfully. He and Sweeney and Lundgren then proceeded out of the building.

Psychotherapy had now begun.

PART III

The Psychodynamics of Murder

From Infanticide to Serial Killing

When Daddy Kills the Dog

Pet Murder and the Infanticidal Attachment

PRELUDE: FROM ANIMAL LOVE TO ANIMAL SACRIFICE

Happily, most human beings adore their pets.

Indeed, since the very inception of civilisation, many people have revered animals deeply. Farm animals have provided food and clothing for thousands of years, while certain domestic animals (whether cats, dogs, rabbits, birds, or fish) have offered joy and comfort, often becoming much cherished members of the family.

The ancient Greeks, for example, regarded dogs as healers and enlisted them as part of the medical cult of Asklepios in Athens, Epidaurus, Lebene, Piraeus, and elsewhere, training their dogs to lick wounds, with reportedly beneficial results, including curing blindness (Dale-Green, 1966; cf. Toynbee, 1973). In ancient Rome, the poet Titus Lucretius Carus, who flourished in the first century B.C.E., wrote a tract, *De rerum natura* [*On the Nature of Things*], in which he discoursed upon the duty of care towards domestic animals. In similar vein, Porphyry of Tyre, a Neoplatonic, Phoenician philosopher of the third century C.E., produced a composition entitled *De abstinentia ab esu animalium* [*On Abstinence from Killing Animals*], advocating vegetarianism. The works of Lucretius and Porphyry provide indisputably powerful evidence of the long history of kindness to animals (cf. Clark, 2011).

In the late eighteenth century and early nineteenth century, animals inspired such awe and reverence that many poets and essayists immortalised them in verse and in prose, most notably Samuel Taylor Coleridge in his poem "To a Young Ass", as well as Robert Southey in his study "The Spider". William Wordsworth paid tribute in his paean on "The Green Linnet", and so, too, did John Keats in his "Ode to a Nightingale", as did Percy Bysshe Shelley in his composition "To a Skylark" (cf. Perkins, 1998).

Nowadays, those humans who share their homes and their lives with pets often report that a cat or a dog has the potential to stave off otherwise unbearable loneliness and, even, to assist their owners through a bereavement. Dogs, in particular, often fulfil many basic attachment needs for humans, as evidenced convincingly in the testimony of some 923 college students examined by Professor Lawrence Kurdek (2008), a developmental psychologist at Wright State University in Dayton, Ohio.

DOI: 10.4324/9781003546245-10

Many people have rejoiced that our animal companions, known more tradition-ally as pets, possess significant healing powers (Serpell, 1986). Indeed, psychother-apists have even begun to use animals as part of the treatment process, as indicated by the rise of P.F.P. (pet-facilitated psychotherapy) and P.F.T. (pet-facilitated ther-apy), also known as A.A.T. (animal-assisted therapy) (e.g., Culliton, 1987; Ser-pell, 1991; Abdill and Juppé, 1997; Allen, Shykoff, and Izzo, 2001; Crawford and Pomerinke, 2003; cf. Calvo, 2017a, 2017b).

Any mental health professional who may doubt the huge benefit that one might derive from pets could do no better than consult the most basic biographical litera-ture about Professor Sigmund Freud. Strikingly, some of Freud's truly notable cases suffered greatly from animal-related fears and symptoms and would often confuse animals with people. Those patients included "kleine Hans" ["Little Hans"], who suffered from a dread of horses (Freud, 1909a), as well as the "Rattenmann" ["Rat Man"], who became terrorised by the prospect of being tortured by rodents (Freud, 1909b), not to mention the "Wolfsmann" ["Wolf Man"], who suffered much tor-ment from his lupine-laden anxiety dream (Freud, 1918). In fact, Sigmund Freud himself adored animals deeply, especially the chow dogs who came to live with him after the onset of his crippling carcinoma in 1923 (Jones, 1957; Schur, 1972; Romm, 1983; cf. Kahr, 2021a). Freud's dogs often sat in his consulting room dur-ing sessions, and, in one of his meetings with the American physician, Dr. Joseph Wortis, Freud exclaimed, "In jeder Beziehung liegt eine Abhängigkeit, selbst mit einem Hund" (quoted in Wortis, 1934b, p. 23). Dr. Wortis (1934b, p. 23), quite struck by Freud's observation, translated these words of wisdom thus: "There is an element of dependence in every relationship, even with a dog."

In 1925, Fräulein Anna Freud acquired a much-loved family pet – an Alsatian called Wolf who would accompany her as a bodyguard on her walks (Molnar, 1996). Freud himself became extremely attached to Wolf, so much so that the Al-satian even sent Freud a special card for the latter's seventieth birthday in 1926, penned, of course, by Anna Freud. Wolf saluted the father of psychoanalysis: "He greets you, despite the transience of every delicacy, / With unchanging doggy fidel-ity" (quoted in Molnar, 1996, p. 273).[1]

Wolf had become such a source of comfort for Freud, not only in the wake of Freud's illness, but, also, in the grieving period following the death of his beloved grandson, Heinz Rudolf Halberstadt (known as "Heinerle"), so much so that Freud (1927c, p. 42) wrote to his Dutch disciple, Dr. Jeanne Lampl-de Groot, "What is it about these little creatures that makes them so charming? After all, we have expe-rienced all sorts of things from them that don't comport with our ideals, and must see them as little animals. But of course, animals seem charming to us and much more attractive than complicated, multistory adult humans. I'm experiencing that right now with our Wolf, who almost replaces our deceased Heinele."[2]

Strikingly, Freud even sided with Wolf against his Welsh-born colleague, Dr. Er-nest Jones. Indeed, during one of Jones's visits to Vienna, Wolf bit the British psy-choanalyst, prompting Freud to lament to his colleague, Dr. Max Eitingon, "I had to punish him for that, but I did so with real reluctance for he – Jones – deserved it" (Freud, 1927e, p. 275).[3]

In 1928, Mrs. Dorothy Burlingham, Anna Freud's close friend, and one of Sigmund Freud's patients, presented her analyst with a chow bitch called Lün Yug. Freud historian Mr. Michael Molnar (1996) has suggested that Burlingham – thought by many to have become Anna Freud's lover, or at least her honorary sister – had purchased Lün Yug for Freud as a replacement for his daughter Anna who had long struggled to separate psychologically from her father. Sadly, Lün Yug died the following year, in the summer of 1929, when Frau Eva Rosenfeld, another of Freud's patients, charged with the responsibility of caring for the dog during a period of vacation, failed to do so with full vigilance, and Lün Yug got run over (Kahr, 1996; cf. Molnar, 1996). In 1930, Anna Freud obtained another Chinese chow for her father, a dog known as Jofi (sometimes rendered as Jo Fie or, even, Jo-fi), who remained with Freud for more than six years, dying of a heart attack following an operation for the removal of ovarian cysts (Molnar, 1996).

Freud even told an American analysand, Dr. Smiley Blanton, that loving a dog might be more straightforward than loving a child. He pontificated that, with a pet, "There is no ambivalence, no element of hostility" (quoted in Blanton, 1929, p. 24). The dogs became constant companions to Freud and, as we know, he kept them in his consulting room during psychoanalytical sessions, often to the chagrin of his patients, some of whom had to endure the dogs either barking at them (Grinker, 1940, 1979) or slobbering on them (Grinker, 1985).

But although the ancient Greeks deployed animals in healing rituals, and the Romantic poets scripted copious eulogies, and Sigmund Freud relished a profound attachment to his dogs, we must remember, of course, that not everyone has regarded animals with such affection, tenderness, or respect. Indeed, throughout history, human beings have also treated animals with tremendous cruelty (Ekroth, 2014; Shelton, 2014). During the Middle Ages and the Renaissance, for instance, large numbers of people entertained themselves with cock-fighting, bear-baiting, and bull-baiting, as well as badger-baiting, and dog-fighting – activities which often resulted in the mutilation or death of the animal (e.g., Ribton-Turner, 1887; Hackwood, 1907). But, often, non-human mammals would be sacrificed outright as part of religious observance, whether as supplications or appeasements, whether as expressions of gratitude to the gods, or whether as part of a prayer for more clement weather. In fact, archaeologists have uncovered a wealth of osteological data, confirming that, throughout the centuries, human beings have performed ritual sacrifices on a wide variety of animals, ranging from horses, sheep, goats, dogs, cattle, lambs, kids, cocks, pigeons, hens, and reindeer, to camels, fowls, doves, donkeys, beavers, hares, sables, squirrels, and elks (Insoll, 2011; cf. Foley, 1985). During the medieval era, animals would be murdered cruelly, often thrown off of buildings as part of rituals, or skinned alive for their pelts, or even executed; in fact, in the early fourteenth century, a French magician called Jean Persant had apparently buried a black cat for use in a sorcery ritual, but this feline survived, and both Persant and the cat then suffered death by burning at the stake, with the cat tied round Persant's neck (Walker-Meikle, 2011).

Cruelty to animals can be detected in a multitude of sources, including in visual imagery. For instance, the famed eighteenth-century illustrator William Hogarth had immortalised the murder and mistreatment of cats and dogs in his printed engraving, *First Stage of Cruelty*, part of a series known as *The Four Stages of Cruelty*, completed in 1751. In chilling fashion, Hogarth depicted male youths sodomising a dog with an arrow, burning the eyes of a bird with a needle, and hanging a pair of cats, among other acts of viciousness.

Sadly, such sadism has persisted throughout the centuries (e.g., Grier, 2002), and many of us know of chilling tales of contemporary violence towards animals.

As psychotherapists, we appreciate only too well how distressed our patients may become when a cherished pet cat or dog passes away from natural causes. For some, the ache may be as great as the loss of a sibling or, even, a child. But what happens to a human being when a pet dies *not* from natural causes such as old age or illness, or even from being run over by a passing vehicle but, rather, from actual *murder*? After all, animal companions can often be very helpless and, consequently, they make excellent victims for those humans who need to perpetrate acts of cruelty. As Professor Hilary Bok (2011, p. 771) remarked in her chapter on "Keeping Pets", which appeared in *The Oxford Handbook of Animal Ethics*, "if we choose to abuse or neglect them, they generally have no recourse."

Over the last forty years or more, I have encountered quite a number of cases in my psychotherapeutic practice of patients who had to endure the death of a treasured family pet, either viscerally or in symbolic form, at the hand of a parent or guardian. Hence, I shall now explore the stories of six patients who had experienced what we might describe as "pet murder" during childhood or adolescence. In each case, the patient in question became clinically psychotic in later life, afflicted by hallucinations and delusions, as well as by extremely self-destructive and other-destructive forms of behaviour. I will thus provide brief encapsulations of these six cases in an effort to explore the impact of parental death wishes, enacted through the family pet or through a soft animal toy – a form of murderousness with which each patient identified profoundly and, I would argue, experienced as an infanticidal attack upon his or her own body and sense of self.

CLINICAL MATERIAL

Case 1: "Ira" and the Murdered Dog

Shortly after his eighteenth birthday, "Ira" decided to enlist in the army. Having had a relatively strained relationship with both his mother and his father, Ira looked forward to an experience of relative independence and to a new set of adventures. He deeply regretted, however, that he would have to leave his beloved pet terrier at home, but he felt confident that his parents, who had always shown affection for his dog, would be more than capable of feeding him and walking him.

After three weeks of basic training, Ira received permission to return to his family house for a brief weekend visit. Upon entering the front door, he greeted his mother and father with hugs and kisses, but he expressed immediate surprise when his terrier, "Buster", failed to appear. Ira knew that Buster would have detected his familiar scent instantly, and he began to worry. Ira called out to Buster, and whistled for him, but when the dog did not materialise, Ira became increasingly concerned. The parents made no comment as they witnessed their soldier son scouring in vain to find his animal. Eventually, the father explained, "He won't come", to which Ira responded, with great concern, "But why not?", whereupon his father announced, quite matter-of-factly, "Buster's dead." Incredulous, Ira inquired as to what had happened; and his father, with a stony face, explained, "Oh, I shot him." Ira nearly collapsed with disbelief as he listened to his father elaborate further, "Oh yes, on the day you left, your mother and I thought to ourselves, well … Ira doesn't need the dog anymore, and *we* didn't want him, so we shot him." Ira's mother, not wishing to be implicated in this extraordinary situation, offered clarification, "Actually, your father shot him. *I* didn't shoot him, obviously." Both parents spoke in an acidic, factual tone, with neither father nor mother expressing contrition for the death of Buster, nor concern that Ira had obviously become extremely distressed.

As nobody could offer comfort or understanding of this brutal act of pet murder, Ira became more and more disorientated, and, towards the end of his weekend of leave, he began to experience auditory hallucinations for the first time. Although Ira had a history of mild and moderate depression during puberty, he had never attempted suicide before, but now, in the wake of the revelation of Buster's assassination, he heard a voice which told him that he must kill himself, and that he must do so with the same weapon that his father had used to shoot the dog.

Ira had no difficulty in locating his father's rifle, which he kept in a cupboard in the garden shed. And, with only an hour remaining of his weekend at home, prior to the departure of his bus back to the army training camp, Ira took his father's weapon, rested the barrel underneath his chin, cocked at a forty-five-degree angle, and fired.

Extraordinarily, in spite of having shot himself, Ira managed to survive this hallucination-driven suicide attempt. The bullet pierced through his jaw, shattering the bone and causing a minor injury to one of his eyes; but otherwise, he escaped physically unscathed. His parents heard the shot and telephoned immediately for an ambulance, which arrived with great speed. But, after Ira recovered medically from this catastrophic act of self-harm, a liaison psychiatrist at the local hospital arranged for him to be admitted to a locked ward with a diagnosis of schizophrenia. He remained a psychiatric in-patient for six years, prior to his discharge into a closely supervised community mental health facility (Kahr, 2012a).

Case 2: "Tamara" and the Intravenous Drip

Throughout her childhood, "Tamara" had to endure a great deal of physical abuse and emotional neglect from both of her parents. She explained that she had begun to dissociate from the age of three or four years and that whenever her parents assaulted her young body, she would imagine herself either floating in outer space, or, alternatively, murdering her parents with a knife. Tamara grew up near the coast; and, consequently, her father – a consummate athlete – spent a great deal of time trying to teach his daughter how to swim in the ocean. Deeply suspicious of her father, and, moreover, knowing of her father's propensity for beating her with his fists and with a belt, Tamara often tried to run away during swimming lessons. On one occasion, shortly after her sixth birthday, Tamara displayed "insolence", and she refused to wade into the ocean for a lesson. Infuriated, Tamara's father grabbed the small child, dragged her several feet from the shore, and then threw her into much deeper water than Tamara had ever experienced hitherto. Tamara struggled to paddle to safety and felt quite certain that she would drown. Her father mocked her and laughed at the frightened child, calling out, "Pretend that you're a fish!"

During her seventh year, Tamara's pet spaniel, "Corky", became fatally ill with cancer, and the veterinarian explained that Corky would have to be put down, as no further medical treatment would be of use. A sensitive and empathic parent would no doubt have found some way to shield his or her child from such a regrettable situation. But, tragically, Tamara's father insisted that the girl should come with him to the veterinarian's office and witness Corky's death by lethal injection. Extraordinarily, the veterinarian agreed to perform the euthanasia with the young Tamara in the room.

Years later, while undergoing psychotherapy, Tamara reported her agony of being forced to watch her pet Corky die in front of her. During this painful session, Tamara railed against her father, as she simply could not understand how a parent could expose a child to such a horrific scene. In recounting the tale, she wept powerfully.

Tamara had embarked upon psychotherapy years previously, after having suffered a psychotic breakdown. She experienced auditory hallucinations and grandiose delusions, and she believed herself to be the child of Her Majesty The Queen (rather than the child of an abusive father). In addition to her florid symptomatology, Tamara had also struggled for many years with an addiction to intravenous drugs. As one might imagine, we spent a great deal of time in psychotherapy discussing how her early experience of watching the veterinarian insert a needle into Corky's vein had contributed to the development of her own propensity to inject herself with a lethal substance in subsequent years. Tamara had, in fact, overdosed on many occasions during her adolescence, and she regarded herself as fortunate to be alive (Kahr, 2012a).

Such a traumatic upbringing contributed not only to the development of psychotic states and to a lengthy period of drug use but, also, to the perpetration of cruelty to animals. It did not surprise me when Tamara confessed that, during her very troubled adolescence, she had killed a pet rabbit, strangling the creature to death, while partying and smoking marijuana with some of her more "rowdy" girlfriends. Regrettably, her teenage companions found this "amusing", and no one could quite appreciate the significance of Tamara's murderous re-enactment of Corky's death, or, indeed, of the infanticidal attacks upon Tamara's own mind and body during childhood.

Case 3: "Vita" and the Surgical Teddy Bear

I first met "Vita" many decades ago while working in a psychiatric hospital. She had suffered from schizophrenia for many years and had spent most of her adolescence and more than half of her adulthood as an in-patient, under section of the Mental Health Act 1959. In addition to the traditional psychotic symptoms of auditory hallucinations, visual hallucinations, and delusions of persecution, Vita also struggled with several comorbidities, including anorexia nervosa, bulimia nervosa, self-harm (such as drug-taking, cutting, and suicidal activities), as well as trichotillomania, which left her virtually bald. When I first met Vita on the psychiatric hospital ward, a senior member of staff – a Consultant Psychiatrist – told me that Vita suffered from the delusion that her parents hoped that she would die. My colleague laughed at the absurdity that a mother or a father might wish a child dead, especially as my colleague had met Vita's parents several times and had found them charming. The psychiatrist regarded Vita as rather less charming, as she would, from time to time, sneak into the hospital kitchen and grab a carving knife, which she would brandish in front of the other patients, necessitating the nurses to restrain Vita and the doctors to increase the dosage of her antipsychotic medication.

During our many conversations together, Vita told me a great deal about her childhood. She enjoyed talking and reminiscing, and she spoke with great fluidity, in spite of her ostensible thought disorder and schizophrenic speech. During one conversation, she recalled that, as a child, she possessed a favourite soft toy – a teddy bear called "Harry" – which, I suppose, functioned as an important transitional object. Having grown up with a sexually abusive father and a cold mother who suffered from lymphoma (and hence had to disappear into hospital for long periods of time), Vita sought comfort from her cuddly toy Harry. With no adult caretaker to whom she could turn for psychological attunement and support, Vita projected her sense of illness into the teddy bear, and, on one occasion during early childhood, she noticed that some of the wire coils inside Harry's tummy had become loose and had begun to stick out through his belly. Vita became distressed and she developed the idea that Harry must be suffering, and so, she brought the teddy into her mother's bedroom and asked for help. In a mocking tone, the mother chimed, "Oh, dear, poor Harry is very ill, isn't he? It looks as though we shall have to operate." A mentally healthy mother would have stroked Harry or would have cuddled him, providing some reassurance that he would be all right; but Vita's mother, in an act of great perversity, took a large knife from the kitchen and sliced open Harry's tummy and performed "surgery" upon him, reinserting the wire coils back inside, and then she sewed up the "wound" that she had thus inflicted. Vita sobbed profusely as she described this episode which had occurred many years previously, sometime during her fifth or sixth year.

One can certainly detect many aspects of Vita's adult behaviours and symptoms in this traumatic incident from early childhood. Just as the mother had gone into the kitchen of the family home to grab a knife, so, too, would Vita sneak into the hospital kitchen from time to time in order to purloin a sharp blade. And just as the mother cut the teddy bear's tummy open, so, too, would Vita take a razor to various parts of her own body (stomach, legs, arms, and even labia), and make tracings, often drawing blood. I would argue that the surgery which her mother had performed on Harry – a screen memory, perhaps, for earlier, comparable traumas – scarred Vita deeply and contributed to a profound sense of unsafety and to the so-called "delusion" that her parents wished her dead.

During the course of a family therapy session, Vita's mother reminisced about her own childhood at my urging, and, to my great astonishment, she told me that she had endured a long history of health problems which had predated her adult-onset lymphoma. In childhood, Vita's mother experienced a very severe appendicitis during a holiday with her own parents on a remote island. In view of the urgency of the situation, her father – a physician – performed the appendectomy himself in shockingly makeshift conditions. Although Vita's mother survived this homemade surgical procedure, one can imagine that such an operation would have exerted quite an impact, and could explain, in part, why, years later, Vita's mother decided to inflict an operation with a knife on her daughter's toy animal! (cf. Kahr, 2007c, 2012a).

Case 4: "Steven" and the Drowning Teddy Bear

Many years ago, while working in a specialist unit for psychotic children, I had the opportunity to meet "Steven", an eight-year-old boy from a broken home who had begun to experience auditory hallucinations. Steven believed that he could hear the voice of Jesus Christ assuring him that he could fly. As Steven ran around the unit pretending to be a bird, he became extremely manic. But, as soon as this boy paused for breath, he worried that he, like Jesus, would be crucified with nails driven through his hands and feet.

I undertook play therapy sessions with Steven. At first, and for several months, he staged the same scenario over and over again, quite compulsively. Steven insisted that we should play a game in which he would be the owner of a sweet shop and I would be the customer. During each of our sessions, I would have to come to his shop and pretend to give Steven all my money for some special sweets, which I would then have to eat in his presence. After I "ate" these imaginary sweets, Steven would confess with chilling glee that he had laced the candies with poison, and that I would soon be dead within a matter of seconds. Although I did not know the deeper meaning of this behaviour during the early months of our work together, I had a sense that someone might have wished Steven dead, and that he had very cleverly attempted to void himself of these feelings by projecting them quite concretely into me during the course of play therapy.

My senior colleague on the unit, Mrs. Valerie Sinason (later Dr. Sinason), a very experienced Consultant Child and Adolescent Psychotherapist, worked with

Steven in parallel in group psychotherapy. As an older woman, she elicited a very particular type of maternal transference which I, as a man, did not experience quite so directly in my own encounters with Steven. During group sessions, Steven would dive into the dressing-up box and don a woman's caftan and then he would pretend to be "mummy". Moreover, he would pick up a teddy bear and begin to stab it with an imaginary knife shouting, "Kill, kill, kill" (quoted in Sinason, 2001, p. 45), and "I'm my mummy" (quoted in Sinason, 2001, p. 45), thus demonstrating his powerful identification with a murderous mother who inflicts a sense of suffering on someone else. In many respects, both Valerie Sinason and I observed the ways in which Steven dealt with his own fear of being murdered by displacing the murderousness on me (forcing me to swallow imaginary poisoned sweets in play therapy) or on a soft toy animal (in group psychotherapy) (cf. Kahr, 2007c, 2012a).

Case 5: "Penelope" and Her Dying Poodle

Unlike the four previous patients described herein, each of whom had to endure the murder of a pet, either concretely or symbolically, "Penelope" reported no such experiences. In contrast to Ira and Tamara and Vita and Steven, this woman did not suffer from schizophrenia. Penelope did, however, exhibit all of the symptoms of a borderline personality organisation, and would, from time to time, experience visual hallucinations which could be contained through psychotherapeutic interpretation and understanding. Moreover, she harboured a deep fear that her beloved pet poodle, "Wallace", would die. Penelope became extremely hypochondriacal on behalf of Wallace, and she would often arrive at her psychotherapy session and spend a great deal of time expressing deep anguish that Wallace might well be dead by the time she returned home. In truth, Wallace seemed very healthy and never had to endure a serious illness, but, even so, Penelope lived in constant fear of his death. In fact, she had ceased to go on travels, as she could not bear the thought of being separated from this poodle in case he should have a sudden heart attack.

Whereas Tamara and Vita had experienced sexual abuse at the hands of parents, and whereas Ira had suffered constant physical abuse, Penelope, by contrast, enjoyed a much more physically protected upbringing. However, in spite of the fact that no one hit her or raped her, she never felt safe, and she always carried the sense that her mother wished her dead, or, at the very least, that her mother had not planned to have a child. Penelope's mother had come to Great Britain during the late 1930s on the *Kindertransport*, fleeing her native Germany. Sadly, Penelope's grandparents did not escape, and both perished in the concentration camp at Theresienstadt. Consequently, although Penelope herself grew up in post-war England, free from bombings and Nazis, the spectre of the Holocaust nevertheless haunted her throughout her life. And although no one had ever abused her in a formal sense, she certainly *felt* abused. Like the psychotic boy Steven, who stabbed the teddy bear in group psychotherapy sessions, Penelope projected her own fear of murder into her pet Wallace as both a creative and a desperate means of managing the situation.

Case 6: "Esther" and the Drowning Puppy

I had the opportunity to interview "Esther" on the geriatric ward of a regional psychiatric hospital, more than forty years ago, during the course of her in-patient admission for schizophrenia. This very persecuted woman, better known to the staff by her nickname Poppy, spent most of her time sitting in a chair, shivering and petrified if anyone approached her.

Although I have carefully disguised the names of all the other patients de-scribed in this chapter, and, likewise, I have disguised the real name of this pa-tient as "Esther", I have, in fact, elected to share the actual *nickname* of this patient – *Poppy* – as it proved to be quite integral to an understanding of her osten-sibly psychotic symptomatology.

A long-stay patient with very poor hygiene, Poppy refused to bathe. Even-tually, out of desperation, some of the female nurses forced her to shower on a twice-weekly basis; and this routine would prompt Poppy to scream, claiming that the staff wished to drown her. The Consultant Psychiatrist dismissed these fears as paranoid delusions.

During my conversations with Poppy, it gradually emerged that, during her childhood, a neighbour's dog gave birth to several puppies and offered one to Poppy, who accepted this wonderful gift with delight. However, when her mother discovered that *Poppy* had brought a *puppy* into the house, she became enraged, scooped up the newborn dog, to whom Poppy had already become quite attached, and placed the little animal in a sack. The mother then dragged both Poppy and the puppy to the river behind their house, and promptly threw the sack into the icy water, and then forced her daughter to watch the puppy drown. Poppy told me that she had never before revealed this story to anyone, and that in view of the similarity of the names "Poppy" and "puppy", she thought that she, too, had drowned.

DISCUSSION: PET MURDER AND PSYCHOTOGENESIS

In each of the six aforementioned life histories, we find a strong correlation between severe psychopathology (four cases of adult schizophrenia, one case of childhood psychosis, and one case of adult borderline personality disorder) and the death of a pet – either real or imaginary. I have also encountered further cases in which a child who has had to suffer from pet murder does not become psychotic himself or herself but eventually marries a person diagnosed as psychotic during later, adult life. Might this close clinical association between psychotic symptomatology and the death or murder of a pet be purely accidental, or might we be able to posit some causal link?

Over several decades, I have published a number of essays on the phenomenon of "*psychological infanticide*" (Kahr, 1993, p. 269) and the "Infanticidal Attach-ment" (Kahr, 2007c, p. 119), which I have defined as a toxic and predominantly unconscious relationship between a parent and an infant in which the mother or father wishes the infant dead. Unlike forensic infanticide or baby murder, which re-sults in the actual bodily death of the child, psychological infanticide kills the soul, and often makes the infant feel internally dead, or deserving of death, and, often, quite suicidal. I have argued that the psychologically infanticidal parent transmits a death wish to the child which then becomes internalised as an "infanticidal introject" (Kahr, 2007c, p. 124), and which the child will then carry throughout the life cycle. Such early experiences contribute to the development of an "infanticidal attachment" (Kahr, 2007c, p. 125) – a type of severely disorganised and chaotic attachment which often accompanies a diagnosis of schizophrenia or other forms of psychosis (e.g., Kahr, 1993, 1994a, 2001d, 2007c, 2007d, 2012a, 2016, 2020a).

Based on my clinical work with psychotic men and women over more than forty years, I have now identified several categories of death wishes which parents can inflict unwittingly upon their offspring, contributing to the development of the infanticidal attachment, and these include actual death attempts, actual death threats, expressions of regret at the birth of a child, and the actual murder or symbolic murder of a pet. Although a mother pretending to perform surgery on a teddy bear – as in the case of Vita – would hardly attract the attention of the police or social services, I wish to argue that such moments create an atmosphere in which the young child feels deeply threatened, even though the parent has done nothing illegal. If a mother can take a large kitchen knife and slice open the stomach of a soft toy, why could the mother not do this to the child as well?

For young boys and girls, the pet functions as an honorary sibling, as a family member, as a companion who protects against loneliness, and as a source of comfort, as well as an expression of one's sense of self. To murder the pet, or to pretend to murder the pet, represents a potential psychological annihilation.

Sigmund Freud understood the child's close unconscious identification with animals very well indeed; and, in his essay, "Eine Schwierigkeit der Psychoanalyse" (Freud, 1917a), known in English as "A Difficulty in the Path of Psycho-Analysis", he observed, "A child can see no difference between his own nature and that of animals" (Freud, 1917b, p. 140).[4]

In a so-called "normal" or neurotic child, an attack on a toy animal in the course of free play might well be an expression of sibling rivalry. Kicking the dog or throwing a stuffed animal across the bedroom could be a very effective way of expressing hatred towards an annoying brother or sister. Freud (1917c) recognised this displacement of rage from the sibling onto the animal only too clearly in his essay on "Eine Kindheitserinnerung aus "Dichtung und Wahrheit" ", known in English as "A Childhood Memory from *Dichtung und Wahrheit*" (Freud, 1917d), in reference to a twenty-seven-year-old male patient from a multi-sibling family. He wrote that, "certain curious fortuitous actions of his (which involved sudden and severe injuries to his favourite animals, like his sporting dog or birds which he had carefully reared,) were probably to be understood as echoes of these hostile impulses against the little brother" (Freud, 1917d, p. 150).[5]

But, when a child attacks an animal more severely, or witnesses a parent assaulting an animal, we often find ourselves, unsurprisingly, in the presence of deeper disruption and trauma. Pet murder might well be an important warning sign that a child may be at great risk for the development of severe mental illness in later life.[6]

The destruction of pets – whether through shooting (as in the case of Ira's dog Buster), through lethal injection (as in the case of Tamara's dog Corky), through actual stabbing (as in the case of Vita's toy Harry), or through pretend-stabbing (as in the case of Steven's group psychotherapy teddy bear) – always occurs in the context of a family. It would be foolhardy to suggest that one act of pet murder results in psychosis. But we might be more justified to wonder whether the destruction of the pet becomes emblematic of a broader familial environment in which the child becomes fearful of his or her sense of safety and must, therefore, resort to hallucinations, delusions, and dissociations as a means of escape from the terrifying realities of daily life.

In the course of investigating the phenomenon of pet murder, I came to learn that the Scottish psychiatrist and sometime psychoanalyst, Dr. Ronald Laing, endured a difficult experience during his own childhood in relation to a favourite rocking horse. Laing's mother, Mrs. Amelia Kirkwood Laing, exerted stern discipline throughout her son's childhood. As Mr. Adrian Laing (1991, p. 27), the son of Ronald Laing, has reported, "The toys which came his way were exceptional treats. There was a wooden horse, for example, which Amelia took away and destroyed when she felt wee Ronald had not only grown out of it but had become 'too attached' to it. For the remainder of his days Ronnie was openly bitter about this wooden horse. To him the destruction of his wooden horse, to which he really had grown very attached, was an act of unmitigated brutality by his mother. Wee Ronald was learning that there was more to his mother than met the eye. Another toy of wee Ronald's was a grand toy car. When this toy was broken Amelia decided to give it away, in its delapidated [*sic*] condition, to a less fortunate lady down the road for her boy to play with."

In reading Adrian Laing's (1991, p. 27) account of his father's childhood experience, we cannot help but be struck by the observation that this event haunted R.D. Laing "For the remainder of his days". In spite of Laing's huge success as a best-selling author and cultural guru, and regardless of the fact that his antipsychiatric work helped to transform the nature of institutional psychiatry around the world, this childhood event still caused him distress. Although Laing never became schizophrenic as such, he did experience a very great deal of anguish throughout much of his life, and he struggled with severe alcoholism and other forms of provocative and aggressive behaviour, often becoming embroiled in fisticuffs and additional destructive activities (e.g., Kahr, 1994b, 2024a; Burston, 1996; Clay, 1996). When I hosted Laing's visit to The Oxford Psycho-Analytical Forum at the University of Oxford, in 1983, one of his teeth fell out in the middle of his lecture at the Department of Experimental Psychology! Only later did I come to discover that, shortly before the talk, Laing had got embroiled in a fight, and his adversary had punched him in the mouth, thus loosening a tooth in the process (Gans, 1992; Kahr, 1994b, 2024a). In view of Ronald Laing's lifetime of destructive and self-destructive activities, one wonders to what extent Amelia Laing's removal of her son's wooden horse might have represented a sense of danger and unsafety which, paradoxically, also allowed Laing to become so exquisitely sensitive to his psychotic patients (e.g., Laing, 1960, 1964, 1971, 1976, 1981, 1985).[7]

CLINICAL IMPLICATIONS

In 1939, Dr. John Bowlby (1939) published the case history of a thirteen-year-old boy who suffered from childhood hysteria. Unlike colleagues who believed that hysteria resulted from constitutional factors, Bowlby investigated the impact of traumatic loss and discovered that one of the patient's hysterical attacks developed in the immediate aftermath of the death of a cherished pet rabbit (cf. Kahr, 2015b, 2019c, 2019d, 2024a).

The loss of a pet from natural causes can produce great devastation for a young person or, indeed, for an adult. But what happens when the pet dies perversely at the hands of parents?

Understanding pet murder in its many forms – whether injecting a dog lethally or whether throwing away a wooden rocking horse – affords us an opportunity to become increasingly sensitised to the impact of animals during the early lives of our clients and patients. Indeed, pets have the potential to become a source for primitive, unconscious identifications in the mind of a young person.

On 7th May, 1934, the Tavistock Clinic hosted a luncheon in the Wharncliffe Rooms of the Hotel Great Central in Marylebone, in North-West London, in order to publicise the work of this pioneering mental health institution. The guests included such distinguished individuals as Geoffrey Shakespeare, Esq., the Parliamentary Secretary to the Ministry of Health, as well as the eminent Viennese physician and psychologist Dr. Alfred Adler, and, also, the Olympic Gold medallist Mr. Harold Abrahams (later immortalised in the film *Chariots of Fire*). Prior to the meal, Dr. John Rawlings Rees, the Medical Director, spoke about the new discipline of dynamic psychotherapy, offered at the Tavistock Clinic. According to contemporary press coverage, Rees described a striking case, that of a little boy who crawled around on all fours, pretending to be a dog. Reared in multiple foster homes, this youngster soon learned that the family dogs received far more affection than the fostered children, and so, in desperation, he developed an unconscious identification with a dog in the hope of gaining more scraps of food and comfort (Anonymous, 1934; cf. Kahr, 2000b).

The psychoanalytical literature brims with case histories of children who, like the boy described by John Rawlings Rees, have identified with animals as a means of psychic survival (e.g., Kupfermann, 1977). The pioneering Viennese psychoanalyst, Dr. Helene Deutsch (1942), noted that ill patients will often identity with animals precisely because they lack the developmental capacity to forge an identification with human beings.

Even Sigmund Freud (1873), during adolescence, impersonated a Spanish dog called "Cipion" [Cipión], immortalised by the seventeenth-century writer Miguel de Cervantes in his short story "El coloquio de los perros" ["The Conversation of the Dogs"], from the *Novelas ejemplares* [*Exemplary Novels*], published in 1613.

In fact, Freud even wrote poetry in Spanish under the pseudonym of this fictional dog. Thus, the identification between humans and animals runs deep throughout the history of psychoanalysis.

In view of the strong potential for young boys and girls to forge identifications with animals, psychological professionals must become increasingly sensitive to any references to pets throughout the course of psychotherapeutic work. It may be that if our patients do not mention pets during the early consultations, we might wish to inquire about any such experiences. Should we hear stories of cruelty to animals, similar to those discussed earlier in this chapter, we must become increasingly alert to the possibility that the patient might have experienced psychological infanticide and might have grown up in the context of an infanticidal attachment relationship with a primary caregiver. We may come to find that pet murder in its many forms might well be pathognomonic of an infanticidal attachment and of the presence of a psychotic personality structure.

As a brief aside, I must mention that two of the patients described in this short contribution remained lifelong vegetarians. There may be many good reasons why a person might wish to become vegetarian, whether out of respect for our fellow creatures, for health reasons, or for religious reasons. But vegetarianism can also develop out of an unconscious identification with animals being slaughtered. Vita, in particular, practised vegetarianism for years, yet she did so in a most uncomfortable manner, and she often tormented herself by reading about abattoirs and wept at the thought of animals being killed in this way. Such a reaction might betoken great sensitivity; but for Vita, I had a strong sense that she could not differentiate her own body from that of the slaughtered animal. Thus, when patients speak of vegetarianism, we should consider the possibility that this lifestyle choice might, in certain cases, have deeper dynamic roots.

Of course, we must investigate not only the impact of pet murder upon the growing child but, also, the reasons why parents or other caregivers may choose to engage in such behaviour in the first place; and this could well be the subject of another study entirely. Clearly, parents kill their children's pets as an act of deferred or displaced infanticide, and as a means of evacuating their own internal horrors into the mind and body of the child through the destruction of a cat or a dog.

Although the roots of such violence in parents and caregivers can be traced back to deeper layers of experience, it might be worth mentioning that a large number of the perpetrators of pet murder in this clinical study had committed acts of pet violence in the immediate aftermath of a bereavement or separation or loss, as we observed, for instance, in the case of Ira's father, who shot Buster the dog the very day after Ira had departed for the army. Similarly, another patient – also a male – told me that his father had suffocated the family hamster on the same day that the mother threw the father out of the house, after having discovered evidence of her husband's many marital infidelities. Thus, the psychology of the parent remains fertile territory for subsequent clinical and theoretical investigations.

In ancient times, our ancestors sacrificed both babies and animals as a tribute to, or an appeasement of, the gods (deMause, 1974, 1982, 1988, 1990, 2002a; Tierney, 1989; Brown, 1991; Kahr, 1994a; Lewis, 2001; Bourget, 2006; Kosken-niemi, 2009; Miles, 2010; Insoll, 2011; cf. Levenson, 1993). In the unconscious mind, the differentiation between killing a pet and killing a human being remains quite murky.

Indeed, during the mid-sixteenth century, the young English monarch, Edward VI, angered at his betrayal by John Dudley, the duke of Northumberland, once snatched a prize falcon from the Privy Chamber and plucked it to death, ripping the bird into pieces. Apparently, the king spoke threateningly about his enemies and, according to Simon Renard (1551, p. 249), the Burgundian-born ambassador to the English court, "He is said to have plucked a falcon, which he kept in his private chamber, and torn it into four pieces, saying as he did so to his governors that he likened himself to the falcon, whom everyone plucked; but that he would pluck them too, thereafter, and tear them into four parts." As we know, Edward VI had no hesitation in assassinating enemies, not least his uncle Edward Seymour, the duke of Somerset, whom he had beheaded on Tower Hill in 1552.

Many centuries later, in 1945, during his time in the *Führerbunker*, none other than Adolf Hitler ordered his personal physician, *Obersturmbannführer* Werner Haase, to kill his dog Blondi with a lethal cyanide tablet in order to test its efficacy (O'Donnell, 1978). Not long thereafter, Hitler took his own life, having of course already orchestrated the deaths of millions upon millions of others.

Thus, these two disparate historical examples underscore, only too chillingly, that pet murder will often serve as a prelude to the murder of men, women, and children.

I wish to hypothesise, therefore, that many of our patients who have grown up in families in which parents have killed off pets will become psychotically fearful of being murdered themselves and, in certain instances, will become violent themselves, through identification. Hopefully, as we cultivate a greater awareness of pet murder and its potential links to the infanticidal attachment, psychological workers can begin to acquire an even clearer insight into, and sensitivity towards, these very complex and very powerful family dynamics and thus not only protect our patients but, also, their own potential victims.

Notes

1 The original German phrase reads: "Er empfiehlt sich, trotz aller guten Bissen Vergänglichkeit, – in hündisch unwandelbarer Anhänglichkeit" (Wolf [Anna Freud], 1926).

2 The original German prose reads: "Woher es kommt, daß diese kleinen Wesen so rei-zend sind? Wir haben doch allerlei von ihnen erfahren, was nicht zu unseren Idealen stimmt, und müssen sie als kleine Tiere ansehen. Aber freilich erscheinen uns auch die Tiere reizend und weit anziehender als die komplizierten, mehrstöckigen erwachsenen Menschen. Ich erlebe das jetzt an unserem Wolf, der mir fast das verlorene Heinerle ersetzt" (Freud, 1927b, pp. 57–58).

3 The original German passage reads: "Ich mußte ihn dafür strafen, aber ich tat es wirklich ungern, denn er – Jones – verdiente es" (Freud, 1927d, p. 550).

4 The original German phrase reads: "Das Kind empfindet keinen Unterschied zwischen dem eigenen Wesen und dem des Tieres" (Freud, 1917a, p. 4).

5 The original German prose reads: "sonderbare Zufallshandlungen, durch die er sonst geliebte Tiere wie seinen Jagdhund oder sorgsam von ihm gepflegte Vögel plötzlich zu schwerem Schaden brachte, waren wohl als Nachklänge jener feindseligen Impulse gegen den kleinen Bruder zu verstehen" (Freud, 1917c, p. 51).

6 Throughout this essay, I have argued that victimised children who witness cruelty to animals will be at greater risk of developing severe mental illnesses in later life. But as for the perpetrators of these crimes, we must recognise that sadism towards non-humans can often be an indication of forensic tendencies. During the 1990s, I had the privilege of serving as a Staff Psychotherapist at the Young Abusers Project – a visionary clinical service created by Dr. Eileen Vizard in the Child and Family Department at the Tavistock Clinic in North-West London. During our work with young sex offenders, my colleagues and I discovered that the torture of animals during early childhood often became a "red flag" warning sign of the development of paedophilia in later life. In recognition of this important clinical discovery and of her pioneering work in the diagnosis and treatment of juvenile offenders, Dr. Vizard eventually received a C.B.E. [Commander of The Most Excellent Order of the British Empire] in recognition of her pioneering work in child and adolescent mental health (Mezey, Vizard, Hawkes, and Austin, 1991; Vizard, Monck, and Misch, 1995; Vizard, Wynick, Hawkes, Woods, and Jenkins, 1996; Vizard, 1997; cf. Kahr, 2004a, 2020a).

7 Many years after having learned about the way in which Mrs. Amelia Laing destroyed her young son's rocking horse, I encountered a very severely psychotic patient who presented with deep regressive behaviour and with suicidality. This young man had hoped to become a professional musician but, regrettably, had never achieved his dream. During his hospitalisation, the patient told me that after he left home in order to attend university, his parents threw away his upright piano without consulting him. Throughout my conversations with the many other psychotic patients with whom I worked over the years, accounts of precisely this sort of symbolic infanticidal attack would often emerge. For instance, another patient revealed that, at one point in his early childhood, the mother would threaten to destroy all of his toys if he did not clean his room sufficiently. Once, his sister neglected to place a particular toy appropriately in the cupboard, and, in consequence, the mother ripped that cherished object to shreds. Both my patient and his sister eventually developed schizophrenia in later years.

Castration Anxiety in Men Who Murder

WHY DO MEN COMMIT MURDER?

Throughout the course of human history, theologians, philosophers, criminologists, and physicians have all endeavoured to answer this complex question, albeit with little success. In 1986, while commenting on the murders perpetrated by serial killers such as Peter Sutcliffe, better known as the "Yorkshire Ripper", and Kenneth Erskine, otherwise known as the "Stockwell Strangler", the distinguished British forensic psychiatrist, Professor John Gunn, lamented, "Apart from the fact that they are all suffering from some form of mental disturbance, there is unfortunately no common thread" (quoted in Berlins, 1986, p. 10). Likewise, the noted American neurologist, Professor Jonathan Pincus (2001, pp. 176–177), who interviewed numerous murderers across the decades, enquired, "Why might one person become a serial murderer and another something else? The truth is we do not know."

Not only do experts struggle with this conundrum, but so, too, do the killers themselves, who invariably fail to offer coherent explanations for their crimes. Indeed, Dennis Nilsen, the British multiple murderer, confessed that, although he considers the infliction of pain to be abhorrent and the practice of necrophilia repellent, he still assassinated some fifteen young men and engaged in sexual relations with the corpses of many of his victims after their decease. This murderer remained quite perplexed by his actions and admitted, "I wish there was a clear view on motive" (Nilsen, 1983, p. 33).

Though once regarded as the work of Satan, the act of murder became increasingly medicalised, particularly during the nineteenth century, as physicians such as Professore Cesare Lombroso (1876) argued that criminality results from degeneration of the brain. This theory of the putative biopathological origins of murderousness has remained extremely popular, having given rise in recent years to the field of neurocriminology, namely, the study of both the neuroanatomy and the neurophysiology of offenders (e.g., Rafter, 2008; Haycock, 2014; Concannon, 2019). As I have already indicated in Chapter 1, contemporary neurocriminologists, including, first and foremost, the British-born researcher Professor Adrian Raine, remain eternally hopeful that they will discover a genetically transmissible form of abnormality that can be easily identified on a functional magnetic

DOI: 10.4324/9781003546245-11

resonance imaging scan and, ultimately, eradicated. Although Raine and his research colleagues have reported such findings as a reduction of volume in the grey matter of the prefrontal cortex (Raine, et al., 2000) and, also, a bilateral reduction of the volume of the amygdala (Yang, et al., 2009) among criminal patients, no investigators have yet identified one reliable, consistent neuropathogen which might explain the aetiology of the most brutal manifestation of human behaviour, namely, murder.

In 1900, Dr. Sigmund Freud – not yet a *Herr Professor* – proposed a radical challenge to psychiatry and to criminology alike. In his magnum opus, *Die Traumdeutung* (Freud, 1900a) – better known as *The Interpretation of Dreams* (Freud, 1900b, 1900c) – the father of psychoanalysis boldly introduced the notion of the "Todeswunsch" (Freud, 1900a, p. 176), namely, the "death wish", explaining that each human being struggles with deeply powerful murderous desires towards parents, siblings and, even, children. Indeed, the very heart of sibling rivalry and, also, of what has come to be known as the Oedipus Complex, rests predominantly on our murderous strivings towards those nearest and dearest to us. By having dared to speak openly about the ubiquity of murderousness as a feature of the ordinary human mind, Freud forced us to consider a very subversive conundrum, namely, not *why* men and women commit murder but, rather, in view of the universality of these deadly fantasies, *why* more men and women *do not*.

Building upon the foundational work of Freud, numerous psychoanalytical practitioners have maintained a very strong interest in the unconscious motivations of killers. For instance, in 1924, several pioneering American psychoanalysts, including Dr. William Healy and Dr. William Alanson White, testified at the trial of the young murderers Nathan Leopold, Jr. and Richard Loeb, who had assassinated a fourteen-year-old boy called Bobby Franks (Kahr, 2005b; Baatz, 2008; cf. Kahr, 2007b). And, in 1940, the psychologically sympathetic Mexican judge, Señor Raúl Carrancá y Trujillo, who had corresponded with Sigmund Freud, collaborated with the criminologist Dr. Alfonso Quiroz Cuarón and the forensic psychiatrist Dr. José Gómez Robleda, a physician who facilitated hundreds of hours of interviews with none other than Jacques Mornard, the man accused of having murdered Leon Trotsky. These Mexican investigators even undertook dream analysis of this criminal as well as a study of his handwriting (Gallo, 2012), in an effort to understand the roots of murder.

In spite of these and many other valiant efforts to establish a field of psychoanalytically orientated criminology, the early Freudians failed to produce a comprehensive and coherent theory of the psychodynamics of murder. Indeed, the Viennese psychoanalytical community, in particular, may have suffered a great setback when, in 1924, a young man broke into the home of Dr. Hermine von Hug-Hellmuth, one of the founders of child psychoanalysis, and strangled her to death. It eventually emerged that the killer, Herr Rudolf Otto Hug, happened to be the nephew of the victim and, also, her sometime patient, whom she had attempted to psychoanalyse, albeit rather unsuccessfully (MacLean, 1986; MacLean and Rappen, 1991). Indeed, after his release from prison, Herr Hug threatened to sue the Wiener Psychoanalytische Vereinigung [Vienna Psycho-Analytical Society], claiming himself to be a victim of the psychoanalytical process (Deutsch, 1973).

With such scandals etched into the public record, those early attempts to apply psychoanalysis to the study of criminology often met with considerable derision. In fact, in 1929, Dr. Franz Alexander, a medical practitioner who had qualified as a psychoanalyst, and Dr. Hugo Staub, a criminologist who had also undertaken psychoanalytical training, reported that many sceptics regarded the psychological approach to the study of offending behaviour as little more than "eine luxuriöse Verschwendung" (Alexander and Staub, 1929 p. [7]) – a luxurious waste.

Sadly, although quite a number of psychodynamically orientated practitioners have written about the inner world of the murderer (e.g., Alexander, 1937; Bromberg, 1951; Hyatt-Williams, 1998), and although many more have facilitated psychotherapeutic treatment of such patients in secure institutions (Williams, 1964; cf. Kahr, 2018c), we still lack a coherent theory of the aetiology of murder.

I will not pretend that any contemporary forensic psychodynamic workers claim to know the deepest and fullest causes of murderous behaviour, but, certainly, we do appreciate that early traumatological experiences will render individuals at far greater risk of enacting their *Todeswunschen*, while those who have enjoyed reasonably robust and securely-attached childhoods will more easily contain and transform their hateful and explosive feelings into *words*, rather than *actions*. But, with reference to those forensic patients – especially males – who actually commit murders, we do not possess sufficient data to identify any particular trauma that might reliably contribute to the perpetration of a killing. We do understand, for instance, that although some murderers will have suffered from sexual abuse as children (Lewis, et al., 1988; Lewis, et al., 1997), not all murderers will have endured such specific bodily attacks (e.g., Pincus, 2001); therefore, we cannot readily foreground one unique intrafamilial pathogen.

As readers will recall, I noted in the introductory chapter of this book that, more than forty years ago, while working on the back wards of a regional psychiatric hospital, I met a patient called "Fred", a sixty-three-year-old man, diagnosed as suffering from paranoid schizophrenia. Decades previously, he had become convinced that his elderly parents planned to poison his soup; consequently, in an act of ostensible self-protection, he shot both his mother and his father in the face at close range, killing them instantly and splattering their brains all over the family kitchen. Naturally, when I first heard the grisly details of what Fred had done, I felt horrified and, indeed, frightened by such unthinkable violence. But, even more so, I found myself quite struck by the very small height of this man – only 5' 1" tall – and by his rather high-pitched, squeaky voice and somewhat traditionally feminine manner. The other male patients on the ward used to tease this man mercilessly, and they referred to him, not as "Fred" but, rather, as "Winifred".

Back then, as a young student, I presumed that anyone capable of two such invasive murders would have to be a large, hulky, deep-voiced brute – a cross between John Wayne and Arnold Schwarzenegger. But "Fred", this double-parental killer, absolutely violated that preconception. In fact, he appeared to be somewhat *castrated* in his demeanour. Perhaps I had encountered merely a rare exception among male murderers.

But, not long thereafter, my interest in the potential role of castration in the minds and histories of male killers became further piqued when I had the privilege of meeting the noted Professor Flora Rheta Schreiber (1973), an American academic who taught at the John Jay College of Criminal Justice at the City University of New York, in Manhattan, and who had already become quite well known for having written the best-selling book *Sybil* – the first modern-day study of multiple personality disorder – in which she demonstrated that the protagonist became dissociative in the wake of numerous early childhood traumata. After the publication of *Sybil*, Professor Schreiber (1983) undertook an even more chilling study, based upon years of interviews with a real-life multiple murderer, Joseph Kallinger – an American shoemaker who, under the influence of persecutory, internal voices, hatched a plot to kill every single member of the world's population, one by one. After having murdered three of his intended victims, the police apprehended Kallinger, and the court arranged for his incarceration in prison, followed sometime thereafter by his admission to a maximum-security psychiatric hospital, where he would remain for the rest of his life.

Having conducted hundreds of hours of tape-recorded interviews with Joseph Kallinger, Professor Schreiber managed to reconstruct his bleak and heart-breaking childhood in exquisitely chilling detail. Hitherto, no researcher had ever written such a comprehensive and nuanced portrait of the early years of a multiple murderer.

In brief, Kallinger, born in 1935, in Philadelphia, Pennsylvania, endured a complex childhood, full of broken attachments. His birth mother placed him for adoption at the age of three weeks and, consequently, this abandoned little baby grew up in a stark orphanage. At twenty-two months, Anna Kallinger and Stephen Kallinger, two childless Austrian émigrés, adopted this much-neglected boy.

The new mother, Anna Kallinger, had survived a traumatic childhood of her own; indeed, at the age of twelve years, her father had died from head injuries, and, as a result, the young girl had to work as a labourer in a factory. In later years, she would inflict head injuries of a different sort upon her own son, explaining to the young boy that she considered him a "disappointment" (Schreiber, 1983, p. 35) and that she wished that she had adopted a girl instead, thus assaulting his young, burgeoning sense of masculinity.

The adoptive father, Stephen Kallinger, struggled with infertility and felt ashamed that he could not inseminate his wife. His failure to reproduce remained a great secret in the family.

Collectively, these two Austrian-born parents treated the young boy roughly and prohibited him from playing with other children. They also subjected him to one particularly cruel and perverse experience.

At the age of six years, little Joseph Kallinger underwent surgery for a hernia, and the physician who performed the operation, Dr. Joseph Daly, inflicted a six-inch scar upon the child's body. *In toto*, the young Joseph spent sixteen days in hospital. After he had returned to the family home, the parents told him that Dr. Daly had not only removed his hernia but, also, that he had extracted a demon which lurked inside his penis and, in consequence, he would become impotent in later life and would never be able to impregnate a girl or get her into trouble. As Anna Kallinger explained to her adopted child, "you won't have no demon in *your* bird because your bird will always be small, small, small, small, small!" (quoted in Schreiber, 1983, p. 28).

The boy became quite preoccupied that the surgeon had performed this procedure with a knife similar to the one used by his adoptive father, Stephen Kallinger – a shoemaker – in his daily work. After this fateful meeting with the parents, the young Kallinger began to hallucinate and imagined that he could see his own penis floating on the tip of a knife (Schreiber, 1983). In every sense, Kallinger experienced multiple assaults on his sense of potency and worth.

Joe Kallinger, the future murderer, suffered so extensively from this symbolic castration that, years hence, when he engaged in sexual intercourse with a woman, he struggled to achieve an erection, and it seems that he could do so only by clutching a knife in his hand, which he had secreted by his bedside. Holding onto a knife brought Kallinger a much-needed sense of temporary sexual potency.

Unsurprisingly, this highly castrated man became so profoundly ashamed and so viciously angry from having endured a psychological castration as a boy that, eventually, he snapped and embarked upon his plan to kill everyone on the planet. His three victims even included his own fifteen-year-old son, Michael Kallinger.

Naturally, it would be far too simplistic to argue that Joseph Kallinger became a murderer solely as a result of the fact that his parents taunted him with a symbolic castration. Innumerable mothers and fathers have shamed their children throughout human history, yet not all of these victims of emotional abuse have actually become killers. Unsurprisingly, Joseph Kallinger endured yet other extreme traumata. For instance, his adoptive parents forced him to pray, while kneeling on sandpaper, causing bruising to his kneecaps. His father beat him all over his body; and his mother hit him on the head with a hammer on several occasions. Furthermore, either father or mother would, at times, also thrust their son's hand into the flames of the burner on the kitchen stove as a particularly cruel punishment, designed to expunge the boy of sin.

Tragically, Kallinger felt unsafe not only inside his childhood home but, also, out on the streets. Indeed, during his eighth year, a group of three older boys subjected him to fellatio at knifepoint, thus placing him in a hugely endangering and frighteningly passive position.

Having endured these multiple traumata, one can certainly appreciate that Kallinger experienced profound death wishes towards his parents, his surgeon and, also, towards the boys in the neighbourhood. But one must wonder whether Sigmund Freud's notion of the "Todeswunsch" – the death wish – might also be underscored by his subsequent concept of the ' "Kastrationskomplex" ' (Freud, 1909a, p. 3) – namely, the castration complex – and whether, among men, in particular, a profound attack on one's psychological sense of potency might contribute in a significant way to the vulnerability towards murderousness in later life (cf. Kahr, 2024b).

Thus far, as a young student of forensic psychology, I had encountered "Fred", known shamingly to the other men on the ward as "Winifred" – a small man who struggled with his masculinity. And through my association with Professor Schreiber, I also had the opportunity to meet Joseph Kallinger at the Farview State Hospital for the Criminally Insane, in Waymart, Pennsylvania. Both of these deadly killers forced me to consider whether castration anxiety could, in any way at all, facilitate the genesis of murders committed by men (Kahr, 2022e).

Let us now meet another life-threatening sadist, albeit a fictional one, namely, "Tom Ripley", the protagonist of Patricia Highsmith's novel *The Talented Mr. Ripley*, a veritable psychological thriller, first published in 1955 and subsequently enshrined in a popular film version of 1999, starring Matt Damon and Jude Law. A homosexual man from a modest background, the young Ripley travels to Italy and encounters a handsome, virile, confident, and wealthy young man, "Richard Greenleaf", known as "Dickie", and falls madly in love with this icon of heterosexual potency. Indeed, on one occasion, Tom Ripley steals into Dickie Greenleaf's bedroom and then dresses himself in Dickie's clothing in an effort to enhance his own flagging virility (cf. Zavitzianos, 1972).

As the film unfolds, Tom Ripley becomes increasingly troubled, owing to the fact that his homoerotic friendship with Dickie Greenleaf begins to flounder and, gradually, the heterosexual character humiliates the young homosexual character more and more, resulting in disastrous consequences. In an effort to restore his injured sense of potency, Tom Ripley grabs an oar, while out boating, and then bashes his rival companion Dickie Greenleaf to death.

Patricia Highsmith's gripping novel and its subsequent film adaptation provide cunning support for the notion that murderers, such as the character Tom Ripley, often feel extremely castrated by more potent men and, in consequence, will search for a phallic substitute, such as a long, pointy knife, or a bullet-firing gun, or even a penile-shaped oar, to attack their rivals.

Many people – even mental health professionals – often snigger at some of Sigmund Freud's original psychoanalytical concepts. Certainly, one must be a very brave person to discuss the notion of "penis envy" in public, lest one be humiliated for even daring to consider that this ancient, seemingly misogynistic Freudian concept might have some validity. Likewise, the idea of "castration anxiety" stimulates similar titters and giggles as, nowadays, few modern parents would ever threaten their sons' genitalia or verbalise injunctions against masturbation as the mothers and fathers of Freud's generation had done (e.g., Freud, 1900a). Indeed, the British psychoanalyst Mrs. Rosemary Davies (2012) even opined that, in recent years, the concept of castration anxiety has, itself, become a bit castrated.

But might the notion of castration anxiety continue to have merit for our understanding of the violent forensic patient?

Certainly, those of us who have worked psychotherapeutically with male genital exhibitionists have drawn richly upon this idea for many decades. As early as 1923, a Hungarian-born psychoanalyst, Dr. Jenö Hárnik (1923), wrote a foundational paper, in German, on the role of castration anxiety in the treatment of exhibitionist patients (as we have indicated in a previous chapter). In that essay – now little-cited in the professional literature – Hárnik argued that the public exposure of the penis provides reassurance to the male flasher who, by shocking his female victims, comes to realise that his genitalia can still exert a potent impact.

Subsequent generations of psychoanalytical practitioners have relied heavily upon the notion of castration anxiety as a means of explaining why men need to display their sexual organs publicly. In 1964, Dr. Ismond Rosen (1964b), a psychoanalyst who worked for many years at the Portman Clinic in London, and who specialised in the treatment of sexual deviations, described the case of a male flasher who feared that sharks would bite off his penis and testicles. Although the likelihood that a landlocked London-based patient would ever be attacked by a shark remains extremely slender, Rosen certainly came to appreciate that the terror of castration invades the mind of the genital exhibitionist quite pervasively.

In 2019, I published a report about a male genital exhibitionist patient with whom I worked psychotherapeutically many years previously (Kahr, 2019e). This young man, who suffered from profound intellectual disabilities, exposed himself to several young females in public and received a caution from the police who, had he not suffered from disabilities, might well have arrested him. During the course of treatment, my patient, "Tobiasz" – also discussed in a previous chapter in this book – eventually revealed that, as a young boy at boarding school, several of his classmates ganged up and began to tug on his penis on a nightly basis, pulling so hard that the patient thought that these lads would actually rip his genitals from his body. With such a traumatic attack on the genital region, Tobiasz experienced a deep sense of shame and assault and, in later years, he exposed his penis publicly in a desperate attempt to receive confirmation that he could still be a potent male. Thus, forensic psychotherapists continue to encounter patients whose criminal acts can be traced to early-life genital trauma.

It will not be widely known or appreciated that one of the most notorious murderers in history, namely, the American necrophile and cannibal, Jeffrey Dahmer, first encountered the police, not for murder but, rather, for displaying his genitalia out of doors, and would be arrested for masturbating in public near the Kinnickinnic River in the city of Milwaukee, Wisconsin, charged with lewd and lascivious behaviour, indecent exposure, and disorderly conduct (Masters, 1993).

Jeffrey Dahmer, once a much-neglected infant, experienced considerable emotional deprivation, in part, due to the fact that his depressed mother refused to breastfeed him; indeed, sometime thereafter, she attempted to commit suicide. As a three-year-old, Dahmer underwent inguinal hernia surgery through his groin. Such early childhood experiences would have predisposed a young boy to huge anger; and consequently, Dahmer murdered a dog and then impaled the animal's skull with a stake. By sixteen years of age, he had already developed necrophilic masturbatory fantasies. And at twenty-two years of age, Jeffrey Dahmer exposed himself before a crowd of some twenty-five women and children at the Wisconsin State Fair Park (Masters, 1993) – in West Allis, a suburb of Milwaukee – thus providing himself with considerable reassurance and relief that the surgeon from his childhood had not eviscerated his genitalia. Across his criminal career, Dahmer enacted the most brutal killings of seventeen young men and boys and, in some cases, he preserved even the penises, the testicles and, also, the pudenda of the victims in his home as macabre souvenirs (Masters, 1993) and, perhaps, as symbols of triumph, having projected castration anxiety into those males whose lives Dahmer cut so tragically short.

Staggeringly, Dahmer engaged not only in necrophilia but, also, in necrophagia, and would, at times, even devour parts of the slaughtered corpses.

Although innumerable psychiatric writers have pontificated about Dahmer, no one, to the best of my knowledge, has considered whether castration anxiety might have contributed to the development of his murderous psychopathology in later years (Kahr, 2001b, 2020b, 2023b).

One need not search very far to discover other cases of murderers who have endured what we might conceptualise as psychologically castrating experiences in childhood. For instance, during his interview on Death Row with the American murderer Leo Murphy, the forensic neurologist Professor Jonathan Pincus (2001) unearthed a great deal of relevant data. Leo Murphy, son of a prostitute mother who struggled with alcoholism, endured many physical and verbal attacks during his early years. Tragically, after the breakup of the marriage of his parents, the father wed an even more vicious woman, and, in due course, the new stepmother would torture him in a far more sinister and castrating fashion.

This deeply sadistic stepmother would actually hang the little boy Leo Murphy by his thumbs; she would also burn his hands on the stove; and she would even singe his lips and his fingers with cigarettes which she would then force him to smoke. Additionally, she would beat her stepson with a wire brush and with a belt and would push him down the stairs of the basement with his hands tied behind his back. Shockingly, this adult woman would also chain the little boy to a pole and would then smear faeces onto his face.

These acts of physical cruelty should be sufficient to induce a lifetime of murderous rage in a young child; but this vicious stepmother humiliated Leo Murphy in even more castrating ways, by treating him as a fully demasculinised object of penetration. The stepmother not only dressed the boy in girls' clothing, but she tied up his penis to hide his genitalia and then inserted enemas and tampons – including her very own used tampons, soiled by her menstrual blood – into his anus. She would also squeeze his testicles painfully and would thrust a thermometer into his urethra, which she would secure with tape, resulting in bleeding and infection. Moreover, she often masturbated the boy to orgasm and covered his face with semen and, further, forced him to perform oral sex upon her own genital region.

Unsurprisingly, this young male victim of such feminising, castrating abuse felt so impotent and so girl-like that he even developed dissociative identity disorder and often imagined himself to be a female. Thus when, in later years, he committed murder, he attempted to reclaim his phallic potency by shooting his victim to death with a gun (Pincus, 2001).

The vast majority of contemporary criminological researchers have attempted to explain the act of murder by recourse to *concretely* identifiable, often visible, aetiological factors, such as brain pathology, socioeconomic status, and gross acts of documentable intrafamilial violence, including rape (e.g., Lewis, 1998). Certainly, many, if not all, of these characteristics and experiences may well have contributed to the genesis of crimes such as murder in years hence.

But, as we know from the work of Sigmund Freud and from the innumerable psychoanalytical practitioners who have followed in his wake, one need not be formally bereaved in order to become melancholic; one need not be bodily violated in order to feel abused; and one need not be surgically castrated in order to become impotent. Slights and other narcissistic injuries will all contribute to our sense of impotency, whether in males or in females, and will often result in deadly rage.

Although the novelist Patricia Highsmith, to the best of our knowledge, never committed a murder, she certainly understood much about Tom Ripley's sense of being demasculinised – castrated, in fact – and she very much appreciated how this fictional character could achieve a sense of psychic equilibrium *only* by clutching a giant, phallic oar and by smashing his infinitely more potent masculine rival to death. Likewise, Joseph Kallinger and Jeffrey Dahmer, both real-life victims of hernia operations as well as many other far more damaging early traumata, turned to the use of the knife in order to commit murders, plunging a phallic substitute into the innocent flesh of their victims, thus reliving early experiences of impotency in their own histories and within their own criminal minds.

Kallinger had come to believe that the surgeon had removed the potency from his penis, and Dahmer had felt abandoned by his depressed mother and thus compelled to expose his own genitals in order to elicit a reaction which resulted in his arrest. Ultimately, both of these men became murderers and attempted to locate their feelings of hopelessness in those whom they killed off most savagely. And by murdering others, both Kallinger and Dahmer endeavoured to reverse the experience of having felt killed themselves.

As I indicated, such seemingly antique Freudian concepts as penis envy and castration anxiety often evoke tremendous suspicion and derision. In his Chichele Lecture on "Freud and Literary Biography", delivered at the University of Oxford, Professor Richard Ellmann (1985) underscored the complicated position of psychoanalytical concepts in popular culture. He mentioned a 1983 newspaper article about an American man who, egged on by his mother, then murdered his father. The reporter who wrote about this crime actually concluded that the killer must have suffered from an Oedipus Complex. Ellmann (1985, p. 58) quipped that it would be very easy to dismiss such a diagnosis as little more than an expression of American "journalistic excess". Thus, in an era of brain scans galore, suggesting that something as diffuse and intangible and unproven as "castration anxiety" could serve as a contributory aetiological factor in the genesis of murder might well seem truly ridiculous.

And yet, those of us who work as clinicians, listening to patients free-associating on the couch on a daily basis over many years, will appreciate, only too clearly, the shame and rage that results when a male patient explains to us that he cannot achieve an erection with his female partner due to the fact that she had irritated or disappointed him in some way. Indeed, we hear stories, quite frequently, of men who fantasise about cruelty towards their spouses or girlfriends as a desperate attempt to locate their castrated feelings elsewhere.

Needless to say, according to the experience of most psychoanalytical workers, castration anxiety represents a universal or near-universal theme in the study of the male mind. Freud had certainly alerted his colleagues to the widespread nature of fears of castration among his male patients and those with whom he consulted (e.g., Freud, 1905a, 1909a, 1918, 1922, 1926, 1937). And, back in the 1920s, Dr. Richard Sterba, then a young psychoanalytical student in Vienna, worked as a physician at an outpatient clinic for children, and, on one occasion, had to examine a little boy who lay naked on a table, covering his genitalia with his hands. According to Sterba, this small child shouted, "Don't cut it off." (quoted in Sterba, 1982, p. 33). The young physician reassured the boy that his genitals would remain unharmed; but such an experience prompted Sterba (1982, p. 33) to comment, "This was a most impressive manifestation of castration anxiety, which we find omnipresent and ubiquitously troubling in the analyses of men."

Nevertheless, in spite of the widespread nature of castration anxiety, the vast majority of men do *not* become forensic patients. It would thus be folly to suggest that castration anxiety *causes* murder. But one need only speak to our venerable American colleague, Professor James Gilligan, who has examined more murderers than perhaps any other living forensic psychiatrist. Gilligan (1996, 2001) has become convinced that the vast majority of murders result not from brain pathology *per se* but, rather, from an experience of being humiliated. As he explained, his patients felt not only shamed and humiliated but, also, "disrespected, dishonored, disgraced, demeaned, defeated, insulted, slighted, rejected, ridiculed, mocked, embarrassed, treated as inferior, unimportant, insignificant or a failure" (Gilligan, 2016, p. 132).

After his arrest for multiple murders in 1983, Dennis Nilsen met with his solicitor, Ronald Moss, to prepare a defence. Moss asked Nilsen why he had committed so many vicious killings. But Nilsen had no clear idea as to what had prompted him to perpetrate such unspeakable crimes. He merely replied, "I am hoping you will tell me" (quoted in Masters, 1985, p. 24). But although Nilsen could not provide a coherent narrative of the motivations for his horrific crimes, he did, however, possess the linguistic capacity to describe himself as an "unhappy, brooding child, secretive and stricken with inferiority" (quoted in Masters, 1985, p. 41).

Perhaps the notion of inferiority in a male, which Freud would have conceptualised as castration anxiety, might have some merit, in spite of its current status as little more than a Woody Allen-esque parody in modern psychology. And perhaps, by recognising the deep sense of castration inferiority experienced by our forensic patients from early childhood and adolescence onwards, we might well be able to raise consciousness more fully about this feature of human development and thus contribute, in some small way, towards the prevention of future grotesque crimes.

PART IV

Forensic Patients in the Community

Sub-Clinical Psychopathy

The Sub-Clinical Psychopath

Committing Crimes Without Breaking the Law

THE SUB-CLINICAL FORENSIC PERPETRATOR

In 1969, Peter Sutcliffe, a twenty-three-year-old sometime gravedigger from the market town of Bingley in the West Riding region of Yorkshire, attacked a female prostitute by hitting her on the head with a stone, wrapped in a sock. The victim did not press charges. Consequently, Sutcliffe remained at liberty. In 1975, some six years later, Sutcliffe attacked another woman, assaulting her with a hammer and, also, slashing her stomach with a knife. Over the next five years, Sutcliffe perpetrated many more offences which became increasingly violent in nature and which resulted in the murders of many innocent women, whom he bludgeoned with hammers and skewered with screwdrivers (Burn, 1984). Regrettably, this extremely dangerous man would not be apprehended until 1981, more than a decade after his first detected offence; and, eventually, after having served several years in Her Majesty's Prison, Parkhurst, on the Isle of Wight, he would ultimately be transferred in 1984 to the high-security Broadmoor Hospital in the village of Crowthorne, in the county of Berkshire, where he remained for many years, prior to his ultimate transfer to a prison in the village of Durham in his native Yorkshire, where he died, in hospital, in 2020, amid the coronavirus pandemic.

When Peter Sutcliffe – reviled in the press as the "Yorkshire Ripper" – stood trial, the court psychiatrists debated the appropriate diagnosis of this multiple murderer. But although those who assessed Sutcliffe clinically may have struggled as to whether they should classify him as suffering from paranoid schizophrenia or from a personality disorder, everyone would have agreed that he certainly merited being described as a forensic patient, namely, someone whose substantial psychological illness will have contributed to the enactment of violent criminality consisting of either the destruction of property or of attacks on the body of another person or persons, or, indeed, upon oneself.

When forensic mental health professionals and members of the public alike encounter multiple murderers, career paedophiles, serial arsonists, and marital rapists, few, if any of us, doubt that these offenders have actually crossed a very dangerous line. Consequently, forensic patients will require special treatment, which invariably consists of confinement in an institutional setting and, wherever

DOI: 10.4324/9781003546245-13

possible, psychological care as well, perhaps even the opportunity to undertake dynamically orientated psychotherapy.

Thankfully, most people who attend for psychoanalysis or psychotherapy have never perpetrated acts of gross, forensic criminality and do not suffer from an overtly diagnosable mental illness. The vast majority of psychological patients conduct their lives with considerable honour and dignity, and most will "contain" their violent impulses with a reasonable degree of success. We might refer to such individuals as "non-forensic" patients.

But although these predominantly law-abiding people will never commit murder, arson, or rape, and will never attack the bodies of small children, many of our otherwise ostensibly "normal" patients have, nevertheless, perpetrated acts of violence, even criminality, which have often remained *undetected*. From time to time, those of us who work as clinical psychotherapists may find ourselves in the truly uncomfortable and morally agonising position of being the only person privy to confessions of such acts of destruction.

Of course, every human being – whether a forensic psychiatric patient or an upstanding member of the community – has the capacity to harbour violent thoughts and fantasies. In 2007, I published a large-scale study of the sexual fantasies of more than 19,000 British adults (Kahr, 2007a). Fully twenty-nine per cent of Britons admitted that they will have experienced sexual fantasies of "Playing a dominant or aggressive role during sex" (Kahr, 2007a, p. 588), while seven per cent had fantasised about "Using a whip or paddle or cane or slipper or strap" (Kahr, 2007a, p. 588) on someone else. Likewise, twenty-three per cent of British adults will have engaged in coital or masturbatory fantasies about "Tying someone up" (Kahr, 2007a, p. 588), and four per cent will have enjoyed "Gagging someone else" (Kahr, 2007a, p. 589). One per cent of the respondents in my study even admitted to having fantasised about "Sex with a child" (Kahr, 2007a, p. 589). While the figure of one per cent may seem mercifully small, we must remember that one per cent of the adult British population represents, nevertheless, nearly half a million individuals.

In 2008, I obtained highly comparable data about the pervasiveness of aggression and cruelty in the sexual fantasies of ordinary American men and women, aged eighteen years and older (Kahr, 2008). Clearly, sadism emerges in quite a widespread manner in the so-called normal population... on both sides of the Atlantic Ocean!

One might assume that my data, though carefully collected through the use of an anonymised and highly respected computer polling research network, might, in fact, have provided only a very conservative estimate of the true state of affairs. After all, many respondents may not have wished to confess their more violent fantasies to a team of researchers. But those who did admit to masturbating about forensic activities did so without restraint. One of the participants in my survey, a man called "Yannis", revealed that he would fantasise about "Taking all my enemies, anyone who's ever been cruel to me, and fucking them until they bleed to death" (quoted in Kahr, 2007a, p. 336).

My own findings on the prevalence of violent sexual fantasies underscore the work published two years earlier by Professor David Buss (2005), an American psychologist, whose large-scale investigation had confirmed that as many as ninety-one per cent of American men and eighty-four per cent of American women have actually experienced vivid, detailed fantasies of committing murder.

Obviously, masturbating about murder or rape in no way guarantees that one will actually perpetrate murder or rape in the forensic sense. But where does one draw the line? And to what extent do violent fantasies place a person at risk for an ultimate forensic enactment at some point in the future?

Over the course of several decades, I have become increasingly aware that many patients undergoing psychotherapy have, often quite unconsciously, progressed beyond the realm of masturbatory or coital fantasy, and have committed acts of violence or have even broken the law. None of these patients had ever, to the best of my knowledge, perpetrated such grotesque acts of murder as the Yorkshire Ripper had done, and none had ever attracted the attention of the police or the courts or even the forensic psychiatrists. But, in certain cases, ordinary, seemingly "normal" or "neurotic" men and women have engaged in acts of violence which, from time to time, have even resulted in the death of another human being.

I have come to think of such individuals as "sub-clinical" forensic patients, whose sadism – often deeply unconscious – has remained undetected for long periods of time.

In this chapter, I shall endeavour to explore the psychodynamics of the so-called "sub-clinical", non-forensic patient, concentrating on how and why such individuals function in this quasi-forensic fashion. I shall also consider what impact this unconscious "criminality" might have upon these patients, upon their intimates and, also, upon the independent psychotherapist, working in a private office, who has undertaken to provide treatment.

In my experience, few, if any, practitioners of psychotherapy would deny that a capacity for violence lies at the very core of the human mind. Each of us has the potentiality to fantasise about murder, but, thankfully, most of us will develop the ability to harness and encapsulate such fantasies, and to neutralise their toxicity through an investment in loving attachments and in creative sublimations.

And yet, in spite of the fact that the vast majority of us will find it very easy to refrain from setting buildings on fire or from assaulting our colleagues with hammers and knives, every single one of us has, at one time or another, committed a crime of some sort.

I shall never forget that, nearly forty years ago, during my very first seminar as a young student at the Portman Clinic in London, Dr. Mervin Glasser, then Medical Director at this specialist institution for the treatment of forensic patients, pontificated to my cohort of trainees that one need not be a murderer or a paedophile in order to be a criminal. As Glasser warned us, anyone who has ever taken a paper clip from his or her clinic office and used it to attach *personal* papers, as opposed to *clinic* papers, has, in point of fact, committed an act of theft. As Dr. Glasser spoke, a shame-filled hush descended over all the students in this seminar on the psychology of violence, as each one of us recalled instances of having rung our spouses from the clinic telephone, having nicked a pencil from the storeroom cupboard, or, worst of all, having used a stapler for private purposes. Technically, we had all engaged in enactments of thievery. But did such activities really qualify us as forensic patients? When I confessed to my own training analyst later that day that I had, over the years, purloined a paper clip here and there, he merely chuckled. After all, he had treated *real* murderers and rapists in his time, and he simply analysed my guilt as a vestige of early childhood fears of having murdered my siblings in my mind: a criminal from a sense of unconscious guilt (Freud, 1916).

But sometimes acts of cruelty and violence among the non-forensic population can be much more extreme, and, over the years, I have encountered numerous instances of such "acting-out" among the seemingly normal, ambulatory patients with whom I have had the privilege of working in a private practice setting in a comfortable part of London.

CLINICAL CASE MATERIAL

"Mrs. A." arrived at my consulting room for a session in a state of fury. Her mother-in-law, whom she hated, had become frail and incapacitated after having broken a hip. Mrs. A.'s husband had hoped that he and his wife might be able to offer the mother a bedroom in their large house, but Mrs. A. told me how she had adamantly refused to do so, because the presence of a mother-in-law would restrict her own social life unduly. Mrs. A. admitted that, although her mother-in-law had never done anything untoward, my patient simply and honestly did not wish to extend herself in this way.

I reminded Mrs. A. that she and I had devoted many previous sessions of psychotherapy to an exploration of her fantasy of being an "unwanted" child, in view of the fact that she had arrived some ten years after all of her other siblings. Consequently, Mrs. A. had come to think of herself as a "mistake" and she thus carried a great deal of rage in her heart at all times.

I wondered whether Mrs. A.'s attack on her fragile mother-in-law might well constitute a displaced attack on *her* own mother of infancy. Perhaps, by denying shelter to her husband's mother, Mrs. A. had succeeded in gratifying an unconscious wish to assault her biological mother. Mrs. A. then spurted out, "Why should I give my mother-in-law a room? I had to sleep on the staircase as a child!" I enquired further and soon discovered that, during Mrs. A.'s very early childhood, her father had lost his job, and, consequently, the family had to move to a much smaller house with fewer bedrooms. And for a period of time, Mrs. A. did, indeed, have to spend the whole night on a mattress placed unceremoniously in the stairwell. In view of this fact, how on earth could Mrs. A. have developed sufficient generosity of spirit to have created a bedroom for her sick mother-in-law decades later?

In spite of my valiant efforts to explore and to interpret the interconnection between Mrs. A.'s early childhood experience and her adult state of mind, she refused to alter her position in regard to her mother-in-law, and she then explained with steely resolution, "I simply refuse to look after that woman. It's not my responsibility." Mrs. A. spoke with such ferocity that I came to regard her decision not as a lifestyle choice or as the assertion of her autonomy but, rather, as an expression of historical cruelty.

But does the refusal to allow one's mother-in-law to sleep in the spare room actually constitute a forensic enactment? After all, Mrs. A. broke no laws. But might she have committed a crime? In many respects, I would argue that for Mrs. A. to have made such a verbal pronouncement, prohibiting her mother-in-law from occupying the spare bedroom, does indeed qualify as a type of forensic gesture.

It saddens me to report that Mrs. A. eventually sent her mother-in-law to a care home, attended by a nurse, and that, six months later, the aged woman suffered a heart attack after falling in the bath, whereupon she died instantly.

Let us also consider the case of "Mr. B.", a generally calm, quiet, creative gentleman who worked long hours in a respectable profession and who would pay all of his bills on time, yet who harboured strong antisemitic sentiments. During the course of a lengthy analysis, Mr. B. wondered on many occasions whether I might be of Jewish origin. Although I never answered him directly, I always explored what possible meaning or meanings such a preoccupation could serve. Mr. B., a Labour Party supporter who read only *The Guardian* newspaper, knew quite well that his hatred of Jews had no rational basis. He even relished the company of many Jewish friends. And yet, secretly, while lying on the couch, he enjoyed indulging in fantasies of Jew-killing.

When, after several years of treatment, I resolved to raise my sessional fee by a relatively tiny amount, Mr. B., a hugely wealthy man, exploded. He simply could not believe that after four years of work I would dare to do something so seemingly cruel, and he then explained that my ostensible outrageousness provided him with proof-positive that I *must* be Jewish. He began to rant with a fury that I had never before encountered in clinical practice, and he delighted in telling me that if he had worked in Auschwitz during the Second World War, he would have escorted me and my entire family personally to the gas chambers and would have poured the Zyklon-B poisonous pellets into the pipes himself, rejoicing in our agonising deaths.

It pleases me to report that Mr. B.'s abusiveness did not result in my death. In this respect, he had not committed a forensic enactment as such. But the quality of cruelty that he displayed in the transference very much mirrored the sadism experienced by his wife, whom he had often insulted viciously and whom he had occasionally struck with his bare hands, causing tremendous marital distress, threats of divorce, and legal consultations. Does Mr. B. qualify, therefore, as a sub-clinical forensic patient? If we should agree to expand our definition of what constitutes the forensic state of mind, then Mr. B. might very well meet the criteria.

"Ms. C.", a highly seductive and flirtatious person, had no difficulty enticing numerous men into her bed. Very physically beautiful and very superficially charismatic, she often identified herself with the siren "Lorelei" who lured sailors unsuspectingly to their doom. For three years, immediately *prior* to the commencement of her psychotherapy, Ms. C. participated in a long and passionate affair with "Mr. D.", a man who had hoped to marry her; but Ms. C. grew tired of this gentleman and she dumped him unceremoniously. Distraught, Mr. D. retreated to a pub and drank himself senseless in order to relieve his unbearable anguish. In a state of great inebriation, Mr. D. tripped and plunged down a flight of stairs, injuring his neck and becoming partially paralysed. In spite of numerous pleas from Mr. D. for a visit, Ms. C. refused to oblige.

Should we, therefore, consider Ms. C. to be a forensic patient? Once again, she broke no laws and perpetrated no crimes that would excite a lawyer or a police officer or a court. In fact, she had remained in her home, with her three flatmates in Highgate in North London, on the evening that Mr. D. became crippled at a pub in Clapham in South-West London. From a legal perspective, she boasted a perfect alibi. And yet, nevertheless, she had unleashed a terrific degree of sadism upon her lover and, one might argue, had stimulated his deep pain and his consequent act of alcoholic self-harm, which resulted in the tragic damage to his spinal cord.

Marital couples, in particular, have a huge capacity to become violent in a sub-clinical manner. Often, each member of the couple will comport himself or herself in life with great compassion and great dignity, but when the two partners interact as a couple, the sadistic underbelly of each spouse becomes infinitely more visible.

"Mr. E." and "Mrs. E.", a long-standing marital couple, had come to consult with me in a state of anguish. Mrs. E. explained that her husband, who had recently turned forty, had begun to drink excessively; and Mrs. E. attributed this sudden increase in her husband's alcohol consumption to a "mid-life crisis". One evening, Mr. E. returned from the pub after having consumed twelve pints of lager – four pints more than his ordinary intake. Feeling sexually aroused, he began to make love to Mrs. E., but, in the middle of intercourse, he vomited all over her face.

How does one conceptualise this act in classificatory terms? To the best of my knowledge, one cannot be convicted of a criminal offence for vomiting on one's spouse as a result of inebriation. Indeed, to the best of my knowledge, no one has ever identified the phenomenon of "forensic vomiting". And yet, Mrs. E. felt painfully attacked and deeply humiliated. Does such an interchange qualify as a sub-clinical forensic enactment? As Mrs. E. exclaimed in the course of one of our marital psychotherapy sessions, "My husband is a thief. He stole my sense of safety." Certainly, this woman experienced her husband's *vomitus* in criminal terms.

"Mr. F." and "Mrs. F." presented for couple psychotherapy after Mrs. F., riddled with ovarian cancer, had discovered that her husband had recently slept with Mrs. F.'s own sister. In fact, Mrs. F., while trawling through her husband's trouser pockets, found a receipt for a hotel room, positioned just round the corner from the hospital, which Mr. F. had rented for his incestuous rendezvous. Damningly, the time of check-in and check-out – printed on the receipt – confirmed that Mr. F. had hired this hotel room during one of Mrs. F.'s chemotherapy treatment sessions. Mr. F. attempted to exculpate himself by claiming that he experienced his wife's ovarian cancer as so unbearably painful that he simply *had* to sleep with his sister-in-law in a desperate attempt to find some respite from the prospect of losing his wife.

Needless to say, this explanation did not satisfy Mrs. F., who felt viciously betrayed and profoundly murderous as a result. Mrs. F. stopped speaking to her sister in consequence, and she eventually kicked her husband out of the house. Two years later, in spite of her valiant struggle against cancer, Mrs. F. passed away. One cannot help but wonder whether Mr. F. considered himself a widower or, in fact, a murderer.[1]

Over the years of working in private practice, I have encountered the most enormous array of acts of cruelty – both conscious and unconscious – committed by otherwise law-abiding and reasonably mentally healthy men and women. Some of these sadistic activities could, one suspects, be subject to prosecution if a member of the law enforcement community should ever have come to know about them. "Mrs. G.", for instance, told me that her ex-husband, whom I never met and whom I certainly never treated, would, when angry, pour a tiny number of drops of acid into shampoo bottles in the bathrooms of his friends' homes each time he attended a dinner party. When Mrs. G. discovered her husband's "sub-clinical" treachery, she knew that she would have to divorce him and, eventually, she did so.

"Mr. H.", a man who consulted with me many years ago, had thrown a kitchen knife and a fork at his wife during a horribly heated marital row. Fortunately, Mr. H. missed "Mrs. H.", albeit by only a few inches. Nevertheless, one wonders what would have occurred if he had thrown with better aim, and whether this action should be considered forensic in nature and, if so, to what extent.

And "Mrs. I.", yet another patient, told me that she had discovered that her fourteen-year-old son had obtained a forged identity card and that he had used this card to purchase alcohol. When I expressed concern, Mrs. I. told me that she proposed to do absolutely nothing about this, explaining that most of her son's friends snorted speed and cocaine and other dangerous drugs; therefore, her son's drinking did not concern her in the least. In fact, she hoped that, by ignoring her son, he might not progress beyond bourbon and vodka.

These aforementioned clinical vignettes – all taken from moments of private psychotherapy practice – raise the most enormous number of deeply disturbing questions. For instance, what might be, or, indeed, *should* be, the responsibility of the mental health clinician when confronted with such data? Do we simply listen to these recitations of cruelty in a "neutral" manner? Do we interpret the unconscious sadism vigorously and risk, potentially, becoming policemen or policewomen in the transference? Do we turn a blind eye ourselves? Or do we step out of our roles as private practitioners and speak to social services or to law enforcement agencies?

I shall never forget that, several decades ago, as a very young student at the Portman Clinic, one of my fellow trainees presented the case of a man who had perpetrated various sexual crimes against children. This budding psychotherapist became understandably agitated, unsure of what her professional obligation might be. The seminar leader – a deeply compassionate and highly experienced psychoanalyst – spoke with resolution. He explained, "You have one responsibility and one responsibility only. You must persevere with the psychoanalytical work and you must do nothing else. If you telephone the authorities, you will cause the patient to flee from treatment, and if that should transpire, then you will never have a chance to work through the patient's paedophilic tendencies."

This remark made a great deal of sense to me and to my fellow students at the time and allowed us to experience some psychological relief, knowing that we would not have to "turn in" our patients to the police. But in the intervening decades, British law has changed dramatically, and different professional bodies have now come to adopt newer rules and regulations about mandatory reporting. It will therefore come as no surprise that most mental health professionals struggle to know whether they can, could, should, or must, report their patients for criminal activities, even though psychotherapy offers – at least in theory – the pledge of complete confidentiality (Bollas and Sundelson, 1995).

Such matters become infinitely more complex, particularly as many psychotherapists and counsellors might have completed a prior training in medicine, in social work, in education, or in psychology – disciplines which do require members to report suspected acts of child abuse and other crimes.

THE CASE OF "MR. J."

Sometimes, the private practitioner will be confronted by a range of particularly complex and challenging sub-clinical forensic enactments.

Many years ago, a local general medical practitioner rang me and explained that she had given my telephone number to a prospective psychotherapy patient in great need of help. She told me his name – "Mr. J." – and she informed me that, in view of the urgency of the situation, this gentleman would ring for an appointment forthwith.

The patient did, indeed, telephone … *two years later*!

In spite of the very long delay between the referral and the first telephone contact, I had indeed remembered Mr. J.'s name from my earlier conversation with his doctor, and I agreed to offer him an appointment for the following week.

I saw Mr. J. for a first consultation in the month of January, on a cold and blustery day. To my surprise, he arrived wearing only a T-shirt and jeans, revealing an overly developed muscular chest, which he displayed prominently. Within minutes, he told me that he had suffered from a deep depression for as long as he could remember. Mr. J. also reported that he had lived with the H.I.V. virus for more than ten years.

Having already undergone psychotherapy many years previously, Mr. J. had no difficulty providing me with a full recitation of his early childhood, during the course of which he had endured extensive traumata.

Towards the end of our first consultation, I asked Mr. J. whether he might find it useful to return for a second consultation. He replied by informing me that he had very much enjoyed our conversation and that he would, indeed, like to see me again, but that he had left his diary at home and that he would have to call me later in the day to discuss his availability.

Mr. J. did, indeed, ring, as promised, but *not* that January afternoon. Instead, he next telephoned me the following October – some *nine months later* – and requested a second consultation.

Naturally, I devoted most of my interpretative efforts to an understanding of the meaning of Mr. J.'s reluctance to engage in human contact and to his profound fear of doing so, as evidenced by the fact that he took two years to call me for his first appointment, and then nine months for his second appointment. Privately, I thought to myself that if we continued at this rate, I might not be alive to see his treatment through to a successful conclusion – no doubt a pertinent countertransferential response, stimulated by the patient's own anxieties about living in the shadow of a potentially deadly illness.

Mr. J. told me without hesitation that he had delayed for nine months before ringing back because he had experienced me as extremely frightening and he thought that I looked like a monster. He explained that he had found my physical appearance – especially my eyes – very, very scary indeed; but he also knew that I had come highly recommended, and so, in desperation, he thought that he would attempt a second consultation. He then stood up from the chair and moved to the far side of the room, near the door, and told me that he would prefer to sit on the floor, approximately nine or ten feet away from me, as he felt very much safer.

I risked a transference interpretation at this point, and I wondered whether he had *really* experienced me as frightening and scary and thus needed to protect himself from me, or whether, perhaps, he actually wanted to protect *me* from *him*.

The patient had certainly not expected such a frank comment; in fact, he admitted that my remark had rather startled him. He then explained that he had no idea how best to respond, and so, instead, he simply sat on the floor, staring at me with discomfort – quite a change from his otherwise free and easy revelatory style.

As the second consultation neared its conclusion, I knew that we would have to address the possibility of a third consultation, and I experienced considerable trepidation, knowing that Mr. J. would find this both desirable and dreadful at the same time. Once again, he promised that he would ring me, and I then asked him how many months he would take to do so. Mr. J. laughed and promised to call me later that day.

He then telephoned for his third appointment in March of the following year, only five months after his second appointment. I took some small sense of satisfaction that the gap between our sessions had begun to narrow and that perhaps Mr. J. could, bit by bit, tolerate an increasing amount of human contact.

Eventually, Mr. J. and I began to develop a deeper rapport, and he confessed that he no longer thought that I resembled a monster but, rather, merely a greedy London psychotherapist who charges high fees.

Although I suspected that Mr. J. would benefit from extensive multi-frequency psychoanalytical treatment, I thought it quite unlikely that he would ever consider such an arrangement, and so, upon discussion, we agreed to embark on once-weekly psychotherapeutic work. I felt quite prepared to fail utterly with Mr. J., knowing his degree of psychopathology. I appreciated that the enforced intimacy of psychotherapy might seem rather like a prison sentence to this very frightened individual who had indulged in thousands of one-night stands with strangers. But, I also appreciated that, in spite of the extremely long gaps between our appointments thus far, Mr. J. also wanted to reach out for help and, to his credit, had refused to kill me off entirely.

To my surprise and delight, Mr. J. did engage with our weekly appointments, but he invariably arrived late. Unlike other patients who might occasionally ring the doorbell two or three minutes tardy, after having rushed through traffic, this man always pressed the buzzer at exactly twenty-five minutes past the hour – precisely halfway through the fifty-minute session. I interpreted to Mr. J. that he really wanted me to know that fifty per cent of him yearned to engage and that the other fifty per cent continued to find both me and this process rather scary. Mr. J. still sat on the floor, explaining that he regarded the patient's chair – some six feet away from mine – as far too intimate.

After one year of late arrivals, cancelled sessions, and "forgotten" appointments, Mr. J. finally began to attend on time, and he did, eventually, return to the chair, which I came to regard as a huge achievement. Moreover, he could now confess two hugely important experiences from his personal biography.

In our very first meeting, Mr. J. had revealed to me that, during his eighth year, his mother had suffered a significant cerebral aneurysm, which resulted in her immediate death. I knew that such a trauma had left Mr. J. alone and isolated, cared for solely by a very bereaved and often absent "macho" father, who hated his feminised son. After his mother's death, Mr. J. used to dress up in his dead mother's clothes in a desperate attempt to bring her back to life. He and I had, of course, talked about the impact of this early, incomparably horrific trauma in virtually every session. But on this occasion, Mr. J. confessed some further, previously unknown, information about his mother's death.

I knew already that the mother had died in the family home at 4.00 p.m., one afternoon, shortly after the eight-year-old Mr. J. had returned from school. But I did not know what had happened in the few moments immediately *prior* to the mother's death.

Apparently, Mr. J. had asked his mother if she could teach him how to bake a cake, but she refused, explaining that she felt unwell. Mr. J. pleaded, but to no avail, and, in a state of protest, he stormed out of the kitchen and began to play in the room next door. Shortly afterwards, he heard an anguished gurgling sound emanating from the kitchen. With no one else in the house, Mr. J. knew that this strangulating noise must have come from his mother's mouth, but little Mr. J., feeling angry and stubborn, did not return to the kitchen to investigate. Approximately one hour later, he did seek out his mother's company, and when he walked into the kitchen, he found her collapsed on the floor. Unable to rouse her, he ran next door to the home of a neighbour who called an ambulance; but, alas, the paramedics pronounced her dead.

Mr. J. related this story with a look of horror upon his face, and then confessed that, through his negligence, he had killed his mother and had sentenced himself to a life of misery with a father who hated him and whom he reviled in return.

Shortly after having told me this deeply painful and highly important story about his mother's death, he also revealed that he wished to disclose yet another secret, namely, that he had a tattoo on his back. Before I could respond in any way, Mr. J. ripped off his T-shirt, exposing a full-length tattoo of a very terrifying sea monster, with gnashing teeth, blood red claws, and fuming smoke, which extended from Mr. J.'s shoulder blades to the very top of his buttocks. As Mr. J. stood before me in a state of semi-nakedness, he smiled, as if taking pride in having shocked me, which he had indeed done, and then he quickly pulled his T-shirt back on over his head and torso.

I commented on the importance of this revelation about his mother's death, and, with sympathy in my voice, I expressed deep concern and sadness, aware that as an eight-year-old boy he had endured an unbearable shock. I then paused and interpreted further that by having just whipped off his T-shirt so abruptly he might have hoped that he could shock me by revealing the monster that he had carried inside himself all this time.

Mr. J. listened carefully to my words but he did not reply in a direct way. Instead, he sat silently, pensively, almost dreamily, listening to my comments. The silence continued. I then made one more remark and reminded him of how monstrous he had found me when he had first stepped into my office more than one year previously. I interpreted that by having carried the guilt of killing his mother – by not having rushed to her side immediately upon hearing her gurgle – he had suffered under the weight of being a murderous monster all of his life. And I underscored that by finding his own scariness unbearable he took secret comfort in locating this frightening feeling into other people.

Mr. J. burst into tears and then told me that he had, in fact, killed not *one* person, but *two*.

Through his sobs, Mr. J. explained that he held himself responsible not only for the death of his mother but, also, for the incipient demise of a former male lover whom he had infected with H.I.V.

The patient reported to me that, ten years previously, not long after he became diagnosed as H.I.V.-positive, his boyfriend at the time, for whom he cared deeply, pleaded with Mr. J. to engage in unprotected anal intercourse. Mr. J. refused to comply with this dangerous request, but the boyfriend kept insisting again … and again … and again. Eventually, Mr. J. succumbed and consented to his partner's pleas for unsafe sex. Some months later, the boyfriend, too, received a similar positive medical diagnosis and, subsequently, became very seriously ill on many occasions.

Although the boyfriend did *not* die, Mr. J. had long carried a terrific sense of guilt that he had, in fact, assassinated this man by having sentenced him to a life afflicted by a serious disease, albeit one that can now be survived due to the heroic advances in modern pharmacology.

I shall refrain from commenting upon the ethics of the increasingly common practice of H.I.V.-negative adults actively seeking to become infected by H.I.V.-positive adults, a phenomenon known as "pozzing" or as "poz-chasing". Some people may well regard such an activity as perfectly justifiable, assuming that the "poz chaser" will have offered "informed consent". But others among us might well regard this behaviour as an unadulterated example of suicidality or as the enactment of unconscious traumatic experiences. Never having met Mr. J.'s boyfriend, I do not know the meaning of his wish to be infected, but I did come to learn more and more about the awful psychological burden which Mr. J. experienced, having agreed to the plan.

In subsequent psychotherapy sessions, we devoted considerable attention to the possible interconnections between the death of Mr. J.'s mother and the "pozzing" of Mr. J.'s boyfriend. I came to hypothesise that by infecting his boyfriend in the 1990s, at a time when effective medications had become more widely available, Mr. J. had succeeded in both killing off his boyfriend by infecting him with a life-threatening illness and, also, at the same time, in bringing him back to life by paying for the boyfriend's private medical care – something which, alas, he could not have done for his dead mother.

Although we could devote infinitely more thought to the case of Mr. J., and although I could describe the subsequent unfolding of his psychotherapy in much greater detail, I have chosen to discuss him in this context primarily as an illustration of the fact that one can be a murderer without having committed any crimes and without having broken the law in any way. Indeed, by having participated in consensual, adult sex with his age-appropriate boyfriend, he violated no laws, in spite of having known that he had already received a diagnosis of H.I.V. And yet, in view of Mr. J.'s traumatic history, and his fear that he had killed his own mother, he lived with the burden of having committed not one murder … but two.

THE PRIVATE FORENSIC PRACTITIONER

Thus far, I have presented a series of vignettes which demonstrate, I trust, that the community-based independent psychotherapy practitioner will often encounter very seriously violent individuals who possess a capacity for great cruelty. But I have not, as yet, offered any indication as to the specificities of providing treatment in such a context.

How, then, does one work with the sub-clinical forensic patient in psychotherapy?

In order to consider the practicalities of psychotherapy for such individuals, we would require a much more extended discussion. But we can, however, consider a small number of key observations and straightforward recommendations.

First and foremost, unlike our colleagues who work in secure or semi-secure forensic institutions, supported by large multi-disciplinary teams of psychiatrists, psychologists, psychiatric nurses, social workers, and creative arts therapists, the independent psychotherapist functions in virtually complete isolation and must, therefore, consider his or her physical safety. When "Verna", the staggeringly beautiful fashion model, dressed in a mini-skirt with stiletto heels – whom I described in the second chapter of this book – arrived in my office and explained to me that her boyfriend suffered from pathological jealousy and had, on many occasions, threatened to kill any man with whom she spent any time, I listened to her cordially, engaged her in discussion, questioned her as to the authenticity of her boyfriend's threats, and then promptly referred her to a Consultant Forensic Psychiatrist who worked in a secure institution. The community-based forensic psychotherapist must always be courteous and professional, but he or she need not be unnecessarily heroic and certainly must never be masochistic.

Not only should the private practitioner consider his or her safety, but also, he or she must maintain very rigorous clinical boundaries in an effort to provide structure and containment for potentially violent patients. For instance, if an ordinary, reliable, neurotic patient with a good track record of attendance asked me in a thoughtful and appreciative manner to reschedule a particular session in order to attend his or her child's play at school, I would not hesitate to be helpful. But if a sub-clinical forensic patient did likewise, I would, in most instances, politely decline to do so and would adhere stringently to the original appointment time. As the psychoanalyst Dr. Hanna Segal (1973) had observed, when working with patients who struggle with timekeeping – an unconscious expression of their state of disorientation and confusion – the clinician must become the reliable clock. In this way, the psychotherapeutic process can begin to serve as something of a secure base (Bowlby, 1988). Whenever the aforementioned Mr. J., the man who infected his boyfriend with H.I.V., asked for changes of appointment time, I invariably declined and found that, by doing so, his attendance record at sessions actually began to improve.

In addition to the insistence upon physical safety and the maintenance of regularity and reliability – essential characteristics of *all* psychotherapeutic work, but of especial importance for the forensic psychotherapist – one must also avail oneself, quite classically, of the rich opportunities for analysis of the transference.

"Mr. K.", a homosexual man, worked in a perfectly respectable profession by day, but in order to make extra money, he established a pornographic video business by night, in which he convinced handsome heterosexual men to masturbate on camera, and then posted these amateur films online. As Mr. K. described to me the ways in which he would entice so many ostensibly consenting adult males to perform sexual acts for him, I became rather concerned as to whether the men in question really understood the ultimate fate of their sex videos and whether Mr. K. had truly offered them the opportunity to provide informed consent. Although Mr. K. had committed no obvious crime – as any consenting adult male may agree to be filmed – this patient certainly flirted with sexual exploitation. As the treatment unfolded, I endeavoured to maintain my analytically neutral position but, also, I continued to express vigilance and concern about Mr. K.'s after-hours business venture.

During the course of a psychotherapy session in which Mr. K. spoke quite painfully about his extremely difficult relationship with his emotionally distant parents, he then began to cry as he recalled certain childhood memories. He told me that although he appreciated having thrice-weekly psychotherapy with me, he found the "exposure" of his mind, while free-associating on the couch, very difficult indeed. I interpreted that perhaps he harboured a wish to sit in the analytical chair himself and to place me on the couch instead, so that he could project the feeling of being exposed into me, just as he did each night when filming these exposed heterosexual men who volunteered to participate in his pornographic videos. My comment rather surprised Mr. K., who began to cry further, and who, some months later, acquired a much better understanding of the potential violence of his film activities. Soon thereafter, the patient shut down his production company completely.

"Mr. L.", a successful businessman, with whom I worked many long years ago, also taught me a great deal about the value of interpreting any signs of "criminality" which might creep into the transference as a creative and effective means of examining the ways in which patients will project their forensic aspects onto or into the psychotherapist. Each month, I would present Mr. L. with a bill, and each month, he would pay me with a wad of cash, sealed in an envelope. When I tried to analyse his motivations for settling his account in this fashion, wondering why a businessman of his stature would not pay by cheque – the traditional payment at that point in time, long before the creation of online banking – he sloughed me off, explaining that he had a bit of spare cash lying around at home and that he needed to use it.

Extraordinarily, on quite a number of occasions, Mr. L. would overpay me by fifty pounds. Consequently, I would then have to return this money to him at the very beginning of the next session. This enactment between us occurred for many months until I interpreted to Mr. L. that perhaps he wanted me to know something about his own anxieties surrounding his business dealings, and that he struggled from a fear of some kind of criminality which he tried to project into me, secretly hopeful that I might pocket the extra fifty pounds in an unethical manner. This interpretation provoked much useful discussion about Mr. L.'s fears of being robbed of money – a metaphor for his memories of being robbed of love by his mentally ill mother decades previously – and of his wish to entrap somebody else and to shame that person, just as he had felt shamed throughout his childhood.

The notion of the sub-clinical forensic psychotherapy patient can hardly be described as a novel idea. Since the very inception of psychoanalysis, practitioners have encountered men and women who have expressed deeply violent conflicts while reclining on the consulting room couch. As early as 1907, Professor Sigmund Freud treated a gentleman called Herr Ernst Lanzer, better known to us as "Der Rattenmann" ["The Rat Man"], who, although described by a friend as "a man of irreproachable conduct" (Freud, 1909c, p. 159),[2] actually considered himself to be a "criminal" (Freud, 1909c, p. 159),[3] tormented by "some criminal impulse" (Freud, 1909c, p. 159),[4] owing to his violent and obsessive murderous thoughts.

Dr. Donald Winnicott also encountered sub-clinical forensic enactments in his private practice in Central London on a regular basis. For instance, Winnicott's patient Dr. Margaret Little, a qualified psychoanalyst in her own right but, also, a very troubled, tormented woman, committed an act of violence at the very outset of her treatment. As Little (1985, p. 20) recalled, "In one early session with D.W. I felt in utter despair of ever getting him to understand anything. I wandered round his room trying to find a way. I contemplated throwing myself out of the window, but felt that he would stop me. Then I thought of throwing out all his books, but finally I attacked and smashed a large vase filled with white lilac, and trampled on it. In a flash he was gone from the room, but he came back just before the end of the hour. Finding me clearing up the mess he said, 'I might have expected you to do that [clear up? or smash?], but later.' Next day an exact replica had replaced the vase and the lilac, and a few days later he explained that I had destroyed something that he valued".

Winnicott tolerated the destruction of objects in the consulting room with grace and equanimity. In fact, during the 1960s, his niece, Miss Celia Britton, and her boyfriend drank tea and ate cucumber sandwiches with Winnicott at the end of a working day, and, while there in his home, the elderly psychoanalyst pointed to a potted plant with a missing leaf. He explained to his niece and to her partner, "that plant saved my life. My last patient this evening tore it apart rather than me" (quoted in Holmes, 2015).

Not only did Donald Winnicott and his fellow psychoanalysts engage with patients of the sub-forensic variety, but even non-psychoanalytical psychologists have come to appreciate the widespread prevalence of so-called "ambulatory psychopathy" or "subcriminal psychopathy". Helpfully, the distinguished American psychopathologist Professor Cathy Spatz Widom (1977) had, as a young researcher, first examined the phenomenon of violence amongst the non-institutionalised population, inaugurating a programme of study into sub-clinical psychopathy.

Thus, mental health professionals have a long familiarity dealing with challenging, violent thoughts and enactments among ordinary psychotherapy patients undergoing treatment in warmly furnished consulting rooms situated in pleasant parts of town.

What, then, might we reasonably conclude from this brief examination of the sub-clinical forensic psychotherapy patient?

First and foremost, we may take great comfort from the knowledge that most human beings manage to contain their more violent impulses quite substantially, and that most psychotherapy patients do *not* enact their destructive, murderous fantasies in a deadly manner. Happily, the vast majority of men and women undergoing psychotherapy would be refused a bed at Broadmoor Hospital or at any other forensic institution.

And yet, many non-forensic patients, by virtue of being human beings who have suffered from impingements, misattunements, and even traumata during infancy and early childhood, carry within their bosoms a smouldering rage, which often provokes aggressive fantasies, and which, from time to time, erupts in sub-clinical forensic enactments. Therefore, every psychotherapist must become increasingly vigilant about the possibility of meeting a sub-clinical forensic patient at one or more points during the course of a clinical career.

Sub-clinical forensic enactments vary in depth, scope, and intensity. While Donald Winnicott had no difficulty surviving the destruction of one of the leaves of the potted plant in his Belgravia consulting room, other practitioners – myself included – have struggled greatly with the complexity and with the ethicality of possessing knowledge about individuals who lace shampoo bottles with acid and who willingly infect their sexual partners with the human immunodeficiency virus. Consequently, ordinary psychotherapeutic practitioners working in the community must come to acquire a strong forensic spine and a sharply focused diagnostic radar. In view of the fact that one will, from time to time, encounter scantily-clad women who claim to have Mafiosi boyfriends, or businessmen who try to entrap one in an act of dishonesty through overpayment in cash, the private psychotherapy practitioner must endeavour at all times to remain within the bounds of professionalism in a rigorous and thoughtful manner and must find a way to create a medium-secure unit of sorts in Hampstead or Harley Street, or in Crouch End or Kensington – pleasant parts of our nation's capital – without the aid of locked wards, teams of doctors and nurses, psychotropic medications, or the protections provided by the Mental Health Act 2007.

The jobbing psychotherapist must seek appropriate clinical supervision from an experienced forensic practitioner when confronted with unexpectedly violent or potentially violent patients and must, if at all possible, avoid the sin of being too naïve. Even the most loyal, honourable, and decent of patients can surprise us with acts of criminality, either symbolic or real.

In summary, I wish to propose that we must begin to think about creative ways in which we might helpfully expand the definition of the forensic patient. Obviously, our community-based patients do not pose a threat to our society in the way that Peter Sutcliffe – the Yorkshire Ripper – had done. No one need fear walking the streets of leafy Bloomsbury and of being assaulted by an accountant leaving my consulting room. But by internalising a forensic lens, the independent practitioner of psychotherapy will have the opportunity to become more sensitive to, and increasingly savvy about, the possible range and meaning of various enactments within daily clinical practice, owing to the fact that our caseloads may contain many more sub-clinically forensic patients than we might, at first, have fully appreciated.

As an independent psychotherapist who, years previously, had worked in forensic settings, and who undertook training in forensic psychotherapy at the Portman Clinic, I confess that I have found such experiences deeply invaluable for my work with more ordinary patients. My immersion in the forensic world, and my continued association with forensic colleagues, has allowed me to become, I trust, more observant and even more suspicious about the potential sadistic underbelly of human behaviour. Such contact with the forensic world has, I believe, helped me to develop a greater awareness of the disturbing fact that every forensic patient had begun life as a "sub-forensic" or, indeed, "pre-forensic" or, even, "non-forensic" patient, prior to committing acts of violence. The community-based, independent psychotherapy practitioner might, therefore, find himself or herself in a valuable position to help identify and treat those patients who have not *yet* exploded and who have not *yet* become full-fledged forensic individuals. The traditional, classical, independent mental health professional working in private practice might, therefore, perform an increasingly important role in terms of prevention.

With greater exposure to forensic psychotherapeutic thinking, every mental health practitioner of whatever core professional background or theoretical orientation will have the opportunity to become more and more sensitised to the nature and scope of violence in its many shapes and forms. Additionally, psychotherapeutic practitioners will develop an improved understanding of the fact that most, if not all, of our forensic and sub-clinical forensic patients have experienced a welter of traumata during the earliest years of life, which will have contributed hugely to the development of violent fantasies and behaviours in years to come.

Psychotherapists must begin to discuss our frightening cases more fully, more regularly, and more honestly, so that we may all help one another to navigate complex ethical problems and, also, to verbalise our own countertransferential hatred (Winnicott, 1949a; Kahr, 2011a, 2015a, 2025b) towards these patients, so that we may become more proficient at facilitating the psychotherapeutic process.

How many of us have ever wondered what might have happened if the young, impecunious Adolf Hitler, during his years as a struggling artist in Vienna, had stumbled into Sigmund Freud's consulting room for treatment? Many dramatists have, in fact, written plays about such an imaginary encounter, for example, the 2007 radio play *Dr Freud Will See You Now Mr Hitler*, penned by Laurence Marks and Maurice Gran. Although one suspects that Freud might well have failed to treat Hitler successfully, we must remember that even the son of Alois Schicklgruber and Klara Pölzl Schicklgruber had begun life as a non-forensic baby who then became a sub-clinical forensic man, prior to his eruption as a full-fledged proto-forensic mass murderer. If we intervene early in our community-based settings, we might, perhaps, be able to contain even just a little bit of the violence which surrounds us all too chillingly.

Notes

1 I shall present a much more detailed version of the case of "Mr. F." and "Mrs. F." in Chapter 9, in which I will refer to the couple as "Lester" and "Martina", and to the sister of "Martina" as "Norma".

2 The original German phrase reads: "ein tadelloser Mensch" (Freud, 1909b, p. 360).

3 The original German word reads: "Verbrecher" (Freud, 1909b, p. 360).

4 The original German phrase reads: "ein verbrecherischer Impuls" (Freud, 1909b, p. 360).

Criminality in the Bedroom
Unconscious Sadism in Non-Forensic Couples

WHEN WEDDING DRESSES CATCH FIRE

Back in the late tenth century, more than 1,000 years ago, an aristocrat named Foulques Nerra – sometimes known as "Fulk the Black" – reigned over the *comté* of Anjou in the heart of France. A devout Christian who had founded numerous abbeys and monasteries, and a patron of architecture who had built many castles, Foulques Nerra had also established a school for the education of the poor. But like many medieval potentates, Foulques dedicated himself not only to charitable works but, also, to violence; and, over many years, he distinguished himself in bloody combat, defeating the forces of Conan, the *duc* de Bretagne, in the battle of Conquereuil in 992, killing his enemy's son Alain.

Foulques Nerra did not, however, confine his murderousness to the battlefield. It seems that he also practised early-medieval siege warfare at home. In the year 999, Foulques had discovered his countess, Élisabeth de Vendôme, *in flagrante* with a goatherd and, desperate for retribution, the nobleman had his wife bedecked in her wedding dress and then burned alive in the marketplace of Angers, the capital of Anjou (Guillot, 1972; Seward, 2014; cf. de Salies, 1874), in an act described by one medieval source as an "*horribili incendio combusta*" (quoted in Guillot, 1972, p. 25, fn. 129), namely, burned by a horrible fire.

It seems uncertain that the fervent French Catholics of the tenth century would have regarded the vicious, unspeakable immolation of the approximately twenty-year-old *comtesse* Élisabeth as an act of domestic violence. Steeped in a climate of spousal abuse and frequent executions, these medieval Angevins might well have conceptualised the burning as justifiable punishment for the countess' adulterous sin. But from our twenty-first-century perspective, it would be impossible to regard this act of brutality as anything other than the most vicious of marital attacks. By setting fire to his wife – a crime that would today land a man in Broadmoor Hospital for the criminally insane – and by having insisted that Élisabeth, little more than a late adolescent, should be burned in the very gown that she had worn on the day of their wedding, Foulques Nerra has become immortalised as one of the most gruesome perpetrators of marital sadism in history.

Although we cannot excuse the murderousness of Foulques for sanctioning this uxoricide, let us not forget that the Angevin count had done so because of his *wife's*

DOI: 10.4324/9781003546245-14

infidelity with a farmhand. This tale from medieval French history serves as a vicious reminder that in many, if not in all, cases of marital explosion, *each* member of the couple might have contributed in some way or ways to the final outcome.

One could of course cite numerous other instances of sexual cruelty between spouses throughout the centuries. In fact, one need not search very far for evidence (e.g., Bloch, 1991; Bourke, 2007; Butler, 2007; Goldberg, 2008).

Consider, for instance, one of the cruellest forms of sexual sadism in marriage, namely, rape. Indeed, for many centuries, men could, and did, readily force themselves sexually upon their spouses, claiming that the mere act of marriage constituted a woman's consent to intercourse in the first place. The eminent American sociologist and traumatologist Professor David Finkelhor studied spousal rape in Boston, Massachusetts; and, in a landmark investigation, he and his colleague Dr. Kersti Yllo discovered that rape occurred in approximately three per cent of these American marriages, and further, that one would be much more likely to be raped by a formally married spouse or by a cohabiting partner than by a stranger (Finkelhor and Yllo, 1985). Extrapolating this data to a British sample, one could estimate that, based on Finkelhor's and Yllo's findings, approximately 600,000 British women might well have suffered formal rape at the hands of their husbands, while countless others will have had to endure unwanted sexual contact of various types. Fortunately, although many countries worldwide have, in recent years, declared spousal rape illegal, including, of course, the United Kingdom, many others have not; and, at the present time, numerous countries and territories, including Afghanistan, Algeria, Bahrain, Bangladesh, Ethiopia, Guinea, Haiti, Iran, Iraq, Libya, Morocco, North Korea, Saudi Arabia, Sri Lanka, Syria, Tuvalu, and the United Arab Emirates, do not prosecute men for raping their wives or for committing other acts of sexual sadism upon their wedded partners.

Gross sexual violence occurs far too frequently within the context of long-term marital relationships, and always with disastrous consequences, including the infliction of physical and psychological damage. Fortunately, most married couples never engage in such clinically sadistic behaviours. Indeed, the vast majority of intimate partners treat one another's physical bodies with a reasonable degree of respect and thus refrain from the use of sexual force.

But one need not be a violent, acting-out, forensic patient, a rapist or a torturer, for instance, to perpetrate deep cruelty upon one's spousal partner. Often, some of the "nicest" people, including those from privileged, well-bred, well-spoken, and well-educated families, and from seemingly progressive, so-called "First World countries", treat their intimates with shocking viciousness, either physically or verbally, during sexual encounters. Many people, in fact, will reserve their most primitive and aggressive urges *specifically*, if not *exclusively*, for their long-term marital partners. And often, in consequence, the bedroom will become a veritable boxing ring in which otherwise normal-neurotic couples might come to concretise some of their most sadistic tendencies.

Although I began my mental health career working in the forensic field with murderers, paedophiles, arsonists, rapists, and others who had committed acts of shocking abuse – many of whom also suffered from psychotic illnesses – I have accumulated far more experience in recent decades with ordinary, warm-hearted, honourable, philanthropic, and civic-minded people who vote for the Labour Party, who read *The Guardian* newspaper, who make charitable contributions to worthwhile organisations, and who volunteer from time to time at the local soup kitchen *by day*, but who, nevertheless, will sometimes – indeed often – become deceptive, contemptuous, humiliating, and vengeful towards their spouses *by night*.

Those of us who work in the arena of marital mental health, either as couple psychotherapists, as couple psychoanalysts, or as couple counsellors, have a unique opportunity to discover the hidden shadows of normal-neurotic marriages at very close range. Indeed, we now understand far more about violence in the ordinary couple than in the forensic couple (cf. Welldon, 2012; Motz, 2014), in large measure because most severe forensic patients live in prisons or hospitals where mental health colleagues have little or no licence or opportunity to work with the spouses.

In view of the increased understanding of violence – especially sexual violence – in non-forensic couples (e.g., Weitzman, 2000), what, precisely, have we come to learn in recent years about the origins of such cruelty, about its function and, also, about its treatment?

In the course of this chapter, I shall offer copious clinical vignettes in an effort to sketch a psychodiagnostic terrain of the different types of sexual hurt inflicted by otherwise ordinary, law-abiding citizens. I shall then provide some thoughts about how the psychological clinician can better engage with these stories while working with both individuals and with couples. In all instances, I have, of course, altered the names and other obvious identifying biographical details of the individuals and couples concerned. Otherwise, I have refrained from any distortion of the data that I have heard over the years in my consulting room.

Violence towards one's spouse will manifest itself in many forms, and will often be underpinned by eroticism. Indeed, in the non-forensic population, spousal sexual sadism exists along a continuum, ranging from seemingly minor acts of unkindness and insensitivity which occur in the marital bedroom, characterised by only small amounts of "acting-out", to those of a more severe nature, marked by a very considerable degree of acting-out and consequent destruction. Let us now explore the panopticon of the different varieties and degrees of sexual sadism in the marital relationship, which might form the template of a veritable typology of sexual cruelty.

BODILY EVACUATION AS A FORM OF SADISM

In the non-forensic sample of individuals and couples that one meets in an out-patient setting – often an independent psychotherapy consulting room – one becomes immediately aware of a vast range of acts of sexual unkindness. At one extreme, I recall the case of "Archibald", a hospital administrator, and "Betty", a nurse: a long-standing married couple, with six children, who generally enjoyed one another's company and who boasted a capacity to make one another laugh. Archibald and Betty presented for couple psychotherapy one year after the death of Betty's mother, a bereavement which had plunged the wife into a state of moderate depression. Betty's mother had provided enormous support to the entire family, helping to look after the six children; consequently, her death left Betty deeply heartbroken. Yet in spite of Betty's melancholia, the couple still enjoyed a vigorous sexual life.

One evening, Archibald returned home from the pub, where this hulking man with broad shoulders had drunk twelve pints of lager in swift succession. Archibald could generally guzzle as many as eight pints without experiencing any adverse effects, but after twelve of these drinks, he felt more than unusually woozy. As he explained to me, Betty's newfound depressed mood states had caused him distress, and, consequently, he consumed four additional pints in order to fortify himself against the gloomy atmosphere at home. Later that evening, after the children had gone to sleep, Archibald and Betty went to bed and began to fondle one another, and soon proceeded to engage in coitus.

However, in the midst of genital penetration, Archibald began to wretch. Fortunately, he removed himself from inside his wife, staggered off the bed, but then vomited profusely on the floor, spewing all over Betty's discarded clothing. Although such an encounter between a drunk husband and a depressed wife would be of little interest to a family lawyer – one certainly cannot sue successfully for divorce as a result of a single episode of vomiting – Archibald's behaviour caused Betty great disgust, and, for several weeks thereafter, she developed a phobic anxiety that her husband might actually vomit upon *her*. In view of Betty's depression, she had *already* begun to feel ugly, dirty, and unwanted. And thus, when her husband discharged himself in this manner during sexual intercourse, Betty felt that the external world of *vomitus* both confirmed and exacerbated what she had already begun to experience in her internal world, soiled by death and by consequent bereavement.

When Betty disclosed this information during a couple psychotherapy session, Archibald – usually quite compassionate – told Betty brusquely, "Oh, for fuck's sake, woman. Get over yourself. I had a few too many drinks. I didn't slap you." This reaction served only to inflame Betty's deep unhappiness in the face of such an unpleasant sexual encounter with her husband, and she then burst into tears. It took a great deal of time as well as much slow, painstaking psychotherapeutic work to help Archibald come to understand the way in which he had felt burdened and resentful about his wife's depression, and how her affective state had made him feel impotent and useless. Gradually, Archibald began to appreciate that he had found a way of concretising his rage through the evacuation of vomit rather than through the expression of angry words, and that he would, in future, become more aware – more conscious – of his tendency to act out in such a manner.

"Cressida" and "Dexter", another normal-neurotic couple, had recently celebrated their silver wedding anniversary. During their very first couple psychotherapy consultation, Dexter, a professional athlete, admitted that he and Cressida, an unemployed artist, had begun to fight "a bit" during recent months, and that their general medical practitioner had recommended "talking therapy". Although Dexter explained that he had agreed to attend for sessions, he had his doubts about psychotherapy, as he believed that he and his wife had only "one little problem." In order to prove to me that he and Cressida had established, essentially, a truly great marriage, Dexter then boasted that he and Cressida would "make love" every single night, and that, consequently, they would enjoy a highly satisfying sexual life. During Dexter's introductory speech, Cressida became increasingly ashen and, in due course, she began to fume. After Dexter paused, I turned in her direction, whereupon she exploded. "A great sex life?", Cressida cried. "You think we have a great sex life?" Dexter then began to stumble over his words, uncertain of how best to reply.

At this point, Cressida erupted fully and explained to me that, in reality, they do not "make love", and have, in fact, *never* made love – quite the contrary. She then elaborated that every night Dexter would take her into the bedroom, undress himself fully, sit astride her naked torso, then masturbate furiously and ejaculate onto her face. By this point, he would have exhausted himself so much that he would generally fall onto the bed and then succumb to deep sleep until the morning. After narrating her account of this nightly scenario, Cressida burst into tears.

Dexter, an often charming man who had many friends and who frequently donated large sums of money to those in need, had absolutely no capacity to express any comfort, tenderness, or regret to Cressida as she cried and screamed in the consulting room. Instead, he explained that he simply could not stop himself ejaculating so quickly because he has always found her so irresistibly beautiful and that he could never imagine being with any other woman. Although Dexter may have intended this as a great compliment, Cressida became even more enraged at this point, and she shouted, "Yes, but why do you have to do it on my face? You make me feel so cheap. It's disgusting. And you never bring *me* to orgasm. You're so selfish. So cruel!"

One need not be a mental health professional to wonder why Dexter restricted his sexual activities to climaxing upon his wife's face and why Cressida – ostensibly horrified by this – had endured such a nightly ritual over so many long years. What then permitted such a complex marito-sexual dynamic to persevere? It might be tempting to describe the couple's night-time ritual as a type of sadomasochism, characterised by Dexter's sadistic ejaculation upon his beautiful partner, and by Cressida's masochistic enjoyment of participating in this situation. But as I began to understand the unconscious life of this couple more fully, I came to realise that sadomasochism does not quite accurately describe the situation.

Dexter grew up in the East End of London as the seventh child of very impoverished parents who lived in a tiny two-bedroom flat on a council estate. Dexter described the estate as "disgusting" and "dirty", but boasted that his mother prided herself on cleanliness and that she had managed to create a completely spotless home in spite of the family's impecuniousness and grubby surroundings. The mother never allowed Dexter and his siblings to play outside for fear that they might muddy their clothing. And in spite of having little money for the water bill, each child had to bathe every single day. Dexter's mother, clearly an obsessional woman, also refused to allow her children to walk barefoot on the beach during rare family holidays at the seaside, in case one of them might happen to step on something "nasty". Chuckling affectionately, Dexter explained, "My mother was such a fierce lady that any germs would have been far too frightened to enter the front door of our home."

Cressida had a rather more complicated childhood, characterised by a neglectful, alcoholic mother, and by a father who treated her with a certain amount of sexual lasciviousness. Although Cressida's father never laid a hand upon her, she recalled that he took an inordinate amount of interest in the size of her growing breasts, and upon the length of her skirts, making daily comments about her physicality, which she found intrusive and infuriating.

As our work progressed, the couple confessed to me that each night, prior to their sexual ritual, they would drink a bottle of very fine wine at dinner, and then they would retire to the sitting room and snort some cocaine. This revelation helped me to understand more fully the way in which such complex, nightly sexual choreography could be performed again and again.

Dexter and Cressida had never produced any children, and they claimed that they had never wished to do so. In view of the frequent facial ejaculations, I wondered whether the couple had *ever* engaged in traditional coitus, and I enquired about this. Dexter replied that he and Cressida had attempted "old-fashioned" intercourse a few times, but that neither of them had really enjoyed it very much, and that he would experience a much more powerful orgasm by masturbating himself.

As our psychotherapeutic work proceeded, and as our shared understanding grew, I became increasingly able to speak quite frankly with this couple. Cressida presented the marital dynamic as a veritable crime scene in which Dexter, the perpetrator, had committed a foul act upon her body, insisting that she had no part to play in this abusive situation whatsoever. Dexter, by contrast, considered himself to be a truly worshipful lover, and would defend himself by explaining that most of his male friends boasted mistresses, or visited sex workers, or watched pornography, but that he never cheated on his wife, and that he still found her so very attractive and hugely exciting.

I offered a rather different conceptualisation, which I shared with the couple in slow, methodical stages.

I hypothesised that the nightly ritual of Dexter masturbating upon Cressida had begun, not in the bedroom but, rather, in the dining room, beforehand, when each kept filling the other's glass with more "fine wine", and then became fuelled further in the sitting room while each of them inhaled cocaine. I compared this routine to that of an athlete warming up before a sporting event, or that of an actor vocalising prior to stepping out on stage. By underscoring this portion of the scenario, I began to explore with Dexter and Cressida whether, in fact, each of them might be more equally complicitous in the unfolding of the sexual scenario which would follow. At first, Cressida refused to consider that she had played any active role in this situation, but, eventually, as her defences began to loosen, both she and Dexter could begin to appreciate more fully the ways in which they had conspired *as a couple* to script such an evening routine *jointly*.

Integrating our growing knowledge of the biographies of both Dexter and Cressida, we then began to consider the ways in which their highly institutionalised nightly sexual ritual might represent *not* a creative engagement of lovemaking but, rather, an instance of what Professor Sigmund Freud (1914, p. 490) had first identified as a "Wiederholungszwang" – a "repetition compulsion" – in which people would restage early childhood experiences relentlessly, without any conscious awareness of doing so.

As our sessions progressed over a period of many months, this couple came to understand more fully that Dexter had suffered from a lifelong obsessional neurosis which he had kept secret from Cressida and, often, from himself as well. It soon transpired that he had internalised so many of his mother's injunctions about germs and filth that he had developed the habit of washing his hands twenty or thirty times per day, and always furtively so. Whenever he touched his genitals, he would skulk away to the bathroom afterwards, ostensibly in order to urinate but, in fact, he did so in order to scrub his organ several times with carbolic soap. Essentially, he found sexual activity particularly dirty, both physically and mentally, and it proved not only shaming but, also, relieving for Dexter to verbalise this secret to me and to his wife at long last. Eventually, he plucked up the courage to inform us that he preferred to ejaculate on Cressida's face rather than to insert his penis inside her vagina, as he regarded the female genitalia as particularly unclean. Naturally, such a confession hurt Cressida deeply, and she began to cry, but, gradually, she came to realise that Dexter's revelation did not surprise her in the least. In many ways, she had already known this about her husband and had already sensed his disgust of bodies in general.

I interpreted that Dexter's struggle to penetrate his wife vaginally stemmed, in part, not only from his fear of maternal disapproval and, also, from a terror of contamination but, moreover, served as an expression of his hateful feelings towards women more generally, starting with his mother, who controlled his mind and body so relentlessly, and ending with his wife, onto whom he transferred these powerful affects. Drawing upon the foundational observations of Dr. Karl Abraham (1917), one of Freud's earliest disciples, I tried to help the couple to understand that the act of ejaculation upon the woman's body might well represent an expression of deep admiration and excitement, but might also constitute a form of angry soiling.

Cressida, too, eventually came to acquire a more sophisticated knowledge of her own role in facilitating what seemed to be, on the surface, an exclusively sadistic sexual interaction, with Dexter as the ejaculating perpetrator and herself as the unwitting collaborator. In fact, by drinking wine and by using cocaine each night – the necessary preparation for the sadomasochistic sexual ritual – Cressida had assisted Dexter in setting the stage for this particular form of erotic theatre, recreating her own role as the passive victim of her father's lecherous and humiliating attentions during her childhood. But, this time, Cressida allowed her husband to ejaculate upon her face, both repeating a most unpleasant experience and, also, allowing herself to attack Dexter afterwards, constantly insulting him, complaining about him, and humiliating him – something which she had never done with her more terrifying father.

Thus, the case of Dexter and Cressida allows us to consider the possibility that the roots of an uncomfortable sexual scenario, laced with hatred, stem from early antecedents, and then become re-enacted inexorably, without conscious understanding. In this instance, both members of the couple deployed the marital bed as a veritable laboratory for discharging, evacuating, and projecting early discomfort and disgust into the other. Dexter did so through ejaculation, and Cressida did so by permitting Dexter to treat her as a dustbin, so that she could then avenge herself upon him with cruel verbal taunts.

Regrettably, I cannot elaborate upon the more detailed development of insights into this couple over the course of time but, fortunately, towards the end of treatment, some three years later, Cressida and Dexter had begun to cultivate a much more loving, much more tender, and much less sadistic style of lovemaking, as well as a much less alcohol-dependent, drug-fuelled approach to interrelating more generally. Neither member of the couple found our psychotherapeutic work particularly easy or enjoyable; and, often, each would take pot-shots at me for "subjecting" them to such an arduous process, which I interpreted as a further expression of their wish to evacuate wounded and hateful feelings into the nearest object to hand.

In the two aforementioned vignettes, that of Archibald and Betty – the couple who turned the bedroom into a *vomitorium* – and that of Cressida and Dexter – the couple whose marital chamber became an *ejaculatorium* – each member of these spousal pairings participated in equal measure in the creation of a sadistic sexual scenario, using the marital bed as a means of evacuating unpleasant, primitive affects rooted in early experiences. Although Archibald vomited on Betty's clothing, and Dexter released his semen on Cressida's face, neither couple, to their credit, "acted out" beyond the confines of the marital relationship. Each of those partners managed to preserve their most particularly noxious feelings exclusively for one another, and did so at the same time, and in the same room. In spite of their difficulties in the bedroom, these couples remained very much faithful and intact.

I wish to propose that such instances of evacuation, confined primarily to the sexual sphere, offer the clinician a great sense of hope, due, in part, to the capability of such couples to communicate hostility in a visible and accessible and engaging style. Prognostically, these couples will manage treatment reasonably well, if not very well indeed, and will usually remain committed to marriage. In my experience, couples of this variety rarely divorce or experience what I have come to refer to as a "conjugal aneurysm" (Kahr, 2014b).

But sexual sadism can become much more complex, and once the enactments of aggressivity begin to emerge outside of the physical bedroom itself, couples will often experience infinitely more distress. Archibald and Betty and, also, Cressida and Dexter remained deeply committed to one another. In more advanced cases of marital infidelity – either psychical or physical in nature, and often both – extramaritality becomes the hallmark of cruelty.

THE INTRA-MARITAL AFFAIR AND THE EXTRAMARITAL AFFAIR

"Elfriede" entered individual psychoanalytical treatment in order to overcome a long-standing inhibition in her professional work. An artist of considerable accomplishment, this woman had begun to "freeze" while in her studio and, for several years, she could produce no work at all. Elfriede, married to her childhood sweetheart "Francis", an ophthalmologist, often smirked with a considerable amount of contempt and would joke that she had married the only blind eye doctor in the United Kingdom, because she believed that Francis simply did not have a clue about his wife and saw nothing of her that would have made her feel recognised.

Indeed, Elfriede led a double life. In spite of her conscious artistic aspirations, she actually spent much of her day chained to a computer for hour after hour, masturbating to internet pornography, immersing herself in cyber-photographs and cyber-films of handsome men. She also frequented clubs and pubs, wearing tight skirts with no underwear beneath, in the hope that some man would notice her and whisk her away, *Madame Bovary*-style, from her bourgeois life as a doctor's wife. As Francis worked incredibly long hours, Elfriede felt extremely abandoned, in spite of the fact that she enjoyed the financial security afforded by her husband's profession.

Often gripped by strong denial, Elfriede devoted a great deal of her session time to boasting that Francis possessed not the slightest inkling about her computer activities or about her many visits to bars; and though she felt triumphant that she could "cheat" on her husband in this way, she also became extremely desolate that her emotionally "blind" ophthalmologist partner could not see the extent of her unhappiness. Interestingly, although Elfriede dedicated much time to the internet and to her erotic forays in the West End of London, she never actually succeeded in sleeping with another man. Various gentlemen had bought her drinks and had made passes at her, but something always stopped her from taking them to bed. Technically, she remained faithful to Francis, but in her private mind she had committed a multitude of infidelities, exemplifying what I have come to refer to as the "intra-marital affair" (Kahr, 2007a, p. 32), as opposed to the more familiar extra-marital variety.

The intra-marital affair – a liaison that unfolds predominantly in the mind – may not leave lipstick stains on the collar or hotel receipts in one's handbag or trouser pockets, but this type of internal enactment can cause great psychological devastation, nonetheless. Intra-marital affairs – these extraordinarily private and deeply consuming sexual fantasy constellations – serve a multiplicity of functions. In my earlier study of the traumatic origins of the sexual fantasy, I identified as many as fifteen possible conscious and unconscious functions of erotic thoughts or intra-marital affairs, including, *inter alia*, that of an unconscious attack on both oneself and upon one's partner (Kahr, 2007a, 2008).

Although sexual fantasies may often provide much private fun and pleasure, and can, frequently, in the context of a healthy marriage, become an additional reservoir of sexual creativity, such intra-marital affairs serve, for the most part, as uncomfortable refuges which help to alienate each spouse from the other. In more extreme cases, especially in those individuals with a pronounced history of emotional and physical trauma, intra-marital affairs often become ossified as "erotic tumours" of the mind, which then dominate all aspects of psychic functioning in much the way that a brain tumour will destroy aspects of healthy cognition. When these erotic tumours erupt, they will often result in what I have earlier identified as the "conjugal aneurysm".

I cannot, on this occasion, provide a more detailed study of either the aetiology or the treatment of Elfriede's intra-marital affair, but I can confirm that she did, indeed, suffer profoundly, and that her private sexual preoccupations, which she had never articulated to anyone prior to the start of her psychoanalytical sessions with me, prevented her from enjoying either her professional work as an artist or her marital relationship with a somewhat emotionally unsophisticated but otherwise loyal and decent husband. Elfriede's intra-marital affairs – an expression of sexual sadism towards Francis – bedevilled her mind; but, fortunately, an immersion in a lengthy period of intensive, multi-frequency psychoanalytical work certainly helped to contain and to work through the force of her intra-marital preoccupations and thus prevent them from becoming ossified as an erotic tumour or from exploding as a conjugal aneurysm.

To her great credit, Elfriede had come to seek help before she could destroy her marriage in a volcanic eruption; and having undergone protracted psychoanalytical treatment, her spousal relationship remains intact and enriched to this day. But other individuals and couples who suffer from the psychopathologies of sexual fantasy will often arrive at our consulting rooms only *after* the conjugal aneurysm has exploded with devastating consequences.

"Gwilym", a successful barrister, devoted his life to public service, and had, as a result of his hard labours, developed a fine reputation in his field of legal expertise. He often lavished his wife "Hester" with expensive pieces of jewellery, and he always made a point of protecting his family diary so that he would never deal with any paperwork at weekends; instead, he spent every Saturday morning playing football with his son, and every Saturday afternoon accompanying his daughter to ballet classes. He devoted Sunday mornings to cooking an enormous roast meal which he and his wife and children enjoyed greatly; and, later in the day, Gwilym would supervise the pleasant ritual of watching a family-friendly film with his loved ones. On paper, he seemed to boast a perfect life.

But, every night, after Hester went to bed, Gwilym would sneak downstairs into his study, lock the door, and masturbate to a particular genre of internet pornography. Although he identified himself as "100 per cent heterosexual", he had become quite obsessed with preoperative transsexuals, and would climax to visual images of men who still retained penises but who also sported newly developed, hormonally-induced breasts, bedecked in lacy lingerie. These internet sessions caused Gwilym a great deal of shame, but they also provided him with a huge degree of unrivalled sexual excitement which eclipsed any pleasure that he had experienced with his otherwise beautiful and loving wife Hester.

As one might imagine, those who perform sexual activities outside of the bedroom will wish to conceal their infidelities – even those of a "virtual" cyber nature – but, at the same time, many will also harbour an unconscious wish to be discovered, in the secret hope that by doing so, a marital crisis may be provoked and then, ultimately, treated. And although Gwilym had already succeeded in arousing suspicion, Hester had eventually become even more aware of her husband's late-night disappearances; and, on one fateful evening, when Gwilym had failed to lock the door to his study, she burst in on him unannounced and found him engaged in a live "cyber-chat" with a male-to-female preoperative transsexual.

At that moment, Hester's world collapsed entirely, and she not only screamed at Gwilym for his tremendous duplicitousness and "perversion", but she also shouted at herself for her naïveté, recognising that she could no longer respect or believe the very special, beloved man in whom she had placed every ounce of her trust. At Hester's insistence, she and Gwilym then arranged a consultation to see me for marital psychotherapy.

In spite of his pornographic predilection, Gwilym explained that he had not ever met a transsexual man in person. In fact, he never exchanged bodily fluids with anyone other than his wife. But his copious cyber activities, indicative of a strong set of intra-marital affairs and erotic tumours, provoked a hugely explosive conjugal aneurysm which made Hester feel that she had lived a lie throughout her entire marriage. I must confess that, upon hearing of this aneurytic spousal relationship, I had initially assumed – quite wrongly, I must confess – that such marital turmoil could never be survived, and that Hester and Gwilym had come to see me in order to find a more human way of divorcing.

But the couple loved each other greatly, and, after five years of psychotherapy, had finally come to enjoy some understanding and even experience some forgiveness. Once again, I cannot discuss the complexities of the treatment itself in the context of such a brief communication, but I can report that, through our work, Gwilym eventually began to conceptualise his need for a fantasied sexual experience with a male-female person as the result of much early deprivation from both his mother *and* his father. And Hester not only developed a greater, more sensitive appreciation of Gwilym's complicated sexual mind but, also, came to realise the ways in which her own infantile rage, never before contained or treated, had helped to provoke Gwilym to seek a Hester-free refuge in his study late at night.

The cases of Elfriede and Francis and, also, of Gwilym and Hester, typify the widespread nature of what we might come to consider as "disorders of sexual fantasy" in otherwise healthy, law-abiding, and compassionate individuals. Neither Elfriede nor Gwilym had ever perpetrated acts of discernible cruelty against their children, their friends, their colleagues, or other members of society. Instead, they reserved their private sadistic attacks solely for their spouses, and ultimately, in view of the consequences, for themselves.

Elfriede and Gwilym – the two fantasists under consideration – differ from Archibald, who vomited on his wife, and from Dexter, who ejaculated on his wife, because the former individuals, Elfriede and Gwilym, "acted out" *beyond* the space of the marital bedroom, *behind* their partners' backs, while the latter, Archibald and Dexter, did so in the *presence* of their spouses. Of course, I do not wish to propose so crude a theory which would suggest that those who perpetrate sadistic acts in front of their partners may be less dangerous than those who do so more secretively. The very reality of marital rape would contradict such an assertion completely. But I do wish to hypothesise that when the sadistic enactment occurs in full view of the partner, then the cry for help becomes more apparent more quickly, and each member of the spousal pair will have a greater opportunity for awareness and for seeking psychological treatment.[1]

SADISTIC ENACTMENTS AS A DEFENCE AGAINST DEATH

Sexual insensitivity, sexual thoughtlessness, sexual narcissism, and sexual cruelty can cause a great deal of distress to partners. Thus far, we have examined what might transpire when partners treat one another's bodies or bodily spaces with unkindness, or when spouses "cheat" on each other in a fantasmatic way, often assisted by the internet. But what happens when infidelity moves beyond the realms of fantasy and into the arena of bodily enactments with another living person outside of the marital home?

For the non-forensic couple – those who never commit arrestable crimes such as rape or murder or domestic violence – sadistic infidelity may well be the most serious expression of cruelty, and it presents far greater challenges to both the couple and to the clinician.

"Isaac" had just turned forty years of age. A successful banker with lots of money to spare, this man travelled extensively for business and, during his frequent trips abroad, he spent many evenings alone in luxury hotels. Separated from his wife "Jessica" and from his four young children, Isaac often arranged for prostitutes to visit him in his hotel suite. After paying these sex workers, he would then engage them in a variety of erotic activities.

Although Isaac explained that he found most of these prostitutes to be "disposable", one young woman in particular, a nineteen-year-old called "Katerina", had really captivated him, and he began to meet with her more frequently, often flying abroad just to see her. Before long, Isaac stopped paying Katerina for sex and he eventually established her as a second spouse, and even purchased a beautiful apartment for her. In due course, Katerina became pregnant with twins, and, soon thereafter, Isaac found himself supporting two wives and six children, as well as both a British household and a Continental household.

Isaac's concretely enacted infidelity can be traced to a multitude of sources. But above all, we must note that the series of visits to sex workers and the creation of a second marriage to Katerina all occurred in the wake of his fortieth birthday. During the course of one-to-one psychotherapy with this man, it did not surprise me to learn that Isaac's father had also experienced a conjugal aneurysm at the age of forty and had decimated Isaac's mother in a most traumatic way. He had simply disappeared, abandoning both wife and son forever. The ten-year-old Isaac never saw his father again.

To Isaac's credit, perhaps, he continued to maintain very regular contact – physical, emotional, as well as financial – with his wife Jessica and with his four British children. He never abandoned them in the completely callous way in which his own father had done. Although Isaac had repeated a parental, intergenerational trauma, he had minimised the extent of the abandonment. But in spite of the fact that he did not disappear from Jessica and his children as his father had disappeared from him, Isaac nonetheless committed an act of great infidelity – a form of sexual sadism – which cost him dearly. Not only did he find himself crippled economically by the cost of maintaining his two wives, six children, and two household establishments, but he ultimately found himself virtually bankrupt after Jessica discovered his "double life" and sued for divorce, winning an impressive settlement which deprived Isaac of millions.

As a man who had only recently entered his fifth decade of life, Isaac began to fear death greatly. Indeed, in the wake of his divorce, he found it extremely difficult to differentiate between the emotional death that he experienced when Jessica took the children and his own sense of having an ageing body, which would someday cease to function. In our psychological work together, we gradually came to appreciate the way in which Isaac's attraction to prostitutes and, in particular, to the youthful continental Katerina, served as a means of eroticisation which then protected him from a sense of deadliness – a common form of "acting-out" in the middle years of life in which one replaces death with sex in the hope that the birth of a new baby will minimise the pain experienced by each of us as we face the severe limitation of time.

Throughout psychotherapy, Isaac struggled to appreciate the full extent of the way in which his deep infidelity and his creation of a second family with Katerina had caused immense pain to his wife Jessica and to his four children. During many sessions, Isaac referred to Jessica as a "fucking bitch" for having hired such a "shark" of a lawyer who kept asking for more and more money in the divorce settlement. Isaac experienced great difficulty appreciating his deep, sadistic betrayal of Jessica. Fortunately, as psychotherapy progressed, Isaac became increasingly sensitive, and he eventually began to realise that his enactments had caused immense pain and suffering.

I shall conclude this section with one further clinical vignette, to which I have already referred quite briefly in the previous chapter of this book, which illustrates, most shockingly, the true depth and the profound viciousness of sexual sadism in spousal relationships. "Lester", a businessman, and "Martina", a schoolteacher, had wed during their early thirties and had remained in a very long marriage of more than twenty-five years; but throughout their time together, Lester had cheated on innumerable occasions. The couple arrived at my office in a dreadful state because, one year previously, Martina had received a diagnosis of lymphoma, and had subsequently undergone several rounds of debilitating chemotherapy and radiotherapy which caused her to lose all of her hair, and which produced great nausea and fatigue. Owing to the gravity of her cancer, Martina had hoped that Lester would cease his infidelities and that he would become a good caretaker instead;

and, indeed, he did promise that he would look after her throughout this dreadful medical ordeal.

Tragically, Lester perpetrated one of the greatest acts of marital sadism that I have encountered in over forty years of clinical practice. It seems that after Lester dropped Martina off at hospital for her chemotherapy sessions, he would then, quite frequently, check into a hotel room round the corner from the hospital in order to indulge in sex with Martina's younger and healthier sister whom he had always fancied. A skilled philanderer, Lester had managed to keep the details of these furtive encounters secret from Martina, but her baby sister, "Norma", riddled with guilt, confessed what had happened in order to clear her troubled conscience. Shockingly, Martina – the wife – also discovered a hotel room receipt in her husband's trousers; thus, she had acquired confirmation from two separate sources that this infidelity had actually occurred. To her great credit, Martina refrained not only from killing herself in desperation but, also, from injuring her husband and her sister, which many other women might have done in such comparable, horrific circumstances.

I could expound at great length on the psychodynamic aspects of this case, and upon the role of the childhood histories of both Lester and Martina, and also of her sister Norma, in creating such an unholy triangle. But, in this context, I have chosen to undertake the more primary task of describing a typology of sadism; and no discussion of the topic would be complete without providing an indication of the magnitude of cruelty in otherwise normal-neurotic marriages between essentially law-abiding, decent citizens. I can report with heavy heart that in the midst of our efforts to unravel and treat this exceptionally painful conjugal explosion, Martina succumbed to her lymphoma, and she died at the age of fifty-six years.

The case of the forty-year-old Isaac, volcanically immersed in a profound mid-life crisis, which prompted him to find a second wife and to create a second family, and, also, the case of Lester, a long-term marital despoiler, who slept with his wife's sister during chemotherapy sessions, each underscore the painful association between sexual infidelity, marital sadism, and the struggle with death anxiety. In both instances, one member of the couple endeavoured in quite a primitive manner to defend against the inevitability of ageing and death by introducing eroticism into the mixture, in the vain hope that, by suddenly becoming sexual, one could deny the reality of an ailing body.[2]

TORCHING THE MARITAL BEDROOM

In 2007, I published the results of a five-year study, the British Sexual Fantasy Research Project, which surveyed and analysed the sexual behaviours and, in particular, the erotic fantasies of a randomised sample of some 13,553 adult Britons (Kahr, 2007a), supplemented by comparable data on some 3,617 American adults, released the following year, in 2008 (Kahr, 2008). The study of British sexuality revealed that as many as thirty-six per cent of adults, aged eighteen or older, will have kissed someone other than a regular spouse or partner, outside of the marital relationship; twenty-five per cent will have fondled someone other than a spouse or partner; eighteen per cent will have engaged in extramarital oral sex; twenty-four per cent will have practised extramarital vaginal sex; and five per cent will have indulged in extramarital anal sex (Kahr, 2007a). In each of these instances, men in partnerships have cheated more frequently than women … but not much more. For instance, although twenty-eight per cent of partnered males boasted one or more experiences of extramarital vaginal sex, as many as twenty per cent of part-nered females did so as well. Translated from percentages into actual figures, this indicates that nearly 11,000,000 British adults will have submitted themselves to extramarital vaginal penetration.

When we examine sexual fantasies, as opposed to sexual behaviours, the inci-dence becomes infinitely greater; and hardly a man or woman alive will not have climaxed to the thought of sexual congress with someone other than his or her long-term partner. This should not surprise us, as the indulgence in sexual fantasy has for many centuries helped to protect us from actual, forensic infidelities. If we take a pretty co-worker or a handsome stranger to bed *in our minds*, we might, perhaps, be less likely to do so in the "outside" world.

But when one explores the content of many of these sexual fantasies, one finds that the average Briton often achieves climax by masturbating about extramari-tal sex, with as many as forty-one per cent of British adults having admitted to the erotic fantasy of sexual relations with someone else's partner. Furthermore, as many as twenty-nine per cent of the adult British sample reported having fantasised about being dominant or aggressive during sexual activity, and thirty-three per cent admitted to comparable fantasies of being submissive or passive during sexual practices, while as many as thirteen per cent have enjoyed the thought of spanking someone else, and twelve per cent have indulged in fantasies of being spanked. As many as twenty-three per cent of adults reported sexual pleasure at the thought of tying up another person, and twenty-five per cent of adults actually admitted to sexual excitement at the prospect of being tied up (Kahr, 2007a). Clearly, the interrelationship between sexuality, aggression, and infidelity remains both hugely intimate and extremely popular.

In the preceding pages, I have endeavoured to outline a typology of sexual sad-ism in the ostensibly non-forensic couple, namely, those partners who constitute the vast majority of the world's population. None of the members of the couples described herein have ever set their spouses on fire as Foulques Nerra, the medieval Angevin *comte*, had done back in the tenth century. Indeed, none of the couples in my clinical survey had ever, to the best of my knowledge, received even so much as a parking ticket from the local traffic warden. Most of the men and women with whom I have worked have led reasonably exemplary lives, have paid their taxes, and have helped old men and women cross the road. They have, indeed, proved to be model citizens except, perhaps, in the bedroom.

And whether by vomiting on each other, by ejaculating on each other, by mas-turbating to internet pornography throughout the small hours of the morning, by keeping a second home, a second wife, and a second child in another country, or by sleeping with one's sister-in-law while one's spouse undergoes chemotherapy, all of the aforementioned couples have found a way of expressing sadism, thus soiling the potentialities of the marital bedroom. In most cases, one partner holds the distinction of being the overt instigator of the cruelty. For example, in the case of Gwilym, the man who spent hours engaged in cyber-chats with preoperative transsexuals, any court of law would describe him as the perpetrator and his wife Hester as the innocent victim. After all, *she* had never masturbated with a stranger over the internet. Only Gwilym had done so. Of course, *in sensu stricto*, Gwilym had actually committed those acts of infidelity, rather than Hester, but those of us who work from a couple psychoanalytical perspective have come to realise that even though one partner engages in the forensic enactment of infidelity, both partners in a marriage may well have contributed to the creation of the unconscious emotional climate in which such enactments become possible, even necessary, in order to maintain psychological equilibrium, and in order to protect the couple from even worse marital violence. When, during couple psychotherapy, Hester screamed at Gwilym, she did so with such ferocity that I often wished that I had brought a pair of ear plugs to the consulting room. I realised of course that any wife who discovered her husband *in flagrante* might yearn to raise her voice in such a pained and anguished way. But as I came to know this couple better, I learned from Gwilym that Hester *had*, indeed, screamed at him night and day, long before he ever had access to something called the internet. I can reveal that the screaming had become so persistent and so penetrative that, on one occasion, a colleague who worked in the adjoining consulting room in my office building complained to me afterwards about the noise level. This vignette helped me to realise that although one member of the couple often commits the "crime", *both* members of the couple will have facilitated its ultimate emergence.

Many people often lambaste Sigmund Freud for having foregrounded the importance of sexuality and, also, aggression as the dominant features of the human unconscious mind. Whether Freud overestimated the role of such basic drives remains a matter for debate. But as a couple mental health worker, I would even be inclined to suggest that Freud might have *underestimated* the impact of destructive sexuality and aggression in the intimate partner relationship, because, as a couple worker, I often see evidence of little else.

In the clinical consulting room, we invariably encounter proof of the painfully close admixture of these two most powerful drives. "Oscar", an elderly man, had developed a severe bronchitis, and he languished for days and days in the marital bed. Once, he asked his wife "Priscilla" to bring him a cup of hot tea to ease his aching throat. Priscilla returned with the tea ... four and a half hours later... claiming that she had forgotten all about her husband's request because she had become so engrossed in watching a film on television. Oscar, too weak to move, could not shout to her for assistance. Even such a seemingly simple example of sadism in the marital bedroom underscores how one need not dress like a dominatrix and whip one's spouse in order to make one's partner feel quite horribly beaten.

In most instances, such enactments in the bedroom might be described as deeply unconscious, and most of my patients have absolutely no idea why they have engaged in sexual cruelty in the bedroom. "Quincy", a man with whom I had worked on a one-to-one basis in individual psychoanalysis, spent months and months explaining how much closer he had become to his wife "Rose", and how their sexual life had improved greatly in recent months. Imagine my surprise when Quincy told me, one day, that he had recently embarked upon an extra-marital affair with a woman called "Saskia". Curiously, each time Quincy took Saskia – the new girlfriend – to bed, he could not attain an erection; but when he had sex with Rose – his wife – he managed to become completely tumescent. This made no sense to Quincy, and he joked that he would be remembered as "the only man in history who could fuck his wife but not his mistress." Through sustained psychoanalytical work, Quincy and I came to realise that this episode of marital enactment – taking a mistress – had occurred in the wake of his ninth wedding anniversary to Rose; and that this might mirror quite precisely the fact that Quincy's father had begun to live with a mistress shortly after Quincy's ninth birthday. Indeed, Quincy found the parallel extremely striking, and he soon came to realise that he had become engulfed in the unconscious re-enactment of an early childhood trauma, without realising that he had done so. A few weeks thereafter, he broke off his affair with Saskia, and he then resumed his very satisfying sexual relationship with Rose!

Marital unkindness appears in many guises, and, on the surface, numerous acts of thoughtlessness seem to be devoid of a sexual substratum. During my very first consultation with "Thérèse" and "Ugo", a continental couple, I took a moment to clarify the correct spelling of their names and to write down their home address and telephone numbers. I turned to Thérèse and asked, "Would I be correct that you spell your name with two accents – an acute accent on the first "e", and a grave accent on the second "e"?" She confirmed this to be the case, whereupon Ugo exclaimed, "My God, I never knew that you had accents on your name." Thérèse became utterly heartbroken that her husband of five years did not seem to know something as fundamental as the spelling of her forename. It then emerged that this couple, in spite of their rows, had sex constantly; and it soon became apparent that their sexual life served primarily as an erotic defence against talking to one another. They managed physicality very well, but they could not relate in any other way, not least in terms of basic literacy, emotional or otherwise.

Sometimes, the unkindness between couples may not seem unkind at all. "Vincent", a young college student, got drunk at a party, and took "Wendy", another inebriated student, to bed. In his psychotherapy session, he boasted to me that as Wendy had imbibed far too much alcohol, he thought it best *not* to penetrate her, in case she might regret this in the morning. Vincent thus presented himself as a true gentleman. But as he lay on the couch in my office, free-associating, he then immediately became reminded of a newspaper article that he had read some years ago about an American university student – a male – who had entered a sorority house and had shot all of the women dead with a machine gun. Although Vincent had, indeed, behaved in a thoughtful manner by not having forced himself upon a drunken female, his free association revealed that he found himself struggling with sadistic desires nonetheless, unsurprisingly so, in view of their ubiquity in psychological life.

In many respects, we save our most unkind components for the person we claim to love above all others. We do so, in part, because we can. If we offend the host or hostess of a dinner party by insulting the food, we know that we will not be invited back again, and thus, we cannot "use" that venue as a vehicle for the discharge of sadism. But if we critique our spouse's food, we know that such an evacuation must be tolerated and will be tolerated; and, therefore, we return again and again and continue to perpetrate the same unconscious crime.

Sometimes, in more cynical moments, having spent long days in the office working with rageful couples, I do wonder whether we marry our partners primarily as an expression of love, or rather, as an opportunity to express hatred. Such a dynamic epitomises the shrewd observation offered many years ago by Dr. Donald Winnicott (1970, p. 262), namely, that, *"What is good is always being destroyed"*, and that we all have a very powerful need to use and abuse objects as a means of equilibrating our own faulty sense of self (cf. Winnicott, 1969a).

In an ideal world, the marital bedroom should be a place in which a couple can experience tenderness, eroticism, bodily safety, and psychological comfort. It could, and should, be a space in which partners can find a refuge from the anxieties of the world, or even dream creatively about how they might change the planet. It might become a venue in which spouses can read a book, watch a film, welcome young children on a Saturday morning, play with the cat and dog, and, of course, sleep in peace. But, owing to the widespread nature of early trauma and the sadism which devolves therefrom, the bedroom often becomes a place of cruelty which can manifest itself in both gross and subtle forms, even among those who have no criminal history in other areas of their lives.

As mental health professionals, we must continue to become more bold, more adept, and more diplomatic at working with couples to help them unearth, and then to articulate, the many ways in which sadism can blight the landscape of an otherwise non-sadistic marital couple. As we know, one need not set one's spouse on fire in order to torch the bedroom. Fortunately, as we become better adept at the art of forensically-informed couple psychoanalysis and couple psychotherapy, we will, one hopes, ultimately prove to be more effective at helping to extinguish these deadly marital flames.

Notes

1 As I have indicated, the disorders of sexual fantasy often serve as the bedrock of infidelity, either in the form of an intra-marital affair or an extramarital affair. When I first presented this essay to a group of mental health colleagues, a member of the audience asked whether I regard all affairs as inherently pathological. This particular individual noted that many couples engage in "swinging" or in "open marriage" and so forth; and other audience members remarked that the partner of a very ill spouse might sometimes take a lover (e.g., as in the case of an elderly man whose wife suffers from Alzheimer's disease in a care home and thus might, unsurprisingly, have another partner for sexual

relationships). One would need a further chapter in order to provide a clearer answer to such a question, which concerns both clinicians and ethicists. On this occasion, I cannot offer a fully articulated position about the inherent pathology or non-pathology of the extramarital affair or the intra-marital affair for that matter; but I can report that in all the couples who have presented for psychotherapeutic treatment, each affair or instance of infidelity certainly caused great pain and suffering to all the people concerned.

2 In the context of such a relatively brief communication, I have elected to focus predominantly on three particular types of sexual cruelty, namely, the use of bodily evacuations, the intra-marital affair and the extramarital affair (or the disorders of sexual fantasy), and finally, the use of cruelty as a defence against death anxiety. But couples have an infinite capacity to express marital sadism in other ways. One could, of course, also examine other varieties of potential sexual cruelty, namely, the withholding of sex as a form of aggression (e.g., Friedman, 1962; Grier, 2001), as well as the practice of bondage and dominance (or "consensual kink") as possible forms of sexual cruelty (Ortmann and Sprott, 2013). These complex subjects deserve much further consideration.

Conclusion

The Future of Forensic Psychoanalysis

While strolling through Central London, many pedestrians will encounter the iconic Marble Arch – that majestic early-nineteenth-century creation designed by the royally appointed architect John Nash. Nowadays, anyone can wander through this remarkable structure, but, at the time of its completion, only members of the Royal Family and their troops would have received permission to pass through this magnificent forty-five-feet-high structure.

It will not be widely appreciated, however, that many centuries previously, the terrain surrounding this region, once known as the village of Tyburn, served as the very epicentre of public executions by dissection, hanging, or burning for over 600 years. Those accused or convicted of criminality would be murdered at Tyburn, at least as early as the twelfth century. For instance, in 1196, William Fitz Osbern, known colloquially as "Longbeard", suffered death by hanging at Tyburn after having organised a revolt of merchants in order to protest a levy of taxes (Bartlett, 2000; Brandon and Brooke, 2007). Many Britons would congregate at Tyburn and revel in these sadistic murders. But, by the early eighteenth century, Bernard Mandeville (1725, p. 20), a Dutch-born philosopher and polemicist, spoke more critically about the "Torrent of Mob" who congregated at Tyburn to witness these brutal executions, which he described as "little better than Barbarity" (Mandeville, 1725, p. 36).

Happily, during the reign of George IV, this spectacularly imposing arch, made of white marble, would eventually come to replace the deadly Tyburn gallows. But, sadly, this transformation from a public execution arena to a royal arch required more than *six centuries*.

In view of the fact that human beings often operate with a vicious degree of sluggishness and lethargy, we must wonder whether, at this point in time, we now possess the passion and the sanity to speed up our understanding, not only of the causes of criminality but, most especially, its treatment. Or will we have to wait yet another 600 years before we begin to witness greater humanisation of the dehumanised?

In the twenty-first century, we no longer rush to execute offender patients in a Tyburnesque manner (e.g., Kahr, 2020b), but we do, however, incarcerate them in secure psychiatric institutions or in prisons, and we frequently ply them with heavy

DOI: 10.4324/9781003546245-15

dosages of medication (e.g., Sheard, Marini, Bridges, and Wagner, 1976). But we have little evidence that such an approach to treatment will prevent criminality in the years to come. Moreover, many psychiatric and penological institutions fail to protect the inmates satisfactorily, and large numbers of those incarcerated therein will continue to be raped (Starchild, 1990), or will still perpetrate violent attacks on other patients (Walker and Seifert, 1994), or upon members of staff (van Leeuwen and Harte, 2017), or, indeed, members of the public (Terranova and Rocca, 2016), or, even, upon themselves through self-mutilation (Wray and Eldridge, 1970; Shea, 1993). Indeed, in previous chapters, I have already summarised the work of the investigative journalist Ms. Alisa Roth (2018), who exposed the horror of American prisons; therefore, in view of her detailed descriptions of those institutions, it would not be unreasonable to wonder whether we have truly progressed beyond the ugliness and the cruelty of medieval prisons (e.g., Bassett, 1943).

In fact, while many would argue that these violent perpetrators deserve to be punished, certain leading psychoanalysts, such as the Hungarian-born, British-based Dr. Michael Balint (1951), actually argued that when we abuse offenders, we do so consciously in order to protect the public but, moreover, we do so *unconsciously*, as an act of revenge and retaliation.

Alas, by imprisoning offenders in cruel institutions, with no access to sophisticated psychological treatment, we not only continue to damage these already traumatised individuals, but we place ourselves at risk as well. In fact, many prisoners, upon release, will perpetrate further crimes in a recidivist manner, while others will kill themselves. The National Institute for Health and Care Excellence has reported that offenders in prison will be approximately 8.6 times more likely to commit suicide than members of the general public (*Preventing Suicide in Community and Custodial Settings: NICE Guideline*, 2018).

The vast majority of contemporary forensic patients will not have access to psychotherapeutic interventions; instead, a significant percentage will be transferred back and forth between custodial settings and psychiatric institutions (e.g., Hill, Mitchell, and Leipold, 2017), while heavily medicated.

As someone who has enjoyed the privilege of working in a calm, quiet, private consulting room in pleasant parts of London for many years, I must offer my deepest admiration to the many men and women who have laboured for lifetimes in ugly, dirty penological and psychiatric buildings, perched alongside the most dangerous criminal offenders in the world. I really do salute these brave colleagues.

But I do believe that we can improve the forensic mental health arena quite significantly by championing the incorporation of depth psychology even more vigorously than ever before.

Back in the early 1990s, I had the great privilege of undergoing clinical supervision with the great Dr. Murray Cox – a brilliant psychiatrist and group analyst who transformed the climate at Broadmoor Hospital, the United Kingdom's leading secure institution – home to many notable multiple murderers – by arranging for members of the Royal Shakespeare Company, not least the highly distinguished actor Mark Rylance, to perform the works of the Bard for the inmates (e.g., Cox, 1992b; cf. Cox, 1992a). A distinguished Shakespeare scholar in his own right,

Murray Cox derived huge pleasure by having facilitated this project, entertaining his patients with some of the best actors in the world and, also, permitting them to discuss the plays in detail – many of which deal with grisly acts of criminality – as part of the psychotherapeutic healing process. By Shakespearanising Broadmoor, the late, great Dr. Cox introduced not only aesthetics but, moreover, humanity into the ethos of this old-fashioned institution.

Following in the footsteps of Murray Cox, the forensic psychiatrist and forensic psychoanalyst Dr. Carine Minne collaborated with Mr. Paul Kassman to inaugurate a project entitled "Changing the Game" at Her Majesty's Prison Grendon, in the village of Grendon Underwood, in the county of Buckinghamshire, providing a group psychotherapeutic intervention for convicted, violent gang members – mostly men from deprived, disadvantaged backgrounds. Through this creative, "blue-sky" project, Minne and Kassman (2018) have provided a setting and a structure which has facilitated this group of once-violent individuals to work through their early-life abuse and traumata by participating in sensitive psychological treatment, thus assisting these men to develop more emotional solidity, so much so that many of the graduates of "Changing the Game" have since embarked upon more healthy, life-enhancing activities, and some have even enrolled for university studies.

Thus, psychoanalytically-trained clinicians have made innumerable contributions to the field of forensic mental health, not only through the provision of traditional talking therapies (as I have described throughout the course of this book), but, also, by having created such innovative programmes as Dr. Murray Cox, Dr. Carine Minne, and Mr. Paul Kassman have done. Regrettably, much of orthodox psychiatry has always regarded psychoanalytical approaches to mental health with considerable suspicion. For instance, Professor Michael Gelder, the quondam Professor of Psychiatry at the University of Oxford, and his colleagues Dr. Dennis Gath and Dr. Richard Mayou – each a Clinical Reader in Psychiatry at the same institution – dismissed psychoanalysis in their influential, best-selling *Oxford Textbook of Psychiatry*. These esteemed psychiatrists noted that, "Nowadays it is generally held that social causes of crime are much more important than psychological causes" (Gelder, Gath, and Mayou, 1983, p. 720).

Fortunately, in spite of the fact that many psychiatric workers have, over the decades, dismissed psychoanalysis in far too cavalier a manner, not least amidst the rise of neurocriminological investigations (e.g., Concannon, 2019; cf. Rafter, 2008; Haycock, 2014), our profession has flourished nonetheless and will continue to do so. Indeed, not only have we made advances in exploring the aetiology of forensic illnesses, but, also, we have achieved huge strides in rehabilitation through psychoanalytically orientated treatment. Moreover, we have also created considerable contributions to the *prevention* of criminality in the first place through the support of disciplines such as psychodynamically orientated child mental health and couple mental health, endeavouring to prepare mothers and fathers for parenthood before any formal abuse or traumatisation can unfold (Acquarone, 2002, 2004, 2008; Kahr, 2012b, 2019h; Abse, 2014).

As someone who has laboured for decades not only as a clinician but, also, as an academic historian, I must urge our psychodynamically-sympathetic colleagues to return to the study of our past so that we can draw upon the wisdom of our ancestors and thus both archive and, moreover, promote the genius find-ings of these remarkable, leading figures of our field. For instance, many years ago, Dr. John Bowlby – a true pioneer of psychoanalytically orientated empirical research – studied the early lives of young people, aged five to sixteen years, who had committed acts of thievery or pilfering. Bowlby (1944a, 1944b, 1945–1946, 1946) and his colleagues investigated the childhood histories of many juvenile de-linquents and reconstructed detailed portraits of the early lives of these individuals, some of whom perpetrated acts of great cruelty, such as pushing a young girl off a tricycle or burning a small girl's leg with intention. In virtually every case, these juvenile forensic patients had endured quite significant bereavements during their earliest years; indeed, many had lost a mother and, also, at times, a father.

One of the children who participated in Bowlby's (1944a, 1944b) study, a young thief called "Edward G.L.", the ninth of eleven children, suffered from a chronic depression, having had to navigate extreme deprivations and bereavements throughout his early years. During Edward's fifth year, his father died in a rail-way accident; and then, some seven years later, during the boy's twelfth year, his mother passed away from consumption. Another one of the children in this study, "Audrey H.", had to endure, at approximately seven years of age, the death of her beloved grandmother, followed not long thereafter by the shocking loss of her five-year-old brother, run over by a lorry in Audrey's presence. It did not surprise Bowlby (1944a, 1944b) that, by the age of ten years, Audrey began to steal coins from the pockets of her school mates.

Some of the youngsters in Bowlby's (1944a, 1944b) research project had to tol-erate even more tragic histories, such as "Arthur L.", an illegitimate child, born to a mother who worked in a tavern, impregnated by a publican whom she barely knew. Arthur spent little time with his mother during his infancy as she had des-patched him to live with various relatives. Indeed, during his first nine years, Ar-thur's mother saw him merely on a fortnightly basis and boasted that Arthur had had to rear himself. Eventually, Arthur became a childhood thief and a truant. In a subsequent publication, Bowlby characterised Arthur thus:

> I have never seen a more isolated boy. I do not think I have ever had the experi-ence of talking to a brick wall so vividly as with this boy over a long period. In fact, I never made any contact with him at all, nor did anyone else (Bowlby, 1945–1946, p. 33).

Such traumata of separation, neglect, and loss proved to be rather commonplace, if not omnipresent, in the early life histories of those boys and girls who ultimately became thieves. Needless to say, not every child who has experienced bereavement will become a criminal, but many will have done, underscoring that the trauma of loss places young people at considerable risk.

During the nineteenth century, delinquent children would be subjected to whip-ping, imprisonment, and neglect (Duckworth, 2002), not to mention confinement in a workhouse and, even, transportation abroad (Shore, 1999). But, Bowlby and his team of colleagues progressed beyond these cruel interventions by having provided psychological treatment for many of these criminal children in the hope of preventing them from becoming career offenders in later life. Such early forensic psychotherapeutic interventions represented a great advance in the history of humanity.

Through his pioneering studies, John Bowlby laid the foundations for an understanding of the role of early trauma and deprivation in the development of criminality. For instance, more than forty years later, two psychopathology researchers, Dr. Matti Huttunen and Dr. Pekka Niskanen (1978), undertook an intensive investigation of the Finnish population registers from 1925 to 1957, and, as a result of their research, they discovered that patients who had perpetrated crimes had actually lost their fathers before birth far more frequently than members of a control group. Trauma certainly places men and women at significant risk of developing criminality in later life.

In the chapters of this book, I have endeavoured to demonstrate, through my own clinical work and through the huge contributions of so many of my predecessors, the very powerful role of loss and deprivation, abuse and cruelty, and trauma of all varieties in the early life histories of future delinquents, paedophiles, and murderers. Trauma has certainly scarred the biography of every single forensic patient whom I have ever encountered. For instance, those who set fire to buildings, namely, arsonists, have also experienced considerable impingements in early life. Dr. Lynn Stewart (1993), a psychologist at Her Majesty's Prison Holloway in London, discovered that many female arsonists had come from broken homes and that as many as sixty-two per cent had suffered from sexual assaults. In a subsequent study, three London-based psychiatrists, Dr. Basant Puri, Dr. Richard Baxter, and Dr. Christopher Cordess (1995), confirmed the frequency of sexual abuse in the histories of fire-setters and, also, noted that many had endured early bereavements and social isolation as well. Thus, psychosocial trauma represents a potentially ubiquitous feature in the backgrounds of forensic patients of every shape and size. Even the most conservative and biologically orientated periodicals, such as *Psychological Medicine*, published by Cambridge University Press, have begun to recognise the role of traumatogenesis in the development of criminality (e.g., Augsburger, Basler, and Maercker, 2019). And we owe this recognition predominantly to Sigmund Freud and to his numerous followers who have come to specialise in forensic psychotherapy and forensic psychoanalysis.

Over the course of human history, we have treated offenders – even those suffering from mental distress or mental illness – with profound cruelty. Often, those who have inflicted legal punishments upon convicted criminals have committed far more ghastly acts than those incarcerated for their crimes. Fortunately, in spite of our dreadful track record, a few glimmers of humanitarian light have begun to appear upon the horizon in recent decades. And psychoanalytical mental health professionals, in particular, may take much pleasure and relief from having made some very important contributions in this respect.

Once we come to appreciate that crime results predominantly from early trauma and loss, rather than from bad genes or from a "neurotic taint" (Levy, 1932, p. 76), we will be much better able to offer appropriate assistance to those who have

perpetrated offences, namely, humane containment in psychologically sophisticated institutions, combined with intensive psychotherapy designed to prevent the
likelihood of recidivism. When I began to train, the phrase "forensic psychotherapy" barely existed, and the phrase "forensic psychoanalysis" did not exist at all.
But now, decades later, we have the possibility of providing a more enlightened
form of relief to both the overtly violent and the covertly violent in our midst.

Back in 1932, Melanie Klein, one of the true pioneers of child psychoanalysis,
argued passionately that if mental health practitioners could intervene early on in
the life cycle of a young person, and could provide psychological treatment, one
might, thereby, be able to prevent future breakdown, hospitalisation and, even,
imprisonment. As Klein exclaimed,

> If every child who shows disturbances that are at all severe were to be analysed
> in good time, a great number of those people who later end up in prisons or lu-
> natic asylums, or who go completely to pieces, would be saved from such a fate
> and be able to develop a normal life (Klein, 1932b, p. 374).[1]

I appreciate that I have already included this quotation from Klein in the "Series
Editor's Foreword" to this book, but, in my estimation, it deserves to be repeated at
the end of this volume, as we need Klein's constant reminder that violence *can* be
prevented with proper intervention.

Other colleagues, too, have championed early diagnosis and intervention as a
means of prevention. Indeed, back in 1944, in his essay on "Forty-Four Juvenile
Thieves: Their Characters and Home-Life (II)", published in *The International
Journal of Psycho-Analysis*, Dr. John Bowlby (1944b, p. 126) – one of Melanie
Klein's quondam clinical supervisees – urged us that, "Well-trained play-analysts
must be provided to give treatment. Medicine must step in and cure these cases
long before they are even eligible to come before a Court of Law."

The criminally insane have haunted humanity since time immemorial. And yet,
in spite of centuries of medical and criminological investigations, we have made
little progress in the cure of such individuals, until, I believe, the discovery and
development of both dynamic psychology and traumatogenesis and, moreover, the
growth of forensic psychotherapy and forensic psychoanalysis.

Thankfully, we have indeed harvested enough evidence to demonstrate that psychoanalytical treatment truly facilitates a cure. Consequently, we now have the
opportunity to apply this knowledge on a much wider canvas, and, by doing so, we
might make a real improvement to our utterly too, too violent world.

Note

1 As I have already indicated in the endnote to the "Series Editor's Foreword", the original
   German phrase reads: "Würde jedes Kind, das ernstere Störungen zeigt, rechtzeitig der
   Analyse unterzogen, dann könnte wohl ein großer Teil jener Menschen, die andernfalls in
   Gefängnissen und Irrenhäusern landen oder sonst völlig scheitern, vor diesem Schicksal
   bewahrt bleiben und sich zu normalen Menschen entwickeln" (Klein, 1932a, p. 293).

Original Sources of Chapters

Many of the contributions published in this book, *Forensic Psychoanalysis: From Sub-Clinical Psychopaths to Serial Killers*, appear here, in print, for the very first time. I have already released earlier versions of some of these chapters in other books or journals; however, in each case, I have updated and restyled each chapter quite considerably. I do wish to convey my warmest thanks to all of the publishers, whom I have identified below, each one of whom had provided me with a most appreciated opportunity in which I could share more initial incarnations of this work.

Preamble: Confessions of a Private Forensic Practitioner

This material appears in print here for the very first time.

Introduction: The Ugly World of Forensic Mental Health

A small portion of this material appeared in a much more expanded form in my book *Dangerous Lunatics: Trauma, Criminality, and Forensic Psychotherapy* (Kahr, 2020b), one of the inaugural titles of Confer Books of London. I have re-written that section considerably. I owe my gratitude to Dr. Stephen Setterberg, the former Publisher of both Confer Books and its sometime sibling press Karnac Books, along with all of the members of that Publishing Team, for their support and expertise. A further portion of this chapter first appeared as a podcast review in *The International Journal of Forensic Psychotherapy* (Kahr, 2020c), published by Phoenix Publishing House of Bicester in Oxfordshire. Likewise, I have edited and rewritten that description specifically for this current book publication. I wish to convey my warmest thanks to the Publisher, Mrs. Kate Pearce, and to the two founding editors-in-chief of the journal, Ms. Jessica Collier and Dr. Carine Minne, for having commissioned that piece. Since the essay first appeared in print, Karnac Books of Bicester in Oxfordshire has now become the new publisher of this important forensic journal.

Chapter 1: "Let the great Axe fall": From Ancient Babylonian Torture to Modern Forensic Psychotherapy

I first presented an abbreviated version of this chapter under the full title, "'Let the Great Axe Fall': From Ancient Babylonian Torture to Modern Forensic Psychotherapy. Freud, Welldon, and the Humanization of Criminality" (Kahr, 2022f), on 13th May, 2022, at B.M.A. House, the London headquarters of the British Medical Association, as the opening Plenary of the special conference on "Violence as a Public Health Emergency: Preventing, Treating and Humanizing the Dangerous Mind. Exploring the Past, Present and Future of Forensic Psychotherapy", designed to mark the thirtieth anniversary of the founding of the International Association for Forensic Psychotherapy, co-sponsored by both the Violence Committee and the Psychoanalysis and Law Committee of the International Psychoanalytical Association. I owe immense gratitude to Dr. Carine Minne, then President of the organisation, for having chaired the plenary session, and for her wonderful innovations in our profession. I also wish to convey my warm appreciation to Ms. Barbara Jacobs, the administrator of the International Association for Forensic Psychotherapy, and to colleagues on the Conference Organising Committee, for such tremendous support. A tiny portion of the material about Dr. Donald Winnicott's achievements in this field first appeared in a much revised form as part of a chapter on "Winnicott's Contribution to the Study of Dangerousness" (Kahr, 2001c), which I wrote for my edited book, *Forensic Psychotherapy and Psychopathology: Winnicottian Perspectives* (Kahr, 2001a), one of the launch titles of the "Forensic Psychotherapy Monograph Series", commissioned by the former owner of Karnac Books, the late Mr. Cesare Sacerdoti. The publishers Routledge / Taylor and Francis Group of London and of Abingdon in Oxfordshire have reprinted this book as the new owners of the "Forensic Psychotherapy Monograph Series", now produced in conjunction with the International Association for Forensic Psychotherapy, thanks to the editorial expertise of Ms. Susannah Frearson (Kahr, 2019a). And further tranches of the chapter appeared in a very revised form in a short essay on "Academic Recognition for Forensic Psychotherapy", published in *The Psychotherapy Review* (Kahr, 2000a), and, also, in my previously unpublished speech, "Dr. Estela Welldon's Contribution to Humanity" (Kahr, 2011b), presented as part of the "Tribute to Dr. Estela Welldon: Twenty Years of the I.A.F.P.", which concluded the conference on "Murder in Mind" – the Twentieth International Conference of the International Association for Forensic Psychotherapy – held at the Apex International Hotel, in Edinburgh, Scotland, on 30th April, 2011. I then published a shortened version of this essay in *The International Journal of Forensic Psychotherapy*, under the title, "'Let the great axe fall': From Ancient Babylonian Torture to Modern Forensic Psychotherapy. Freud, Welldon, and the Humanisation of Criminality" (Kahr, 2022d). I extend much appreciation to the Editor-in-Chief, Dr. Carine Minne, and to the Managing Editor, Ms. Annie Pesskin, and, of course, to the Publisher, Mrs. Kate Pearce of Phoenix Publishing House, in Bicester, Oxfordshire – who has now become the new Publisher of Karnac Books – and to our impressive copyeditor, Mrs. Anita Mason, and our most pleasant administrator, Ms. Anita Higgins Taylor – now retired – for their highly collaborative capacities.

Chapter 2: Explosive Patients: Surviving Petrifying Psychotherapeutic Experiences

Portions of this chapter have appeared in significantly revised versions in my book, *Bombs in the Consulting Room: Surviving Psychological Shrapnel* (Kahr, 2020a), published by Routledge / Taylor and Francis Group of London and Abingdon in Oxfordshire, and, also, in an essay entitled, "On Patients Who Explode: Surviving Petrifying Psychotherapeutic Experiences" (Kahr, 2021d), first produced in *The International Journal of Forensic Psychotherapy* due to the kindness of Phoenix Publishing House of Bicester in Oxfordshire. A further rendering of the tale of "Albertina", enhanced with illustrations and detailed references (Kahr 2022a, 2022b), appeared in a wonderfully innovative book, edited by my former student, Ms. Raffaella Hilty (2022) – now an esteemed colleague – entitled, *Primitive Bodily Communications in Psychotherapy: Embodied Expressions of a Disembodied Psyche*, published by Karnac Books of London. I extend my warm thanks to the Publishing Team at Karnac Books for having released such a beautiful text, in particular, Dr. Stephen Setterberg, the previous Publisher.

Much of the material contained in those various texts derived, initially, from two presentations, namely, a lecture entitled "On Patients Who Explode: Surviving Petrifying Psychotherapeutic Experiences" (Kahr, 2018h), first delivered at a conference on "Bombs in the Consulting Room: How to Survive Hostile Transference and Relational Dynamics", sponsored by Confer, based in Tunstall, in Woodbridge, in the county of Suffolk, held at the N.C.V.O. headquarters in London, on 9th June, 2018, at the kind invitation of Ms. Jane Ryan, and, subsequently, I offered an identically entitled version of that paper at a conference on "Working with Hostility in the Consulting Room: A Special One-day Event with Brett Kahr and Dr. Carine Minne" (Kahr, 2019i), hosted by Confer, in conjunction with Confer Ireland, in Dublin, Ireland, at the Palatine Room / Seomra Palatine, National Museum of Ireland – Decorative Arts and History / Ard Mhúsaem na hÉireann, at the Collins Barracks, in Dublin, on 7th December, 2019, pleasantly introduced by Ms. Donna Redmond. On both occasions, I had the honour to share clinical material alongside Dr. Carine Minne, who proved the most gracious of collaborators.

I presented a further version of this talk to a group of mental health professionals at Rafan House in London, via Zoom, on 9th June, 2021, at the kind invitation of Mrs. Sue Schraer (Kahr, 2021f); and then, on 19th June, 2021, I had the privilege of delivering a further incarnation of this paper, entitled, "Взрывоопасные пациенты: как пережить шокирующее психотерапевтическое взаимодействие" ["On Patients Who Explode: Surviving Petrifying Psychotherapeutic Experiences"] (Kahr, 2021g), to the Общество психоаналитической психотерапии [Society of Psychoanalytic Psychotherapy], in Moscow, in Russia, also via Zoom, thanks to the generous request of Dr. Konstantin Nemirovskiy and his colleagues, who hosted an event on "35 конференция, Общество психоаналитической психотерапии, 125-летию со дня рождения Дональда Винникотта и полувековому юбилею его работы 'Игра и реальность'" ["35th Conference of The Society of Psychoanalytic Psychotherapy: 'Playing and Reality': For Donald Woods Winnicott's 125th Birthday"]. I delivered yet another version of "On Patients Who Explode: Surviving Petrifying Psychotherapeutic Experiences" (Kahr, 2021h), at a conference entitled, "A Day with Professor Brett Kahr: 'Bombs in the Consulting Room. Surviving Attacks and Facilitating Cures'", sponsored by the Basingstoke Counselling Service, based in Basingstoke, Hampshire, delivered via Zoom, and hosted from the Meadow Suite in Park House in the University of Reading, on the Whiteknights Campus, in Reading, Berkshire, on 6th November, 2021, due to the gracious request of Ms. Catherine Butler.

Chapter 3: Why Do Men Expose Their Genitals?: The Unconscious Origins of Exhibitionism

A portion of the material contained within this chapter first appeared in a shortened form in my book on *Exhibitionism* (Kahr, 2001b), one of the titles in a special series on "Ideas in Psychoanalysis", published by Icon Books, then based in Duxford in Cambridge, in the county of Cambridgeshire, on behalf of the Freud Museum, London, under the series editorship of Mr. Ivan Ward. I owe particular thanks to the staff members at Icon Books, especially Mr. Jeremy Cox, Mr. Andrew Furlow, Mr. Duncan Heath, and Ms. Jennifer Rigby, and to the copyeditor, Ms. Alison Foskett, for their vigilant publishing contributions. I elaborated upon this work in a lecture on "Male Genital Exhibitionism", delivered at a conference on "Indecent Exposure?: Exhibitionism, Art, Media and Psychoanalysis", held on 9th February, 2002, at the Starr Auditorium at the Tate Modern in London (Kahr, 2002).

Chapter 4: From Penile Trauma to Flashing: A Case of Forensic Disability Psychotherapy

I first published a much earlier incarnation of this clinical material in an essay on "Penile Trauma and Genital Exhibitionism: From Castration Anxiety to Verbal Potency" (Kahr, 2019e), which appeared in *The International Journal of Forensic Psychotherapy*, due to the courtesy of the editors-in-chief at that time, Ms. Jessica Collier and Dr. Carine Minne, and the Publisher of Phoenix Publishing House, Mrs. Kate Pearce. I then produced a more elaborated version as a chapter entitled "Insults and Spears: The Tribulations of Forensic Disability Psychotherapy" (Kahr, 2021c), released in a book edited by Professor Nigel Beail, Dr. Patricia Frankish, and Dr. Allan Skelly (2021), entitled *Trauma and Intellectual Disability: Acknowledgement, Identification and Intervention*, published by Pavilion / Pavilion Publishing and Media in Shoreham by Sea in West Sussex. I owe my gratitude to all of these colleagues and publishers for having kindly facilitated these important projects. I have since rewritten and updated these previous versions most considerably.

Chapter 5: Fragile Monster: How to Make a Paedophile Talk

This material appears here in print for the very first time.

Chapter 6: When Daddy Kills the Dog: Pet Murder and the Infanticidal Attachment

This material appears here in print for the very first time.

Chapter 7: Castration Anxiety in Men Who Murder

I presented a much earlier version of this article, entitled "Castration Anxiety in Men Who Murder" (Kahr, 2018i), on 11th December, 2018, at a panel on "Criminal Minds", part of the Seminar Series on "Spotlight on the Archive: Film and Psychoanalysis in Focus", organised by Professor Caroline Bainbridge, and chaired by Professor Candida Yates, designed to celebrate the centenary of *The International Journal of Psychoanalysis*. This event, held quite appropriately in the Sigmund Freud Room at Byron House, headquarters of the British Psychoanalytical Society in London, and co-sponsored by Media and the Inner World – a joint research network based at the School of Arts at the University of Roehampton in London, and at the Faculty of Media and Communication at Bournemouth University, in Ferne Barrow, in Poole, in the county of Dorset – provided us all with an opportunity to examine severe forensic psychopathology, aided by insights from the cinema. I wish to convey my thanks not only to Professor Bainbridge and Professor Yates but, also, to the late Dr. Dana Birksted-Breen and to Dr. Cleo Van Velsen for their comments. Additionally, I wish to communicate my deep appreciation to Dr. Carine Minne, Chair of the Sohn Seminar at the British Psychoanalytical Society, for having kindly invited me to speak with forensic psychoanalytical colleagues about "The Case of Joseph Kallinger: My Reminiscences of a Multiple Murderer", on 8th March, 2022, via Zoom (Kahr, 2022e). Dr. Minne, as ever, offered many extremely helpful insights about this patient, whom I had the privilege of meeting in 1985. And I owe many thanks to the highly experienced members of the Sohn Seminar, a unique, monthly space in which forensic psychoanalytical practitioners enjoy the rich opportunity to share clinical material in a confidential manner. A shorter version appeared in print in *The International Journal of Forensic Psychotherapy* (Kahr, 2024b). I express immense gratitude to Dr. Carine Minne, the Editor-in-Chief, and to Ms. Annie Pesskin, the Managing Editor, and of, course, to Mrs. Kate Pearce, the Publisher, and to Mrs. Anita Mason, the copyeditor, and to Ms. Anita Higgins Taylor, the journal's former administrator, for their warm encouragement of this essay.

Chapter 8: The Sub-Clinical Psychopath: Committing Crimes Without Breaking the Law

I published an earlier version of this chapter under the title "Committing Crimes without Breaking the Law: Unconscious Sadism in the 'Non-Forensic' Patient"

(Kahr, 2018d), which appeared in the *Festschrift* which I had the honour of editing about the life and work of the esteemed founder of modern forensic psychotherapy, Profesora Estela Valentina Welldon, entitled *New Horizons in Forensic Psychotherapy: Exploring the Work of Estela V. Welldon* (Kahr, 2018a), first published by Karnac Books of London in the "Forensic Psychotherapy Monograph Series", and now published by Routledge, part of the Taylor and Francis Group of London and Abingdon, Oxfordshire, in a hardback edition (Kahr, 2019b). I then presented an expanded version of this material under the title "Sub-Clinical Psychopathy" (Kahr, 2020e), one of the lectures for the "Diploma in Psychopathology: Theory and Practice" course, sponsored by Confer of Woodbridge, Suffolk, at the Theatre Showroom, in the October Gallery, at Lundonia House, in Holborn, in Central London, on 5th March, 2020. Quite poignantly, this happened to be the very last lecture that I ever delivered *in-person* prior to the outbreak of the dreadful COVID-19 pandemic in the United Kingdom. For the next two years, I delivered all of my subsequent presentations via Zoom, before resuming my in-person lectures – a forensic talk, in fact – in May, 2022 (Kahr, 2022f).

Chapter 9: Criminality in the Bedroom: Unconscious Sadism in Non-Forensic Couples

An earlier version of this chapter appeared as a text entitled, "Sexual Cruelty in the Marital Bed: Unconscious Sadism in Non-Forensic Couples" (Kahr, 2018e), published in a book edited by Dr. Amita Sehgal (2018) on *Sadism: Psychoanalytic Developmental Perspectives*, commissioned for the "Forensic Psychotherapy Monograph Series", originally published by Mr. Oliver Rathbone of Karnac Books and now released by Routledge / Taylor and Francis Group, under the welcome supervision of Ms. Susannah Frearson. I extend my thanks to each of these individuals for having cared for this project with such thoughtfulness. I based this material upon a presentation which I delivered on "Sexual Cruelty in the Marital Bed: Unconscious Sadism in Non-Forensic Couples" (Kahr, 2014c), part of a series of evening events on "Working Psychotherapeutically with Sadism: A Seminar Series for Psychotherapists and Psychologists", organised by Ms. Jane Ryan of Confer in London.

Conclusion: The Future of Forensic Psychoanalysis

Several of the discussion points and hypotheses and recommendations contained within this final section first appeared in a chapter in my book, *Dangerous Lunatics: Trauma, Criminality, and Forensic Psychotherapy* (Kahr, 2020b), published by Confer Books of London, to which I have already made reference (see above). Once again, I thank the former Publisher, Dr. Stephen Setterberg, for his visionary contributions. Since the appearance of my book, I have enjoyed the honour of having corresponded with Dr. Setterberg about global violence, amid the horrors of the atrocities in Ukraine; and those conversations have enhanced my understanding of the need for greater preventative work.

Professor Brett Kahr's Selected Forensic Publications: 1985–2025

1985

A Taste for Murder. Book Review of Brian Masters. *Killing for Company: The Case of Dennis Nilsen*. *Broadsheet*. 27th April–3rd May, pp. 10–11.

1989

Historical Perspectives on Incest. Q.E.D. Audio Cassette. London: Q.E.D. Recording Services Limited.

1991

The Sexual Molestation of Children: Historical Perspectives. *Journal of Psychohistory*, *19*, 191–214.

1994

The Historical Foundations of Ritual Abuse: An Excavation of Ancient Infanticide. In Valerie Sinason (Ed.). *Treating Survivors of Satanist Abuse*, pp. 45–56. London: Routledge.
Sadomasochism and Child Sexual Abuse: A Response to Man Cheung Chung. *Journal of the Society for Existential Analysis*, *5*, 121–124.
A.P.P. Conference on Satanist Abuse: Psychodynamic Perspectives. 4th December 1993. *Bulletin of the Association of Child Psychotherapists*, *34*, 13–15.
Child Abuse Has an Ancient History. *The Independent*. 2nd May, p. 19.

1996

Visions of Horror. Book Review of Valerie Sinason (Ed.). *Treating Survivors of Satanist Abuse*. *Tavistock and Portman Gazette*. Autumn, pp. 69–70.

1997

From the Treatment of a Compulsive Spitter: Semen, Saliva, and Alcohol Equivalents. *Intoxication, Crime and the Forensic Patient: Abstracts*, p. 10. Conference on "Intoxication,

Crime and the Forensic Patient". Sixth International Conference of the International Association for Forensic Psychotherapy. Regent's College Conference Centre, Regent's College, Inner Circle, Regent's Park, London.

Book Review of Valerie Sinason (Ed.). *Treating Survivors of Satanist Abuse. Journal of Psychohistory*, *24*, 417–421.

Book Review of Martin Obler and Thomas Clavin. *Fatal Analysis: A True Story of Professional Privilege and Murder*, p. 13. In Brett Kahr. The Psychotherapist's Library. *Newsletter. School of Psychotherapy and Counselling*. Spring Term, pp. 12–14.

Book Review of Graham J. Towl and David A. Crighton. *The Handbook of Psychology for Forensic Practitioners*, p. 14. In Brett Kahr. The Psychotherapist's Library. *Newsletter. School of Psychotherapy and Counselling*. Spring Term, pp. 12–14.

1998

The Forensic Psychotherapy Book Series. *I.A.F.P. Newsletter*. [Newsletter of the International Association for Forensic Psychotherapy], *2*, 5.

In Memory of Judith Swindells. *I.A.F.P. Newsletter*. [Newsletter of the International Association for Forensic Psychotherapy], *2*, 20.

1999

Sigmund Freud and the Case of the Paedophile. *Psychotherapy Review*, *1*, 89–90.

The Adventures of a Psychotherapist: Reminiscences of Flora Rheta Schreiber. *Psychotherapy Review*, *1*, 148–150.

2000

In Memoriam: Dr. Murray Cox. *Psychotherapy Review*, *2*, 214–215.

Academic Recognition for Forensic Psychotherapy. *Psychotherapy Review*, *2*, 261.

2001

Forensic Psychotherapy and Psychopathology: Winnicottian Perspectives. London: H. Karnac (Books), and New York: Other Press.

Exhibitionism. Duxford, Cambridgeshire: Icon Books.

Winnicott's Contribution to the Study of Dangerousness. In Brett Kahr (Ed.). *Forensic Psychotherapy and Psychopathology: Winnicottian Perspectives*, pp. 1–10. London: H. Karnac (Books), and New York: Other Press.

The Legacy of Infanticide. *Journal of Psychohistory*, *29*, 40–44.

Series Foreword. In Sandra L. Bloom (Ed.). *Violence: A Public Health Menace and a Public Health Approach*, pp. vii–x. London: H. Karnac (Books).

Series Foreword. In Jessica Williams Saunders (Ed.). *Life within Hidden Walls: Psychotherapy in Prisons*, pp. vii–x. London: H. Karnac (Books).

Series Foreword. In Brett Kahr (Ed.). *Forensic Psychotherapy and Psychopathology: Winnicottian Perspectives*, pp. ix–xii. London: H. Karnac (Books), and New York: Other Press.

Acknowledgements. In Brett Kahr (Ed.). *Forensic Psychotherapy and Psychopathology: Winnicottian Perspectives*, pp. xvii–xviii. London: H. Karnac (Books), and New York: Other Press.

2002

Kennedy, Roger; Abel-Hirsch, Nicola; Pajaczkowska, Claire, and Kahr, Brett (2002). *Témata psychoanalýzy II: Libido, Eros, Perverze, Exhibicionismus*. Jiří Papoušek (Transl.). Prague: Portál / Edice Spektrum.

Exhibicionismus. In Roger Kennedy, Nicola Abel-Hirsch, Claire Pajaczkowska, and Brett Kahr. *Témata psychoanalýzy II: Libido, Eros, Perverze, Exhibicionismus*. Jiří Papoušek (Transl.), pp. 113–154. Prague: Portál / Edice Spektrum.

Multiple Personality Disorder and Schizophrenia: An Interview with Professor Flora Rheta Schreiber. In Valerie Sinason (Ed.). *Attachment, Trauma and Multiplicity: Working with Dissociative Identity Disorder*, pp. 240–264. Hove, East Sussex: Brunner-Routledge / Taylor and Francis Group.

New Developments in Forensic Psychotherapy. *Frame: The Newsletter for the International Association for Forensic Psychotherapy*, *6*, 84.

2004

Juvenile Paedophilia: The Psychodynamics of an Adolescent. In Charles W. Socarides and Loretta R. Loeb (Eds.). *The Mind of the Paedophile: Psychoanalytic Perspectives*, pp. 95–119. London: H. Karnac (Books).

Series Foreword. In Charles W. Socarides and Loretta R. Loeb (Eds.). *The Mind of the Paedophile: Psychoanalytic Perspectives*, pp. xi–xiv. London: H. Karnac (Books).

2005

Exibicionismo. Carlos Mendes Rosa (Transl.). São Paulo: Viver Mente e Cérebro / T.T. Duetto / Segmento-Duetto, and Rio de Janeiro: Relume Dumará Editora.

Series Foreword. In Lynn Greenwood (Ed.). *Violent Adolescents: Understanding the Destructive Impulse*, pp. xiii–xvi. London: H. Karnac (Books).

2006

Ekshibicionizam. Predrag Raos (Transl.). Zagreb: Naklada Jesenski i Turk.

Winnicott's Contribution to the Study of Dangerousness. [Revised Version]. In Rod Morgan and Sheila Hollins. *Young People and Crime: Improving Provision for Children Who Offend*, pp. 39–47. London: Karnac (Books), and Ruislip, Middlesex: Winnicott Clinic of Psychotherapy.

2007

The Infanticidal Attachment. *Attachment: New Directions in Psychotherapy and Relational Psychoanalysis*, *1*, 117–132.

The Infanticidal Attachment in Schizophrenia and Dissociative Identity Disorder. *Attachment: New Directions in Psychotherapy and Relational Psychoanalysis*, *1*, 305–309.

2008

Psychological Necrophilia: On Couples Wedded to Deadliness. *Psychoanalytic Perspectives on Couple Work*, *4*, 68–76.

Series Foreword. In Rosemary Campher (Ed.). *Violence in Children: Understanding and Helping Those Who Harm*, pp. xi–xiv. London: Karnac Books.

Series Foreword. In Ronald Doctor (Ed.). *Murder: A Psychotherapeutic Investigation*, pp. ix–xii. London: Karnac Books.

Series Foreword. In John Gordon and Gabriel Kirtchuk (Eds.). *Psychic Assaults and Frightened Clinicians: Countertransference in Forensic Settings*, pp. ix–xii. London: Karnac Books.

Series Foreword. In Adah Sachs and Graeme Galton (Eds.). *Forensic Aspects of Dissociative Identity Disorder*, pp. xiii–xvi. London: Karnac Books.

Prefacio. In Lynn Greenwood (Ed.). *Adolescentes violentos: La comprensión del impulso destructivo*. Tamega Viñes Barrobés (Transl.), pp. 11–16. Madrid: Neo Person.

2010

Exibicionismo. Miguel Serras Pereira (Transl.). Coimbra: Almedina.

Defending Lady Macbeth: Testimony of an Expert Witness. *American Imago*, *67*, 453–462.

2011

Multiple Personality Disorder and Schizophrenia: An Interview with Professor Flora Rheta Schreiber. [Revised Version]. In Valerie Sinason (Ed.). *Attachment, Trauma and Multiplicity: Second Edition. Working with Dissociative Identity Disorder*, pp. 204–214. London: Routledge / Taylor and Francis Group, and Hove, East Sussex: Routledge / Taylor and Francis Group.

Dr Paul Weston and the Bloodstained Couch. *International Journal of Psychoanalysis*, *92*, 1051–1058.

An Interview with Estela V. Welldon, July 1996. In Estela V. Welldon. *Playing with Dynamite: A Personal Approach to the Psychoanalytic Understanding of Perversions, Violence, and Criminality*, pp. 1–24. London: Karnac Books.

An Interview with Estela V. Welldon, July 1999. In Estela V. Welldon. *Playing with Dynamite: A Personal Approach to the Psychoanalytic Understanding of Perversions, Violence, and Criminality*, pp. 98–107. London: Karnac Books.

An Interview with Estela V. Welldon, November 2010. In Estela V. Welldon. *Playing with Dynamite: A Personal Approach to the Psychoanalytic Understanding of Perversions, Violence, and Criminality*, pp. 252–262. London: Karnac Books.

Series Foreword. In Estela V. Welldon. *Playing with Dynamite: A Personal Approach to the Psychoanalytic Understanding of Perversions, Violence, and Criminality*, pp. xiii–xvi. London: Karnac Books.

Foreword. In Estela V. Welldon. *Playing with Dynamite: A Personal Approach to the Psychoanalytic Understanding of Perversions, Violence, and Criminality*, pp. xx–xxii. London: Karnac Books.

2012

The Infanticidal Origins of Psychosis: The Role of Trauma in Schizophrenia. In Judy Yellin and Kate White (Eds.). *Shattered States: Disorganised Attachment and its Repair. The John Bowlby Memorial Conference Monograph 2007*, pp. 7–126. London: Karnac Books.

Le Divan taché de sang du Dr Paul Weston. Marcel Hudon (Transl.). In Louis Brunet, Jean-Michel Quinodoz, Pierre Dajez, Danielle Goldstein, François Gross, Florence Guignard, Céline Gür, Marcel Hudon, Luc Magnenat, Diana Messina Pizzuti, André Renaud, Michel Sanchez-Cardenas, and Patricia Waltz (Eds.). *L'Année psychanalytique internationale: 2012. Traduction en langue française d'un choix de textes publiés en 2011 dans* The International Journal of Psychoanalysis, pp. 199–210. Paris: Éditions In Press.

Series Foreword. In Timothy Keogh. *The Internal World of the Juvenile Sex Offender: Through a Glass Darkly then Face to Face*, pp. xi–xiv. London: Karnac Books.

2014

Una entrevista con Estela V. Welldon: Julio de 1996. In Estela V. Welldon. *Jugar con dinamita: Una comprensión psicoanalítica de las perversiones, la violencia y la criminalidad.* Loida Díez Jiménez (Transl.), pp. 45–72. Madrid: Psimática Editorial.

Entrevista con Estela V. Welldon: Julio de 1999. In Estela V. Welldon. *Jugar con dinamita: Una comprensión psicoanalítica de las perversiones, la violencia y la criminalidad.* Loida Díez Jiménez (Transl.), pp. 161–172. Madrid: Psimática Editorial.

Entrevista con Estela V. Welldon: Noviembre de 2010. In Estela V. Welldon. *Jugar con dinamita: Una comprensión psicoanalítica de las perversiones, la violencia y la criminalidad.* Loida Díez Jiménez (Transl.), pp. 335–347. Madrid: Psimática Editorial.

Prólogo de la serie. In Estela V. Welldon. *Jugar con dinamita: Una comprensión psicoanalítica de las perversiones, la violencia y la criminalidad.* Loida Díez Jiménez (Transl.), pp. 15–18. Madrid: Psimática Editorial.

Prólogo. In Estela V. Welldon. *Jugar con dinamita: Una comprensión psicoanalítica de las perversiones, la violencia y la criminalidad.* Loida Díez Jiménez (Transl.), pp. 31–33. Madrid: Psimática Editorial.

Series Editor's Foreword: Towards Forensic Disability Psychotherapy. In Alan Corbett. *Disabling Perversions: Forensic Psychotherapy with People with Intellectual Disabilities*, pp. xiii–xxii. London: Karnac Books.

Una entrevista con Estela V. Welldon: Julio de 1996. In Estela V. Welldon. *Jugar con dinamita: Una comprensión psicoanalítica de las perversiones, la violencia y la criminalidad.* [Revised Edition]. Loida Díez Jiménez (Transl.), pp. 45–72. Madrid: Psimática Editorial.

Entrevista con Estela V. Welldon: Julio de 1999. In Estela V. Welldon. *Jugar con dinamita: Una comprensión psicoanalítica de las perversiones, la violencia y la criminalidad.* [Revised Edition]. Loida Díez Jiménez (Transl.), pp. 161–172. Madrid: Psimática Editorial.

Entrevista con Estela V. Welldon: Noviembre de 2010. In Estela V. Welldon. *Jugar con dinamita: Una comprensión psicoanalítica de las perversiones, la violencia y la criminalidad.* [Revised Edition]. Loida Díez Jiménez (Transl.), pp. 335–347. Madrid: Psimática Editorial.

Prólogo de la serie. In Estela V. Welldon. *Jugar con dinamita: Una comprensión psicoanalítica de las perversiones, la violencia y la criminalidad.* [Revised Edition]. Loida Díez Jiménez (Transl.), pp. 15–18. Madrid: Psimática Editorial.

Prólogo. In Estela V. Welldon. *Jugar con dinamita: Una comprensión psicoanalítica de las perversiones, la violencia y la criminalidad*. [Revised Edition]. Loida Díez Jiménez (Transl.), pp. 31–33. Madrid: Psimática Editorial.

2016

"Happy Birthdeath to Me": Surviving Death Wishes in Early Infancy. In Stella Acquarone (Ed.). *Surviving the Early Years: The Importance of Early Intervention with Babies at Risk*, pp. 57–84. London: Karnac Books.

Cruauté sexuelle dans le lit conjugal: Sadisme inconscient des couples ordinaries. Bernadette Legrand (Transl.). *Dialogue: Familles et couples*, Number *212*, 25–37.

Series Editor's Foreword. In Barry Maletzky. *Sexual Abuse and the Sexual Offender: Common Man or Monster?*, pp. xi–xiv. London: Karnac Books.

Series Editor's Foreword. In Alan Corbett. *Psychotherapy with Male Survivors of Sexual Abuse: The Invisible Men*, pp. xiii–xviii. London: Karnac Books.

On Forensic Psychotherapy. Saturday Forensic Forum: Psychotherapy with Complex Patients in Difficult Settings. [http://saturdayforensicforum.com/2016/01/08/on-forensic-psychotherapy/].

Book Review of Alan Corbett. *Psychotherapy with Male Survivors of Sexual Abuse: The Invisible Men*. In Brett Kahr. Top 10 Books: Brett Kahr's Top Ten Psychotherapy Books – 2016. Confer. [http://www.confer.uk.com/booksof2016.html].

Book Review of Estela V. Welldon. *Sex Now Talk Later*. In Brett Kahr. Top 10 Books: Brett Kahr's Top Ten Psychotherapy Books – 2016. Confer. [http://www.confer.uk.com/booksof2016.html].

2017

An Interview with Estela V. Welldon, July 1996. In Estela V. Welldon. *Playing with Dynamite: A Personal Approach to the Psychoanalytic Understanding of Perversions, Violence, and Criminality*. [Russian Translation]. Konstantin Nemirovskiy (Transl.), pp. 39–69. Moscow: Publisher "Peyeero".

An Interview with Estela V. Welldon, July 1999. In Estela V. Welldon. *Playing with Dynamite: A Personal Approach to the Psychoanalytic Understanding of Perversions, Violence, and Criminality*. [Russian Translation]. Konstantin Nemirovskiy (Transl.), pp. 164–176. Moscow: Publisher "Peyeero".

An Interview with Estela V. Welldon, November 2010. In Estela V. Welldon. *Playing with Dynamite: A Personal Approach to the Psychoanalytic Understanding of Perversions, Violence, and Criminality*. [Russian Translation]. Konstantin Nemirovskiy (Transl.), pp. 353–365. Moscow: Publisher "Peyeero".

Untitled Remarks, pp. 139–142, 143–144, 147, 148–149. In Identity Theft in the Talented Mr. Ripley: Panel Discussion. In A Psychoanalytic Discussion of *The Talented Mr. Ripley*: (The Faction, New Diorama Theatre. London, February 2015). Based on a Panel Discussion Organized by The Faction and Media and the Inner World. *Free Associations*, Number *70*, 135–150. *Free Associations*. [http://freeassociations.org.uk/FA_New/OJS/index.php/fa/article/view/156/172].

Identity Theft in the Talented Mr. Ripley: Panel Discussion. In A Psychoanalytic Discussion of *The Talented Mr. Ripley*: (The Faction, New Diorama Theatre. London, February 2015). Based on a Panel Discussion Organized by The Faction and Media and the

Inner World. *Free Associations*, Number *70*, 135–150. *Free Associations*. (Co-authored by Mark Leipacher, Christopher Hughes, Iain MacRury, and Candida Yates). [http://freeassociations.org.uk/FA_New/OJS/index.php/fa/article/view/156/172].

Alan Corbett: 1963–2016. *British Journal of Psychotherapy*, *33*, 262–263.

Dr Alan Corbett: (1963–2016). Champion of Disabled People. *The Psychotherapist*, Number *65*, p. 26.

Series Foreword. In Estela V. Welldon. *Playing with Dynamite: A Personal Approach to the Psychoanalytic Understanding of Perversions, Violence, and Criminality*. [Russian Translation]. Konstantin Nemirovskiy (Transl.), pp. 15–19. Moscow: Publisher "Peyeero".

Foreword. In Estela V. Welldon. *Playing with Dynamite: A Personal Approach to the Psychoanalytic Understanding of Perversions, Violence, and Criminality*. [Russian Translation]. Konstantin Nemirovskiy (Transl.), pp. 23–26. Moscow: Publisher "Peyeero".

Dr Alan Corbett: In Praise of an Outstanding Psychotherapist. Confer. [http://www.confer.uk.com/blogs/blog-corbett.html].

Dr. Alan Corbett: A Man Enormously Loved. Karnacology / Karnac Books. [https://karnacology.com/hall-of-fame/alan-corbett/].

Dr. Alan Corbett: A Man Enormously Loved. Karnacology / Karnac Books. [http://karnacbooks.com/blog/post-alan-corbett/202].

Remembering Alan Corbett. International Association for Forensic Psychotherapy. [http://forensicpsychotherapy.com/latest-news/remembering-alan-corbett].

Book Review of Estela V. Welldon. *Sex Now Talk Later*. In Brett Kahr. Top 10 Books: Brett Kahr's Top Ten Psychotherapy Books – 2017. Confer. [http://www.confer.uk.com/booksof2017.html].

2018

New Horizons in Forensic Psychotherapy: Exploring the Work of Estela V. Welldon. London: Karnac Books.

Introduction: Estela at La Scala. In Brett Kahr (Ed.). *New Horizons in Forensic Psychotherapy: Exploring the Work of Estela V. Welldon*, pp. 1–14. London: Karnac Books.

"No Intolerable Persons" or "Lewd Pregnant Women": Towards a History of Forensic Psychoanalysis. In Brett Kahr (Ed.). *New Horizons in Forensic Psychotherapy: Exploring the Work of Estela V. Welldon*, pp. 17–87. London: Karnac Books.

Committing Crimes without Breaking the Law: Unconscious Sadism in the "Non-Forensic" Patient. In Brett Kahr (Ed.). *New Horizons in Forensic Psychotherapy: Exploring the Work of Estela V. Welldon*, pp. 239–261. London: Karnac Books.

Sexual Cruelty in the Marital Bed: Unconscious Sadism in Non-Forensic Couples. In Amita Sehgal (Ed.). *Sadism: Psychoanalytic Developmental Perspectives*, pp. 93–117. London: Routledge / Taylor and Francis Group, and Abingdon, Oxfordshire: Routledge / Taylor and Francis Group.

Acknowledgements. In Brett Kahr (Ed.). *New Horizons in Forensic Psychotherapy: Exploring the Work of Estela V. Welldon*, pp. xv–xvi. London: Karnac Books.

Series Editor's Foreword. In Brett Kahr (Ed.). *New Horizons in Forensic Psychotherapy: Exploring the Work of Estela V. Welldon*, pp. xi–xiii. London: Karnac Books.

Series Editor's Foreword. In Amita Sehgal (Ed.). *Sadism: Psychoanalytic Developmental Perspectives*, pp. ix–xi. London: Routledge / Taylor and Francis Group, and Abingdon, Oxfordshire: Routledge / Taylor and Francis Group.

Book Review of Alisa Roth. *Insane: America's Criminal Treatment of Mental Illness.* In Brett Kahr. Brett Kahr's Top Five Books for 2018: A Mid-Year Round-Up. *Autumn Programme 2018: Celebrating 20 Years of Confer*, p. 31. London: Confer.

Book Review of Alisa Roth. *Insane: America's Criminal Treatment of Mental Illness.* In Brett Kahr. Top 10 Books: Brett Kahr's Top Ten Psychotherapy Books – 2018. Confer. [www.confer.uk.com/booksof2018.html].

2019

Forensic Psychotherapy and Psychopathology: Winnicottian Perspectives. [Hardback Edition]. London: Routledge / Taylor and Francis Group, and Abingdon, Oxfordshire: Routledge / Taylor and Francis Group.

New Horizons in Forensic Psychotherapy: Exploring the Work of Estela V. Welldon. [Hardback Edition]. London: Routledge / Taylor and Francis Group, and Abingdon, Oxfordshire: Routledge / Taylor and Francis Group.

Winnicott's Contribution to the Study of Dangerousness. In Brett Kahr (Ed.). *Forensic Psychotherapy and Psychopathology: Winnicottian Perspectives*, pp. 1–10. [Hardback Edition]. London: Routledge / Taylor and Francis Group, and Abingdon, Oxfordshire: Routledge / Taylor and Francis Group.

Introduction: Estela at La Scala. In Brett Kahr (Ed.). *New Horizons in Forensic Psychotherapy: Exploring the Work of Estela V. Welldon*, pp. 1–14. [Hardback Edition]. London: Routledge / Taylor and Francis Group, and Abingdon, Oxfordshire: Routledge / Taylor and Francis Group.

"No Intolerable Persons" or "Lewd Pregnant Women": Towards a History of Forensic Psychoanalysis. In Brett Kahr (Ed.). *New Horizons in Forensic Psychotherapy: Exploring the Work of Estela V. Welldon*, pp. 17–87. [Hardback Edition]. London: Routledge / Taylor and Francis Group, and Abingdon, Oxfordshire: Routledge / Taylor and Francis Group.

Committing Crimes without Breaking the Law: Unconscious Sadism in the "Non-Forensic" Patient. In Brett Kahr (Ed.). *New Horizons in Forensic Psychotherapy: Exploring the Work of Estela V. Welldon*, pp. 239–261. [Hardback Edition]. London: Routledge / Taylor and Francis Group, and Abingdon, Oxfordshire: Routledge / Taylor and Francis Group.

Romans Wewnątrzmałżeński: Erotzysm I Sadyzm w Sypialni. In *Twórcze Związki Miłości i Nienawiści: 6.04.2019. Warszawa. IV Konferencja Pracując Psychoanalitycznie z Parami*. Jacek Mądry (Transl.), pp. 13–38. Warsaw: Specjalistyczna Poradnia Rodzinna dz. Bemowo m.st. Warszawy / Polskie Towarzystwo Psychoterapii Psychoanalitycznej.

The Intra-Marital Affair: Eroticism and Sadism in the Bedroom. In *Twórcze Związki Miłości i Nienawiści: 6.04.2019. Warszawa. IV Konferencja Pracując Psychoanalitycznie z Parami*, pp. 41–63. Warsaw: Specjalistyczna Poradnia Rodzinna dz. Bemowo m.st. Warszawy / Polskie Towarzystwo Psychoterapii Psychoanalitycznej.

'Slashing the Teddy Bear's Tummy with a Carving Knife': The Infanticidal Roots of Schizophrenia. *British Journal of Psychotherapy*, *35*, 399–416.

Penile Trauma and Genital Exhibitionism: From Castration Anxiety to Verbal Potency. *International Journal of Forensic Psychotherapy*, *1*, 93–108.

Professor Estela V. Welldon: Recipient of the Lifetime Achievement Award of the British Psychoanalytic Council. Presented on Saturday, 16th November, 2019, at the British Library, London. *International Journal of Forensic Psychotherapy*, *1*, 171–172.

Rosemary Assunta Campher (1962–2018). *New Psychotherapist*, Number 70, p. 10.

Rosemary Assunta Campher (1962–2018). *New Psychotherapist*, Number 70, p. 10. United Kingdom Council for Psychotherapy. [https://www.psychotherapy.org.uk/wp-content/uploads/2019/11/70_New_Psychotherapist_spring_2019.pdf].

Series Editor's Foreword. In Pamela Windham Stewart and Jessica Collier (Eds.). *The End of the Sentence: Psychotherapy with Female Offenders*, pp. ix–xiv. [Hardback Edition]. London: Routledge / Taylor and Francis Group, and Abingdon, Oxfordshire: Routledge / Taylor and Francis Group.

Series Editor's Foreword. In Pamela Windham Stewart and Jessica Collier (Eds.). *The End of the Sentence: Psychotherapy with Female Offenders*, pp. ix–xiv. [Paperback Edition]. London: Routledge / Taylor and Francis Group, and Abingdon, Oxfordshire: Routledge / Taylor and Francis Group.

Series Foreword. In Brett Kahr (Ed.). *Forensic Psychotherapy and Psychopathology: Winnicottian Perspectives*, pp. ix–xii. [Hardback Edition]. London: Routledge / Taylor and Francis Group, and Abingdon, Oxfordshire: Routledge / Taylor and Francis Group.

Acknowledgements. In Brett Kahr (Ed.). *Forensic Psychotherapy and Psychopathology: Winnicottian Perspectives*, pp. xvii–xviii. [Hardback Edition]. London: Routledge / Taylor and Francis Group, and Abingdon, Oxfordshire: Routledge / Taylor and Francis Group.

Series Editor's Foreword. In Brett Kahr (Ed.). *New Horizons in Forensic Psychotherapy: Exploring the Work of Estela V. Welldon*, pp. xi–xiii. [Hardback Edition]. London: Routledge / Taylor and Francis Group, and Abingdon, Oxfordshire: Routledge / Taylor and Francis Group.

Acknowledgements. In Brett Kahr (Ed.). *New Horizons in Forensic Psychotherapy: Exploring the Work of Estela V. Welldon*, pp. xv–xvi. [Hardback Edition]. London: Routledge / Taylor and Francis Group, and Abingdon, Oxfordshire: Routledge / Taylor and Francis Group.

Professor Estela V. Welldon: Recipient of the Lifetime Achievement Award of the British Psychoanalytic Council. Presented on Saturday, 16th November, 2019, at the British Library, London. International Association for Forensic Psychotherapy. [https://www.forensicpsychotherapy.org/news-events-1].

2020

Bombs in the Consulting Room: Surviving Psychological Shrapnel. London: Routledge / Taylor and Francis Group, and Abingdon, Oxfordshire: Routledge / Taylor and Francis Group.

Dangerous Lunatics: Trauma, Criminality, and Forensic Psychotherapy. London: Confer / Confer Books.

Banged Up: A Chilling Glimpse into British Prisons. *International Journal of Forensic Psychotherapy*, 2, 173–176.

Professor Estela V. Welldon: Recipient of the Lifetime Achievement Award of the British Psychoanalytic Council. Presented on Saturday 16 November 2019, at the British Library, London. *New Associations*, Number 30, pp. 10–11.

Book Review of David Livingstone Smith. *On Inhumanity: Dehumanization and How to Resist It*. In Brett Kahr. Brett Kahr's Top Ten Books of 2020. Confer. [https://www.confer.uk.com/brett-kahrs-books-of-2020.html].

2021

Freud's Pandemics: Surviving Global War, Spanish Flu, and the Nazis. London: Karnac / Karnac Books, Confer.

Insults and Spears: The Tribulations of Forensic Disability Psychotherapy. In Nigel Beail, Patricia Frankish, and Allan Skelly (Eds.). *Trauma and Intellectual Disability: Acknowledgement, Identification and Intervention*, pp. 175–188. Shoreham by Sea, West Sussex: Pavilion / Pavilion Publishing and Media.

Death Wishes Towards Babies: The Unconscious Roots of Schizophrenia. *Division / Review: A Quarterly Psychoanalytic Forum*, Number *23*, 14–15, 17–19, 21–23.

Did the Nazi Holocaust Cause Schizophrenia? *Attachment: New Directions in Psychotherapy and Relational Psychoanalysis*, *15*, 67–87.

On Patients Who Explode: Surviving Petrifying Psychotherapeutic Experiences. *International Journal of Forensic Psychotherapy*, *3*, 93–112.

Jeannie Milligan (1949–2021). *British Psychoanalytic Council eNewsletter*. June. E-Mail to Registrants of the British Psychoanalytic Council. 1st July.

Jeannie Milligan (1949–2021). *Couple and Family Psychoanalysis*, *11*, 219.

Jeannie Milligan (1949–2021): A Pioneer of Forensic Adolescent Psychotherapy. *International Journal of Forensic Psychotherapy*, *3*, 158–162.

Professor Sir Michael Peckham: A Memorial Tribute. *International Journal of Forensic Psychotherapy*, *3*, 163–165.

Jeannie Milligan. Deprivation and Delinquency in the Adolescent Forensic Patient. Brett Kahr (Ed.). *International Journal of Forensic Psychotherapy*, *3*, 133–140.

Abstract, p. 133. In Jeannie Milligan. Deprivation and Delinquency in the Adolescent Forensic Patient. Brett Kahr (Ed.). *International Journal of Forensic Psychotherapy*, *3*, 133–140.

Keywords, p. 133. In Jeannie Milligan. Deprivation and Delinquency in the Adolescent Forensic Patient. Brett Kahr (Ed.). *International Journal of Forensic Psychotherapy*, *3*, 133–140.

Editorial Introduction, pp. 133–134. In Jeannie Milligan. Deprivation and Delinquency in the Adolescent Forensic Patient. Brett Kahr (Ed.). *International Journal of Forensic Psychotherapy*, *3*, 133–140.

Book Review of Gwen Adshead and Eileen Horne. *The Devil You Know: Stories of Human Cruelty and Compassion*. In Brett Kahr. Brett Kahr's Top Ten Books of 2021. Confer. [https://www.confer.uk.com/brett-kahrs-books-of-2021.html].

Book Review of David Livingstone Smith. *Making Monsters: The Uncanny Power of Dehumanization*. In Brett Kahr. Brett Kahr's Top Ten Books of 2021. Confer. [https://www.confer.uk.com/brett-kahrs-books-of-2021.html].

2022

The Spitting Patient: Speaking with Sputum and Free-Associating with Saliva. In Raffaella Hilty (Ed.). *Primitive Bodily Communications in Psychotherapy: Embodied Expressions of a Disembodied Psyche*, pp. 1–49. London: Karnac / Karnac Books, Confer.

Chapter 1. In Raffaella Hilty (Ed.). *Primitive Bodily Communications in Psychotherapy: Embodied Expressions of a Disembodied Psyche*, pp. 201–207. London: Karnac / Karnac Books, Confer.

Foreword. In Masud Khan. *Diary of a Fallen Psychoanalyst: The Work Books of Masud Khan. 1967–1972*. Linda Hopkins and Steven Kuchuck (Eds.), pp. vii–xii. London: Karnac / Karnac Books, Confer.

Book Review of George Makari. *Of Fear and Strangers: A History of Xenophobia. International Journal of Forensic Psychotherapy*, 4, 74–77.

"Let the great axe fall": From Ancient Babylonian Torture to Modern Forensic Psychotherapy. Freud, Welldon, and the Humanisation of Criminality. *International Journal of Forensic Psychotherapy*, 4, 89–118.

"Let the Great Axe Fall": From Ancient Babylonian Torture to Modern Forensic Psychotherapy. Freud, Welldon, and the Humanization of Criminality. Plenary 1. *30th Annnual [sic] Conference: 13–14 May 2022. Violence as a Public Health Emergency: Preventing, Treating and Humanizing the Dangerous Mind. Exploring the Past, Present and Future of Forensic Psychotherapy*. Conference Programme [p. 12]. International Association for Forensic Psychotherapy. [https://www.forensicpsychotherapy.org/_files/ugd/ad20f2_871776fd509a4a118b6c453c1e15e06d.pdf].

2023

Filing Psychoanalytical Complaints: From Verbal Assaults to the Crushing of the Larynx. In Adah Sachs and Valerie Sinason (Eds.). *The Psychotherapist and the Professional Complaint: The Shadow Side of Therapy*, pp. 71–87, 220–222. London: Karnac / Karnac Books, Confer.

Chapter 6. In Adah Sachs and Valerie Sinason (Eds.). *The Psychotherapist and the Professional Complaint: The Shadow Side of Therapy*, pp. 220–222. London: Karnac / Karnac Books, Confer.

Intervista con Estela V. Welldon, luglio 1996. In Estela V. Welldon. *Giocando con la dinamite: Un personale approccio nella comprensione psicoanalitica della Perversione, Violenza e Criminalità*. Caterina Marchetti (Ed.). Marianna Caserio (Transl.), pp. 35–58. Turin: Kemet / Kemet Edizioni.

Intervista con Estela Welldon, luglio 1999. In Estela V. Welldon. *Giocando con la dinamite: Un personale approccio nella comprensione psicoanalitica della Perversione, Violenza e Criminalità*. Caterina Marchetti (Ed.). Marianna Caserio (Transl.), pp. 129–138. Turin: Kemet / Kemet Edizioni.

Un'intervista con Estela V. Welldon, novembre 2010. In Estela V. Welldon. *Giocando con la dinamite: Un personale approccio nella comprensione psicoanalitica della Perversione, Violenza e Criminalità*. Caterina Marchetti (Ed.). Marianna Caserio (Transl.), pp. 281–291. Turin: Kemet / Kemet Edizioni.

Jeffrey Dahmer: From Neurocriminology to Castration Anxiety. Netflix Series Released on 21 September 2022. *International Journal of Forensic Psychotherapy*, 5, 71–76.

Prefazione della collana Karnac. In Estela V. Welldon. *Giocando con la dinamite: Un personale approccio nella comprensione psicoanalitica della Perversione, Violenza e Criminalità*. Caterina Marchetti (Ed.). Marianna Caserio (Transl.), pp. 17–20. Turin: Kemet / Kemet Edizioni.

Prefazione. In Estela V. Welldon. *Giocando con la dinamite: Un personale approccio nella comprensione psicoanalitica della Perversione, Violenza e Criminalità*. Caterina Marchetti (Ed.). Marianna Caserio (Transl.), pp. 24–26. Turin: Kemet / Kemet Edizioni.

2024

Hidden Histories of British Psychoanalysis: From Freud's Death Bed to Laing's Missing Tooth. Bicester, Oxfordshire: Karnac / Karnac Books.

Castration Anxiety: A Neglected Aetiological Factor in the Male Murderer. *International Journal of Forensic Psychotherapy*, 6, 1–15.

Sira Dermen. Psychoanalytic Perspectives on Traumatised Children: The Armenian Experience. Brett Kahr (Ed.). *International Journal of Forensic Psychotherapy*, 6, 72–85.

Abstract, p. 72. In Sira Dermen. Psychoanalytic Perspectives on Traumatised Children: The Armenian Experience. Brett Kahr (Ed.). *International Journal of Forensic Psychotherapy*, 6, 72–85.

Keywords, p. 72. In Sira Dermen. Psychoanalytic Perspectives on Traumatised Children: The Armenian Experience. Brett Kahr (Ed.). *International Journal of Forensic Psychotherapy*, 6, 72–85.

Editorial Introduction: The Earthquake as a Forensic Patient, pp. 72–73. In Sira Dermen. Psychoanalytic Perspectives on Traumatised Children: The Armenian Experience. Brett Kahr (Ed.), pp. 72–73. *International Journal of Forensic Psychotherapy*, 6, 72–85.

Pet Murder and the Infanticidal Attachment. *International Journal of Forensic Psychotherapy*, 6. [In Press].

References

Abdill, Margaret N., and Juppé, Denise (Eds.). (1997). *Pets in Therapy*. Ravensdale, Washington: Idyll Arbor.

Abel, Gene G., and Osborn, Candice (1992). The Paraphilias: The Extent and Nature of Sexually Deviant and Criminal Behavior. *Psychiatric Clinics of North America*, *15*, 675–687.

Abraham, Karl (1917). Über Ejaculatio praecox. *Internationale Zeitschrift für ärztliche Psychoanalyse*, *4*, 171–186.

Abraham, Karl (1919). Erstes Korreferat. In Sigmund Freud, Sándor Ferenczi, Karl Abraham, Ernst Simmel, and Ernest Jones. *Zur Psychoanalyse der Kriegsneurosen*, pp. 31–41. Vienna: Internationaler Psychoanalytischer Verlag.

Abraham, Karl (1924). Letter to Sigmund Freud. 25th May. In Sigmund Freud and Karl Abraham (2009). *Briefwechsel 1907–1925: Vollständige Ausgabe. Band 2: 1915–1925*. Ernst Falzeder and Ludger M. Hermanns (Eds.), pp. 765–766. Vienna: Verlag Turia und Kant.

Abse, Leo (1973). *Private Member*. London: Macdonald London / Macdonald and Company (Publishers).

Abse, Leo (1989). *Margaret, Daughter of Beatrice: A Politician's Psycho-biography of Margaret Thatcher*. London: Jonathan Cape.

Abse, Leo (1994). *Wotan, My Enemy: Can Britain Live with the Germans in the European Union?* London: Robson Books.

Abse, Leo (1996). *The Man Behind the Smile: Tony Blair and the Politics of Perversion*. London: Robson Books.

Abse, Susanna (2014). Psychoanalysis, the Secure Society and the Role of Relationships. *Psychoanalytic Psychotherapy*, *28*, 295–303.

Acquarone, Stella (2002). Mother-Infant Psychotherapy: A Classification of Eleven Psychoanalytic Treatment Strategies. In Brett Kahr (Ed.). *The Legacy of Winnicott: Essays on Infant and Child Mental Health*, pp. 50–78. London: H. Karnac (Books) / Other Press.

Acquarone, Stella (2004). *Infant-Parent Psychotherapy: A Handbook*. London: H. Karnac (Books).

Acquarone, Stella M. (2008). Violence and Babies. In Rosemary Campher (Ed.). *Violence in Children: Understanding and Helping Those Who Harm*, pp. 95–127. London: Karnac Books.

Adshead, Gwen (2016). Making Minds More Secure: Remembering Gill McGauley. *Psychoanalytic Psychotherapy*, *30*, 298–299.

Adshead, Gwen (2018). Mothers-in-Law: Maternal Function and Child Protection. In Brett Kahr (Ed.). *New Horizons in Forensic Psychotherapy: Exploring the Work of Estela V. Welldon*, pp. 110–123. London: Karnac Books.

Adshead, Gwen, and Horne, Eileen (2021). *The Devil You Know: Stories of Human Cruelty and Compassion*. London: Faber / Faber and Faber.

Aichhorn, August (1925). *Verwahrloste Jugend: Die Psychoanalyse in der Fürsorgeerziehung. Zehn Vorträge zur ersten Einführung*. Vienna: Internationaler Psychoanalytischer Verlag.

Aichhorn, August (1932). Treatment Versus Punishment in the Management of Juvenile Delinquents. Frederick M. Sallagar (Transl.). In *Proceedings of the First International Congress on Mental Hygiene: Volume One*, pp. 582–598. New York: International Committee for Mental Hygiene.

Alabaster, Ernest (1899). *Notes and Commentaries on Chinese Criminal Law and Cognate Topics: With Special Relation to Ruling Cases. Together with a Brief Excursus on the Law of Property Chiefly Founded on the Writings of the Late Sir Chaloner Alabaster, K.C.M.G., etc., Sometime H.B.M. Consul-General in China*. London: Luzac and Company.

Alexander, Franz (1937). A Double Murder Committed by a Nineteen Year Old Boy. *Psychoanalytic Review*, *24*, 113–124.

Alexander, Franz, and Staub, Hugo (1929). *Der Verbrecher und seine Richter: Ein psychoanalytischer Einblick in die Welt der Paragraphen*. Vienna: Internationaler Psychoanalytischer Verlag.

Allen, Clifford (1962). *A Textbook of Psychosexual Disorders*. London: Oxford University Press.

Allen, Karen; Shykoff, Barbara E., and Izzo, Joseph L., Jr. (2001). Pet Ownership, but Not ACE Inhibitor Therapy, Blunts Home Blood Pressure Responses to Mental Stress. *Hypertension*, *38*, 815–820.

Alper, Mariel; Durose, Matthew R., and Markman, Joshua (2018). *2018 Update on Prisoner Recidivism: A 9-Year Follow-up Period (2005–2014)*. Washington, D.C.: Bureau of Justice Statistics, Office of Justice Programs, U.S. Department of Justice. Bureau of Justice Statistics. [https://www.bjs.gov/content/pub/pdf/18upr9yfup0514.pdf; Accessed on 9th March, 2019].

Anonymous (1868). Case of Mrs. Elizabeth Heggie. *American Journal of Insanity*, *25*, 1–51.

Anonymous (1871). The McFarland Trial. *American Journal of Insanity*, *27*, 265–273.

Anonymous (1926). Indian Psycho-Analytical Society: Annual Report, 1925, pp. 291–293. In Max Eitingon (Ed.). *Bulletin of the International Psycho-Analytical Association. International Journal of Psycho-Analysis*, *7*, 285–295.

Anonymous (1934). A "Harley Street" for the Anxious Poor: Treatment of "Frightening Illnesses". *Banffshire Advertiser*. 17th May, n.p. Box 1. Folder 1. Tavistock Clinic Archives. Library, Tavistock Centre, Tavistock and Portman NHS Trust, Belsize Park, London.

Anonymous (1995). Personal Communication to the Author. 19th February.

Anonymous (2024). Black Versace Dress of Elizabeth Hurley. Wikipedia. [https://en.wikipedia.org/wiki/Black_Versace_dress_of_Elizabeth_Hurley#Background; Accessed on 1st June, 2024].

Augsburger, Mareike; Basler, Kayley, and Maercker, Andreas (2019). Is There a Female Cycle of Violence After Exposure to Childhood Maltreatment?: A Meta-analysis. *Psychological Medicine*, *49*, 1776–1786.

Baatz, Simon (2008). *For the Thrill of It: Leopold, Loeb, and the Murder that Shocked Chicago*. New York: Harper / HarperCollins Publishers.

Balint, Michael (1951). On Punishing Offenders. In George B. Wilbur, Warner Muensterberger, and Lottie M. Maury (Eds.). *Psychoanalysis and Culture: Essays in Honor of Géza Róheim*, pp. 254–279. New York: International Universities Press.

Bartlett, Robert (2000). *England Under the Norman and Angevin Kings: 1075–1225*. Oxford: Clarendon Press / Oxford University Press.

Bassett, Margery (1943). Newgate Prison in the Middle Ages. *Speculum, 18*, 233–246.

Beail, Nigel; Frankish, Patricia, and Skelly, Allan (Eds.). (2021). *Trauma and Intellectual Disability: Acknowledgement, Identification and Intervention*. Shoreham by Sea, West Sussex: Pavilion / Pavilion Publishing and Media.

Beccaria, Cesare (1764). *Dei delitti e delle pene*. Brescia: Nicoló Bettoni, 1807.

Berlins, Marcel (1986). Portrait of a Serial Killer. *The Times*. 28th July, p. 10.

Bertin, Célia (1982). *La Dernière Bonaparte*. Paris: Librairie Académique Perrin.

Binion, Rudolph (1975). Hitler Looks East. In Lloyd deMause (Ed.). *The New Psychohistory*, pp. 181–198. New York: Psychohistory Press, Division of Atcom.

Binion, Rudolph (1976). *Hitler Among the Germans*. New York: Elsevier Scientific Publishing Company.

Blanton, Smiley (1929). Diary Entry. 2nd September. In Smiley Blanton (1971). *Diary of My Analysis with Sigmund Freud*, pp. 22–25. New York: Hawthorn Books.

Bloch, R. Howard (1991). *Medieval Misogyny and the Invention of Western Romantic Love*. Chicago, Illinois: University of Chicago Press.

Bloom, Sandra L. (Ed.). (2001). *Violence: A Public Health Menace and a Public Health Approach*. London: H. Karnac (Books).

Bollas, Christopher, and Sundelson, David (1995). *The New Informants: The Betrayal of Confidentiality in Psychoanalysis and Psychotherapy*. London: H. Karnac (Books).

Bonaparte, Marie (1927). Le Cas de Madame Lefebvre. *Revue Française de Psychanalyse, 1*, 149–198.

Bok, Hilary (2011). Keeping Pets. In Tom L. Beauchamp and Raymond G. Frey (Eds.). *The Oxford Handbook of Animal Ethics*, pp. 769–795. Oxford: Oxford University Press.

Bose, Girindrashekhar (1945). *Everyday Psycho-Analysis*. Calcutta: Susil Gupta.

Bourget, Steve (2006). *Sex, Death, and Sacrifice in Moche Religion and Visual Culture*. Austin, Texas: University of Texas Press.

Bourke, Joanna (2007). *Rape: A History from 1860 to the Present Day*. London: Virago / Virago Press.

Bowlby, John (1939). Hysteria in Children. In Ronald G. Gordon (Ed.). *A Survey of Child Psychiatry*, pp. 80–94. London: Humphrey Milford / Oxford University Press.

Bowlby, John (1944a). Forty-Four Juvenile Thieves: Their Characters and Home-Life. *International Journal of Psycho-Analysis, 25*, 19–53.

Bowlby, John (1944b). Forty-Four Juvenile Thieves: Their Characters and Home-Life (II). *International Journal of Psycho-Analysis, 25*, 107–128.

Bowlby, John (1945–1946). Childhood Origins of Recidivism. *Howard Journal, 7*, 30–33.

Bowlby, John (1946). *Forty-Four Juvenile Thieves: Their Characters and Home-Life*. Covent Garden, London: Baillière, Tindall and Cox.

Bowlby, John (1988). *A Secure Base: Clinical Applications of Attachment Theory*. London: Routledge.

Bowlby, John; Miller, Emanuel, and Winnicott, Donald W. (1939). Evacuation of Small Children. *British Medical Journal*. 16th December, pp. 1202–1203.

Brandon, David, and Brooke, Alan (2007). *Marylebone and Tyburn Past*. London: Historical Publications.

Brennan, Brenda (1944). Letter to Donald W. Winnicott. 23rd July. PP/DWW/B/D/21. Donald Woods Winnicott Collection. Archives and Manuscripts, Rare Materials Room, Wellcome Library, Wellcome Collection, The Wellcome Building, London.

Breuer, Josef (1895). Beobachtung I. Frl. Anna O … In Josef Breuer and Sigmund Freud. *Studien über Hysterie*, pp. 15–37. Vienna: Franz Deuticke.

Bromberg, Norbert, and Small, Verna Volz (1983). *Hitler's Psychopathology*. New York: International Universities Press.

Bromberg, Walter (1951). A Psychological Study of Murder. *International Journal of Psycho-Analysis*, *32*, 117–127.

Brouardel, Paul (1897). *L'Infanticide*. Paris: Librairie J.-B. Baillière et Fils.

Brown, Shelby (1991). *Late Carthaginian Child Sacrifice and Sacrificial Monuments in Their Mediterranean Context*. Sheffield: JSOT Press / Sheffield Academic Press.

Burlingham, Dorothy, and Freud, Anna (1942). *Young Children in War-Time: A Year's Work in a Residential War Nursery*. London: George Allen and Unwin.

Burn, Gordon (1984). *'… somebody's husband, somebody's son.': The Story of Peter Sutcliffe*. London: Heinemann / William Heinemann.

Burston, Daniel (1996). *The Wings of Madness: The Life and Work of R.D. Laing*. Cambridge, Massachusetts: Harvard University Press.

Buss, David M. (2005). *The Murderer Next Door: Why the Mind is Designed to Kill*. New York: Penguin Press / Penguin Group, Penguin Group (USA).

Butler, Sara M. (2007). *The Language of Abuse: Marital Violence in Later Medieval England*. Leiden: Brill / Koninklijke Brill.

Calvo, Amanda (2017a). Puppy Love: Therapy Pooches Bring Peace of Mind at Spanish Psychiatric Center. Medscape. [http://www.medscape.com/viewarticle/877301?nild=113 514_1842&src=WNL_mdsplsfeat_170321_mscpedit_wir&spon=17&implD=1312706& faf=1; Accessed on 25th March, 2017].

Calvo, Amanda (2017b). Puppy Love: Therapy Pooches Bring Peace of Mind at Spanish Psychiatric Center. Reuters. [https://uk.reuters.com/article/us-spain-health-widerimage/ puppy-love-therapy-pooches-bring-peace-of-mind-at-spanish-psychiatric-center-id UKKBN16N1I9; Accessed on 21st July, 2020].

Canter, David (1994). *Criminal Shadows: Inside the Mind of the Serial Killer*. Hammersmith, London: HarperCollins Publishers.

Caprio, Frank S. (1948). A Case of Exhibitionism with Special Reference to the Family Setting. *American Journal of Psychotherapy*, *2*, 587–602.

Caprio, Frank S., and Brenner, Donald R. (1961). *Sexual Behavior: Psycho-Legal Aspects*. New York: Citadel Press.

Cassity, John Holland (1927). Psychological Considerations of Pedophilia. *Psychoanalytic Review*, *14*, 189–199.

Cawthorne, Nigel (2006). *Public Executions*. London: Arcturus / Arcturus Publishing Company, and Cippenham, Slough, Berkshire: Foulsham / W. Foulsham and Company.

Charcot, Jean-Martin (1887). *Leçons du mardi à la Salpêtrière: Policliniques. 1887–1888. Notes de cours de M.M. Blin, Charcot et Colin*. Paris: Bureaux du Progrès Médical / Librairie A. Delahaye et Émile Lecrosnier.

Chessick, Richard D. (2018). *Apologia Pro Vita Mea: An Intellectual Odyssey*. London: Routledge / Taylor and Francis Group, and Abingdon, Oxfordshire: Routledge / Taylor and Francis Group.

Christoffel, Hans (1936). Exhibitionism and Exhibitionists. *International Journal of Psycho-Analysis*, *17*, 321–345.

Christoffel, Hans (1956). Male Genital Exhibitionism. In Sandor Lorand and Michael Balint (Eds.). *Perversions: Psychodynamics and Therapy*, pp. 243–264. New York: Random House.

Church, Archibald (1893). Removal of Ovaries and Tubes in the Insane and Neurotic. *American Journal of Obstetrics and Diseases of Women and Children, 28*, 491–498.

Claridge, Mary (1966). *Margaret Clitherow (1556?–1586)*. London: Burns and Oates.

Clark, Stephen R.L. (2011). Animals in Classical and Late Antique Philosophy. In Tom L. Beauchamp and Raymond G. Frey (Eds.). *The Oxford Handbook of Animal Ethics*, pp. 35–60. Oxford: Oxford University Press.

Clarke, Charles K. (1886). The Case of William B. – Moral Imbecility. *American Journal of Insanity, 43*, 83–103.

Clay, John (1996). *R. D. Laing: A Divided Self.* London: Hodder and Stoughton / Hodder Headline.

Clouston, Thomas S. (1870). "The McFarland Trial". *Journal of Mental Science, 16*, 420–424.

Cohn, Haim Hermann (1971). Capital Punishment. In *Encyclopaedia Judaica: Volume 5. C-Dh*, pp. 142–145. Jerusalem: Encyclopaedia Judaica / Keter Publishing House.

Coleman, Mary (1985). Shame: A Powerful Underlying Factor in Violence and War. *Journal of Psychoanalytic Anthropology, 8*, 67–79.

Collier, Jessica (2015). 3 Man Unlock: Out of Sight, Out of Mind. Art Psychotherapy with a Woman with Severe and Dangerous Personality Disorder in Prison. *Psychoanalytic Psychotherapy, 29*, 243–261.

Collier, Jessica (2019). Trauma, Art and the "Borderspace": Working with Traumatic Re-enactments. In Pamela Windham Stewart and Jessica Collier (Eds.). *The End of the Sentence: Psychotherapy with Female Offenders*, pp. 164–182. London: Routledge / Taylor and Francis Group, and Abingdon, Oxfordshire: Routledge / Taylor and Francis Group.

Concannon, Diana M. (2019). *Neurocriminology: Forensic and Legal Applications, Public Policy Implications*. Boca Raton, Florida: CRC Press / Taylor and Francis Group.

Conolly, John (1856). *The Treatment of the Insane without Mechanical Restraints*. London: Smith, Elder and Company.

Corbett, Alan (2014). *Disabling Perversions: Forensic Psychotherapy with People with Intellectual Disabilities*. London: Karnac Books.

Corbett, Alan (2018). Extraordinary Therapy: On Splitting, Kindness, and Handicapping Mothers. In Brett Kahr (Ed.). *New Horizons in Forensic Psychotherapy: Exploring the Work of Estela V. Welldon*, pp. 205–218. London: Karnac Books.

Cormack, Una M. (1942). Interviewing and the Bombed. *Social Work, 2*, 178–184.

Coventry, Charles B. (1844). Medical Jurisprudence of Insanity. *American Journal of Insanity, 1*, 134–144.

Coward, Noël (1941). Diary Entry. 19th April. In Noël Coward (1982). *The Noel Coward Diaries*. Graham Payn and Sheridan Morley (Eds.), p. 6. London: Weidenfeld and Nicolson / George Weidenfeld and Nicolson.

Cox, Murray (Ed.). (1992a). *Shakespeare Comes to Broadmoor: 'The Actors are Come Hither'. The Performance of Tragedy in a Secure Psychiatric Hospital*. London: Jessica Kingsley Publishers.

Cox, Murray (1992b). Forensic Psychiatry and Forensic Psychotherapy. In Murray Cox (Ed.). *Shakespeare Comes to Broadmoor: 'The Actors Are Come Hither'. The Performance of Tragedy in a Secure Psychiatric Hospital*, pp. 253–258. London: Jessica Kingsley Publishers.

Cox, Murray (2001). On the Capacity for Being Inside Enough. In Brett Kahr (Ed.). *Forensic Psychotherapy and Psychopathology: Winnicottian Perspectives*, pp. 111–123. London: H. Karnac (Books), and New York: Other Press.

Crawford, Jacqueline J., and Pomerinke, Karen A. (2003). *Therapy Pets: The Animal-Human Healing Partnership*. Amherst, New York: Prometheus Books.

Culliton, Barbara J. (1987). Take Two Pets and Call Me in the Morning: The Benefits of Pets as Therapy for a Whole Host of Ills from Hypertension to Depression Were Discussed at an NIH Conference to Evaluate Current Data. *Science*. 25th September, pp. 1560–1561.

Curen, Richard (2009). 'Can They See in the Door?': Issues in the Assessment and Treatment of Sex Offenders Who Have Intellectual Disabilities. In Tamsin Cottis (Ed.). *Intellectual Disability, Trauma and Psychotherapy*, pp. 90–113. London: Routledge / Taylor and Francis Group, and Hove, East Sussex: Routledge / Taylor and Francis Group.

Curen, Richard (2018). Responses to Trauma, Enactments of Trauma: The Psychodynamics of an Intellectually Disabled Family. In Brett Kahr (Ed.). *New Horizons in Forensic Psychotherapy: Exploring the Work of Estela V. Welldon*, pp. 219–235. London: Karnac Books.

Dale-Green, Patricia (1966). *Dog*. London: Rupert Hart-Davis.

Daube, David (1947). *Studies in Biblical Law*. Cambridge: University Press / Cambridge University Press.

Davies, Rosemary (2012). Anxiety: The Importunate Companion. Psychoanalytic Theory of Castration and Separation Anxieties and Implications for Clinical Technique. *International Journal of Psychoanalysis*, *93*, 1101–1114.

de Salies, Alexandre (1874). *Histoire de Foulques-Nerra: Comte d'Anjou. D'Après les chartres contemporaines et les anciennes chroniques. Suivie de l'office du Saint-Sépulcre de l'abbaye de Beaulieu dont les leçons forment une chronique inédite. Avec 12 planches et une grande carte*. Paris: J.-B. Dumoulin, Libraire, and Angers: E. Barassé, Imprimerie-Libraire.

deMause, Lloyd (1973). The History of Childhood: The Basis for Psychohistory. *History of Childhood Quarterly*, *1*, 1–3.

deMause, Lloyd (1974). The Evolution of Childhood. In Lloyd deMause (Ed.). *The History of Childhood*, pp. 1–73. New York: Psychohistory Press.

deMause, Lloyd (1982). *Foundations of Psychohistory*. New York: Creative Roots.

deMause, Lloyd (1984). *Reagan's America*. New York: Creative Roots.

deMause, Lloyd (1988). On Writing Childhood History. *Journal of Psychohistory*, *16*, 135–171.

deMause, Lloyd (1990). The History of Child Assault. *Journal of Psychohistory*, *18*, 1–29.

deMause, Lloyd (1991). The Gulf War as a Mental Disorder. *Journal of Psychohistory*, *19*, 1–22.

deMause, Lloyd (2002a). *The Emotional Life of Nations*. New York: Karnac / Other Press.

deMause, Lloyd (2002b). The Childhood Origins of Terrorism. *Journal of Psychohistory*, *29*, 340–348.

deMause, Lloyd (2006). "If I Blow Myself Up and Become a Martyr, I'll Finally Be Loved". *Journal of Psychohistory*, *33*, 300–307.

deMause, Lloyd (2012a). The Long History of Europeans Slaughtering Jews. *Journal of Psychohistory*, *39*, 170–174.

deMause, Lloyd (2012b). Wars as Sacrifices to Reduce Guilt. *Journal of Psychohistory*, *39*, 249–252.

Deutsch, Helene (1942). Some Forms of Emotional Disturbance and Their Relationship to Schizophrenia. *Psychoanalytic Quarterly*, *11*, 301–321.

Deutsch, Helene (1973). *Confrontations with Myself: An Epilogue*. New York: W.W. Norton and Company.

Dickens, Charles (1842). *American Notes for General Circulation: In Two Volumes. Vol. I.* London: Chapman and Hall.

Dicks, Henry V. (1970). *Fifty Years of the Tavistock Clinic.* London: Routledge and Kegan Paul.

Doctor, Ronald (2018). Brain, Womb, and Will: A Lethal Cocktail or a Grand Affair? In Brett Kahr (Ed.). *New Horizons in Forensic Psychotherapy: Exploring the Work of Estela V. Welldon*, pp. 127–143. London: Karnac Books.

Duckworth, Jeannie (2002). *Fagin's Children: Criminal Children in Victorian England.* London: Hambledon and London.

East, William Norwood (1936). *Medical Aspects of Crime.* London: J. and A. Churchill.

Eichholz, Enid (1944). Londoners and the Flying Bomb: (From the Point of View of the C.A.B. Worker.). *Social Work*, *3*, 91–95.

Ekroth, Gunnel (2014). Animal Sacrifice in Antiquity. In Gordon Lindsay Campbell (Ed.). *The Oxford Handbook of Animals in Classical Thought and Life*, pp. 324–354. Oxford: Oxford University Press.

Ellmann, Richard (1985). Freud and Literary Biography. In Peregrine Hordern (Ed.). *Freud and the Humanities*, pp. 58–74. London: Duckworth / Gerald Duckworth and Company.

Fallon, James (2013). *The Psychopath Inside: A Neuroscientist's Personal Journey into the Dark Side of the Brain.* New York: Current / Penguin Group, Penguin Group (USA), Penguin Random House Company.

Farber, Stephen, and Green, Marc (n.d.). Interview with Martin Grotjahn. n.d. Cited in Stephen Farber and Marc Green (1993). *Hollywood on the Couch: A Candid Look at the Overheated Love Affair Between Psychiatrists and Moviemakers*, p. 319. New York: William Morrow and Company.

Fenichel, Otto (1945). *The Psychoanalytic Theory of Neurosis.* New York: W.W. Norton and Company.

Ferenczi, Sándor (1915). Spektrophobie. *Internationale Zeitschrift für ärztliche Psychoanalyse*, *3*, 293.

Ferenczi, Sándor (1919a). Pszichoanalizis és kriminológia. In *A pszichoanalizis haladása: Ertekezések*, pp. 126–128. Budapest: Dick Manó Kiadása.

Ferenczi, Sándor (1919b). Die Nacktheit als Schreckmittel. *Internationale Zeitschrift für Psychoanalyse*, *5*, 303–305.

Ferenczi, Sándor (1922). *Populäre Vorträge über Psychoanalyse.* Vienna: Internationaler Psychoanalytischer Verlag.

Finkelhor, David, and Yllo, Kersti (1985). *License to Rape: Sexual Abuse of Wives.* New York: Holt, Rinehart and Winston.

Flor-Henry, Pierre (1987). Cerebral Aspects of Sexual Deviation. In Glenn D. Wilson (Ed.). *Variant Sexuality: Research and Theory*, pp. 49–83. Beckenham, Kent: Croom Helm.

Flor-Henry, Pierre, and Lang, Reuben (1988). Qualitative EEG Analysis in Genital Exhibitionists. *Annals of Sex Research*, *1*, 48–62.

Flügel, John C. (1932). *An Introduction to Psycho-Analysis.* London: Victor Gollancz.

Foley, Helene P. (1985). *Ritual Irony: Poetry and Sacrifice in Euripides.* Ithaca, New York: Cornell University Press.

Frankl, Viktor E. (1995). *Was nicht in meinen Büchern steht: Lebenserinnerungen. 2. Auflage.* Munich: Quintessenz / MMV Medizin Verlag.

Frankl, Viktor E. (1997). *Viktor Frankl Recollections: An Autobiography.* Joseph Fabry and Judith Fabry (Transls.). New York: Insight Books / Plenum Press, Plenum Publishing Corporation.

Freud, Anna (1973). Letter to Ishak Ramzy. 20th December. Cited in Elisabeth Young-Bruehl (1988). *Anna Freud: A Biography*, p. 491, n. 47. New York: Summit Books / Simon and Schuster.

Freud, Anna (1974). Diagnosis and Assessment of Childhood Disturbances. *Journal of the Philadelphia Association of Psychoanalysis*, *1*, 54–67.

Freud, Anna, and Burlingham, Dorothy (1941). Monthly Report: February, 1941, pp. 3–10. In Anna Freud and Dorothy Burlingham (1939–1945). Monthly Reports (February, 1941 – December, 1945). In Anna Freud and Dorothy Burlingham (1973). *Infants without Families: Reports on the Hampstead Nurseries. 1939–1945*. In Anna Freud (1973). *The Writings of Anna Freud: Volume III*, pp. 3–540. New York: International Universities Press.

Freud, Sigmund (1873). Letter to Eduard Silberstein. 20th August. In Sigmund Freud (1989). *Jugendbriefe an Eduard Silberstein: 1871–1881*. Walter Boehlich (Ed.), pp. 49–51. Frankfurt am Main: S. Fischer / S. Fischer Verlag.

Freud, Sigmund (1886). "Bericht.": Ueber meine mit Universitäts-Jubiläums-Reisestipendium unternommene Reise nach Paris und Berlin. Oktober 1885 – Ende März 1886. In Josef Gicklhorn and Renée Gicklhorn (1960). *Sigmund Freuds akademische Laufbahn im Lichte der Dokumente*, pp. 82–89. Vienna: Verlag Urban und Schwarzenberg.

Freud, Sigmund (1895). (Manuskript H): Paranoia. In Sigmund Freud (1950). *Aus den Anfängen der Psychoanalyse: Briefe an Wilhelm Fliess, Abhandlungen und Notizen aus den Jahren 1887–1902*. Marie Bonaparte, Anna Freud, and Ernst Kris (Eds.), pp. 106–112. London: Imago Publishing Company.

Freud, Sigmund (1896a). L'Hérédité et l'étiologie des névroses. *Revue Neurologique*, *4*, 161–169.

Freud, Sigmund (1896b). Heredity and the Aetiology of the Neuroses. James Strachey (Transl.). In Sigmund Freud (1962). *The Standard Edition of the Complete Psychological Works of Sigmund Freud: Volume III. (1893–1899). Early Psycho-Analytic Publications*. James Strachey, Anna Freud, Alix Strachey, and Alan Tyson (Eds. and Transls.), pp. 143–156. London: Hogarth Press and the Institute of Psycho-Analysis.

Freud, Sigmund (1900a). *Die Traumdeutung*. Vienna: Franz Deuticke.

Freud, Sigmund (1900b). *The Interpretation of Dreams*. James Strachey (Transl.). In Sigmund Freud (1953). *The Standard Edition of the Complete Psychological Works of Sigmund Freud: Volume IV. (1900). The Interpretation of Dreams. (First Part)*. James Strachey, Anna Freud, Alix Strachey, and Alan Tyson (Eds. and Transls.), pp. xxiii–338. London: Hogarth Press and the Institute of Psycho-Analysis.

Freud, Sigmund (1900c). *The Interpretation of Dreams*. James Strachey (Transl.). In Sigmund Freud (1953). *The Standard Edition of the Complete Psychological Works of Sigmund Freud: Volume V. (1900–1901). The Interpretation of Dreams. (Second Part) and On Dreams*. James Strachey, Anna Freud, Alix Strachey, and Alan Tyson (Eds. and Transls.), pp. 339–621. London: Hogarth Press and the Institute of Psycho-Analysis.

Freud, Sigmund (1905a). *Drei Abhandlungen zur Sexualtheorie*. Vienna: Franz Deuticke.

Freud, Sigmund (1905b). *Three Essays on the Theory of Sexuality*. James Strachey (Transl.). In Sigmund Freud (1953). *The Standard Edition of the Complete Psychological Works of Sigmund Freud: Volume VII. (1901–1905). A Case of Hysteria. Three Essays on Sexuality and Other Works*. James Strachey, Anna Freud, Alix Strachey, and Alan Tyson (Eds. and Transls.), pp. 130–243. London: Hogarth Press and the Institute of Psycho-Analysis.

Freud, Sigmund (1909a). Analyse der Phobie eines 5jährigen Knaben. *Jahrbuch für psychoanalytische und psychopathologische Forschungen*, *1*, 1–109.

Freud, Sigmund (1909b). Bemerkungen über einen Fall von Zwangsneurose. *Jahrbuch für psychoanalytische und psychopathologische Forschungen*, *1*, 357–421.

Freud, Sigmund (1909c). Notes Upon a Case of Obsessional Neurosis. Alix Strachey and James Strachey (Transls.). In Sigmund Freud (1955). *The Standard Edition of the Complete Psychological Works of Sigmund Freud: Volume X. (1909). Two Case Histories ('Little Hans' and the 'Rat Man')*. James Strachey, Anna Freud, Alix Strachey, and Alan Tyson (Eds. and Transls.), pp. 155–249. London: Hogarth Press and the Institute of Psycho-Analysis.

Freud, Sigmund (1910a). Letter to Sándor Ferenczi. 13ᵗʰ February. In Sigmund Freud and Sándor Ferenczi (1993). *Briefwechsel: Band I / 1. 1908–1911*. Eva Brabant, Ernst Falzeder, Patrizia Giampieri-Deutsch, and André Haynal (Eds.), pp. 212–214. Vienna: Böhlau Verlag / Böhlau Verlag Gesellschaft.

Freud, Sigmund (1910b). Letter to Sándor Ferenczi. 13ᵗʰ February. In Sigmund Freud and Sándor Ferenczi (1993). *The Correspondence of Sigmund Freud and Sándor Ferenczi: Volume I, 1908–1914*. Eva Brabant, Ernst Falzeder, Patrizia Giampieri-Deutsch, and André Haynal (Eds.). Peter T. Hoffer (Transl.), pp. 136–138. Cambridge, Massachusetts: Belknap Press of Harvard University Press.

Freud, Sigmund (1914). Weitere Ratschläge zur Technik der Psychoanalyse: II. Erinnern, Wiederholen und Durcharbeiten. *Internationale Zeitschrift für ärztliche Psychoanalyse*, *2*, 485–491.

Freud, Sigmund (1916). Einige Charaktertypen aus der psychoanalytischen Arbeit. *Imago*, *4*, 317–336.

Freud, Sigmund (1917a). Eine Schwierigkeit der Psychoanalyse. *Imago*, *5*, 1–7.

Freud, Sigmund (1917b). A Difficulty in the Path of Psycho-Analysis. Joan Riviere and James Strachey (Transls.). In Sigmund Freud (1955). *The Standard Edition of the Complete Psychological Works of Sigmund Freud: Volume XVII. (1917–1919). An Infantile Neurosis and Other Works*. James Strachey, Anna Freud, Alix Strachey, and Alan Tyson (Eds. and Transls.), pp. 137–144. London: Hogarth Press and the Institute of Psycho-Analysis.

Freud, Sigmund (1917c). Eine Kindheitserinnerungen aus "Dichtung und Wahrheit". *Imago*, *5*, 49–57.

Freud, Sigmund (1917d). A Childhood Recollection from *Dichtung und Wahrheit*. Caroline J.M. Hubback and James Strachey (Transls.). In Sigmund Freud (1955). *The Standard Edition of the Complete Psychological Works of Sigmund Freud: Volume XVII. (1917–1919). An Infantile Neurosis and Other Works*. James Strachey, Anna Freud, Alix Strachey, and Alan Tyson (Eds. and Transls.), pp. 147–156. London: Hogarth Press and the Institute of Psycho-Analysis.

Freud, Sigmund (1918). Aus der Geschichte einer infantilen Neurose. In *Sammlung kleiner Schriften zur Neurosenlehre: Vierte Folge*, pp. 578–717. Vienna: Hugo Heller und Compagnie.

Freud, Sigmund (1919). "Ein Kind wird geschlagen": Beitrag zur Kenntnis der Entstehung sexueller Perversionen. *Internationale Zeitschrift für ärztliche Psychoanalyse*, *5*, 151–172.

Freud, Sigmund (1922). Über einige neurotische Mechanismen bei Eifersucht, Paranoia und Homosexualität. *Internationale Zeitschrift für Psychoanalyse*, *8*, 249–258.

Freud, Sigmund (1924a). Das ökonomische Problem des Masochismus. *Internationale Zeitschrift für Psychoanalyse*, *10*, 121–133.

Freud, Sigmund (1924b). Letter to George Seldes. 29ᵗʰ June. In George Seldes (1953). *Tell the Truth and Run*, p. 107. New York: Greenberg: Publisher.

Freud, Sigmund (1924c). Letter to George Seldes. 29th June. In Ernest Jones (1957). *The Life and Work of Sigmund Freud: Volume 3. The Last Phase. 1919–1939*, p. 103. New York: Basic Books.

Freud, Sigmund (1925a). Sigmund Freud. In Ludwig R. Grote (Ed.). *Die Medizin der Gegenwart in Selbstdarstellungen*, pp. 1–52. Leipzig: Verlag von Felix Meiner.

Freud, Sigmund (1925b). Geleitwort. In August Aichhorn. *Verwahrloste Jugend: Die Psychoanalyse in der Fürsorgeerziehung. Zehn Vorträge zur ersten Einführung*, pp. 3–6. Vienna: Internationaler Psychoanalytischer Verlag.

Freud, Sigmund (1926). *Hemmung, Symptom und Angst*. Vienna: Internationaler Psychoanalytischer Verlag.

Freud, Sigmund (1927a). Fetischismus. *Internationale Zeitschrift für Psychoanalyse, 13*, 373–378.

Freud, Sigmund (1927b). Letter to Jeanne Lampl-de Groot. 22nd February. In Sigmund Freud (2017). *Briefe an Jeanne Lampl-de Groot: 1921–1939*. Gertie F. Bögels (Ed.), pp. 57–58. Gießen: Psychosozial-Verlag.

Freud, Sigmund (1927c). Letter to Jeanne Lampl-de Groot. 22nd February. In Sigmund Freud (2023). *The Letters of Sigmund Freud to Jeanne Lampl-de Groot, 1921–1939: Psychoanalysis and Politics in the Interwar Years*. Gertie Bögels (Ed.). Kenneth Kronenberg (Transl.), p. 42. London: Routledge / Taylor and Francis Group, and Abingdon, Oxfordshire: Routledge / Taylor and Francis Group.

Freud, Sigmund (1927d). Letter to Max Eitingon. 13th September. In Sigmund Freud and Max Eitingon (2004). *Briefwechsel: 1906–1939. Zweiter Band*. Michael Schröter (Ed.), pp. 549–552. Tübingen: edition diskord.

Freud, Sigmund (1927e). Letter to Max Eitingon. 13th September. Michael Molnar (Transl.), p. 275. Excerpted in Michael Molnar (1996). Of Dogs and Doggerel. *American Imago, 53*, 269–280.

Freud, Sigmund (1930a). Nächstenliebe und Aggressionstrieb. *Die psychoanalytische Bewegung, 2*, 5–13.

Freud, Sigmund (1930b). Diary Entry. 3rd February. In Sigmund Freud (1992). *The Diary of Sigmund Freud: 1929–1939. A Record of the Final Decade*. Michael Molnar (Ed. and Transl.), p. 2. New York: Charles Scribner's Sons, and Toronto: Maxwell Macmillan Canada, and New York: Maxwell Macmillan International, and New York: Charles Scribner's Sons / Macmillan Publishing Company, Maxwell Communication Group of Companies, and Don Mills, Ontario: Maxwell Macmillan Canada.

Freud, Sigmund (1930c). Diary Entry. 26th February. In Sigmund Freud (1992). *The Diary of Sigmund Freud: 1929–1939. A Record of the Final Decade*. Michael Molnar (Ed. and Transl.), p. 2. New York: Charles Scribner's Sons, and Toronto: Maxwell Macmillan Canada, and New York: Maxwell Macmillan International, and New York: Charles Scribner's Sons / Macmillan Publishing Company, Maxwell Communication Group of Companies, and Don Mills, Ontario: Maxwell Macmillan Canada.

Freud, Sigmund (1931a). Die Fakultätsgutachten im Prozeß Halsmann. *Psychoanalytische Bewegung, 3*, 32–34.

Freud, Sigmund (1931b). Geleitworte: Prof. Dr. S. Freud, Wien. In Georg Fuchs. *Wir Zuchthäusler: Erinnerungen des Zellengefangenen Nr. 2911*, pp. x–xi. Munich: Albert Langen.

Freud, Sigmund (1931c). Letter to Georg Fuchs. James Strachey (Transl.). In Sigmund Freud (1964). *The Standard Edition of the Complete Psychological Works of Sigmund Freud: Volume XXII. (1932–36). New Introductory Lectures on Psycho-Analysis and Other*

Works. James Strachey, Anna Freud, Alix Strachey, and Alan Tyson (Eds. and Transls.), pp. 251–252. London: Hogarth Press and the Institute of Psycho-Analysis.

Freud, Sigmund (1933). Letter to Grace Pailthorpe. 8th November. Box 38. Folder 10. Sigmund Freud Papers. Sigmund Freud Collection. Manuscript Reading Room, Room 101, Manuscript Division, James Madison Memorial Building, Library of Congress, Washington, D.C., U.S.A.

Freud, Sigmund (1937). Die endliche und die unendliche Analyse. *Internationale Zeitschrift für Psychoanalyse*, *23*, 209–240.

Friedman, Leonard J. (1962). *Virgin Wives: A Study of Unconsummated Marriages*. London: Tavistock Publications, and Springfield, Illinois: Charles C Thomas, Publisher.

Gallo, Rubén (2012). A Wild Freudian in Mexico: Raúl Carrancá y Trujillo. *Psychoanalysis and History*, *14*, 253–268.

Gans, Steven (1992). Personal Communication to the Author. 5th December.

Gansberg, Alan L.; Wallace, Irving; Wallace, Amy; Wallechinsky, David; and Wallace, Sylvia (1981). In Like Flynn: Errol Flynn (June 20, 1909 – Oct. 14, 1959). In Irving Wallace, Amy Wallace, David Wallechinsky, and Sylvia Wallace (Eds.). *The Intimate Sex Lives of Famous People*, pp. 17–19. New York: Delacorte Press.

Gardiner, Muriel (1978). In Wien vom 12. Februar 1934 bis zum Anschluß. In Muriel Gardiner and Joseph Buttinger. *Damit wir nicht vergessen: Unsere Jahre 1934–1947 in Wien, Paris und New York*, pp. 31–72. Vienna: Verlag der Wiener Volksbuchhandlung.

Gardiner, Muriel (1983). *Code Name "Mary": Memoirs of an American Woman in the Austrian Underground*. New Haven, Connecticut: Yale University Press.

Geary, Laurence M. (1990). O'Connorite Bedlam: Feargus and His Grand-Nephew, Arthur. *Medical History*, *34*, 125–143.

Gelder, Michael; Gath, Dennis, and Mayou, Richard (1983). *Oxford Textbook of Psychiatry*. Oxford: Oxford University Press.

Gilligan, James (1996). *Violence: Our Deadly Epidemic and Its Causes*. New York: G.P. Putnam's Sons.

Gilligan, James (2001). *Preventing Violence*. London: Thames and Hudson.

Gilligan, James (2016). Can Psychoanalysis Help Us to Understand the Causes and Prevention of Violence? *Psychoanalytic Psychotherapy*, *30*, 125–137.

Glasser, Mervin (1978). The Role of the Superego in Exhibitionism. *International Journal of Psychoanalytic Psychotherapy*, *7*, 333–353. New York: Jason Aronson.

Goldberg, Jeremy (2008). *Communal Discord, Child Abduction, and Rape in the Later Middle Ages*. New York: Palgrave Macmillan / St. Martin's Press.

Golden, Charles J., Jackson, Michele L., Peterson-Rohne, Angela, and Gontkovsky, Samuel T. (1996). Neuropsychological Correlates of Violence and Aggression: A Review of the Clinical Literature. *Aggression and Violent Behavior*, *1*, 3–25.

Gomes, Michele (2018a). The Clinical Moment, pp. 246–251. In Michele Gomes. Considering Third Parties: The Question of Allegiance. In Richard Tuch and Lynn S. Kuttnauer (Eds.). *Conundrums and Predicaments in Psychotherapy and Psychoanalysis: The Clinical Moments Project*, pp. 242–261. London: Routledge / Taylor and Francis Group, and Abingdon, Oxfordshire: Routledge / Taylor and Francis Group.

Gomes, Michele (2018b). My Intervention, pp. 259–261. In Michele Gomes. Considering Third Parties: The Question of Allegiance. In Richard Tuch and Lynn S. Kuttnauer (Eds.). *Conundrums and Predicaments in Psychotherapy and Psychoanalysis: The Clinical Moments Project*, pp. 242–261. London: Routledge / Taylor and Francis Group, and Abingdon, Oxfordshire: Routledge / Taylor and Francis Group.

Goodman, Sydney V.C. (n.d.). *Plymouth: The Reconstruction of a Blitzed City*. Plymouth, Devon: P.D.S. Printers.

Gray, John P. (1857). Homicide in Insanity. *American Journal of Insanity, 14*, 119–145.

Grayzel, Susan R. (2012). *At Home and Under Fire: Air Raids and Culture in Britain from the Great War to the Blitz*. Cambridge: Cambridge University Press.

Greenhalgh, Izzy (2021). A Day in the Life of a Prison Mental Health Social Worker. *International Journal of Forensic Psychotherapy, 3*, 77–79.

Grier, Francis (2001). No Sex Couples, Catastrophic Change and the Primal Scene. *British Journal of Psychotherapy, 17*, 474–488.

Grier, Katherine C. (2002). "The Eden of Home": Changing Understandings of Cruelty and Kindness to Animals in Middle-Class American Households, 1820–1900. In Mary J. Henninger-Voss (Ed.). *Animals in Human Histories: The Mirror of Nature and Culture*, pp. 316–362. Rochester, New York: University of Rochester Press, and Woodbridge, Suffolk: Boydell and Brewer.

Grinker, Roy R. (1940). Reminiscences of a Personal Contact with Freud. *American Journal of Orthopsychiatry, 10*, 850–854.

Grinker, Roy R., Sr. (1979). *Fifty Years in Psychiatry: A Living History*. Springfield, Illinois: Charles C Thomas, Publisher.

Grinker, Roy, Sr. (1985). A Memoir of My Psychoanalytic Education. Jay Martin (Ed.). *Psychoanalytic Education, 4*, 3–12.

Grob, Charles S. (1985). Female Exhibitionism. *Journal of Nervous and Mental Disease, 173*, 253–256.

Grotjahn, Martin (1987). *My Favorite Patient: The Memoirs of a Psychoanalyst*. Frankfurt am Main: Verlag Peter Lang.

Grünhut, Max (1941). John Howard. *Howard Journal, 6*, 34–44.

Guillot, Olivier (1972). *Le Comte d'Anjou et son entourage au XIe siècle: Tome I. Étude et appendices*. Paris: Éditions A. et J. Picard.

Gürisik, Ü. Elif (1997). The Flasher. In Estela V. Welldon and Cleo Van Velsen (Eds.). *A Practical Guide to Forensic Psychotherapy*, pp. 155–160. London: Jessica Kingsley Publishers.

Hackwood, Frederick W. (1907). *Old English Sports*. London: T. Fisher Unwin.

Hárnik, Jenö (1923). Schicksale des Narzißmus bei Mann und Weib. *Internationale Zeitschrift für Psychoanalyse, 9*, 278–296.

Harper, Robert Francis (Transl.). (1904). *The Code of Hammurabi: King of Babylon. About 2250 B.C. Autographed Text. Transliteration. Translation. Glossary. Index of Subjects. Lists of Proper Names. Signs. Numerals. Corrections and Erasures with Map. Frontispiece and Photograph of Text*. Chicago, Illinois: University of Chicago Press / Callaghan and Company, and London: Luzac and Company.

Hartnack, Christiane (2001). *Psychoanalysis in Colonial India*. New Delhi: Oxford University Press.

Haycock, Dean A. (2014). *Murderous Minds: Exploring the Criminal Psychopathic Brain: Neurological Imaging and the Manifestation of Evil*. New York: Pegasus Books.

Hill, Simon A., Mitchell, Paul, and Leipold, Alexandra (2017). Transfers of Mentally Disordered Adolescents from Custodial Settings to Psychiatric Hospital in England and Wales 2004–2014. *Journal of Forensic Psychiatry and Psychology, 28*, 1–9.

Hilty, Raffaella (Ed.). (2022). *Primitive Bodily Communications in Psychotherapy: Embodied Expressions of a Disembodied Psyche*. London: Karnac / Karnac Books, Confer.

Hirning, L. Clovis (1947). Genital Exhibitionism, an Interpretive Study. *Journal of Clinical Psychopathology*, *8*, 557–564.

Hollender, Marc H., Brown, C. Winston, and Roback, Howard B. (1977). Genital Exhibitionism in Women. *American Journal of Psychiatry*, *134*, 436–438.

Hollins, Sheila (2019). Forensic Groupwork and *Books Beyond Words*: Valerie Sinason as Colleague, Co-author, and Friend. In Alan Corbett and Tamsin Cottis (Eds.). *Intellectual Disability and Psychotherapy: The Theories, Practice and Influence of Valerie Sinason*, pp. 70–80. London: Routledge / Taylor and Francis Group, and Abingdon, Oxfordshire: Routledge / Taylor and Francis Group.

Holmes, Jeremy (2015). E-Mail to the Author. 26th September.

Holtzman, Deanna, and Kulish, Nancy (2012). Female Exhibitionism: Identification, Competition and Camaraderie. *International Journal of Psychoanalysis*, *93*, 271–292.

Howard, Derek L. (1958). *John Howard: Prison Reformer*. London: Christopher Johnson.

Huttunen, Matti O., and Niskanen, Pekka (1978). Prenatal Loss of Father and Psychiatric Disorders. *Archives of General Psychiatry*, *35*, 429–431.

Hyatt-Williams, Arthur (1998). *Cruelty, Violence, and Murder: Understanding the Criminal Mind*. Paul Williams (Ed.). Northvale, New Jersey: Jason Aronson.

Insoll, Timothy (2011). Sacrifice. In Timothy Insoll (Ed.). *Oxford Handbook of the Archaeology of Ritual and Religion*, pp. 151–165. Oxford: Oxford University Press.

Institute Board Meetings: 16.1.1925 to 30.4.1945 (1925–1945). Archives of the British Psychoanalytical Society, British Psychoanalytical Society, Byron House, Maida Vale, London.

Iremonger, Lucille (1970). *The Fiery Chariot: A Study of British Prime Ministers and the Search for Love*. London: Martin Secker and Warburg.

Iremonger, Lucille (1984). *Orphans of the Heart*. London: Martin Secker and Warburg.

Johns, Claude H.W. (1914). *The Relations Between the Laws of Babylonia and the Laws of the Hebrew Peoples: The Scheich Lectures. 1912*. London: Humphrey Milford / Oxford University Press.

Jones, Ernest (1953). *The Life and Work of Sigmund Freud: Volume 1. The Formative Years and the Great Discoveries. 1856–1900*. New York: Basic Books.

Jones, Ivor H., and Frei, Dorothy (1979). Exhibitionism: A Biological Hypothesis. *British Journal of Medical Psychology*, *52*, 63–70.

Joseph, Betty (1987). Projective Identification: Clinical Aspects. In Joseph Sandler (Ed.). *Projection, Identification, Projective Identification*, pp. 65–76. Madison, Connecticut: International Universities Press.

Jung, Carl Gustav (1941). Letter to Mary Mellon. 7th January. Jung Archive. Zürich, Switzerland. Cited in William Schoenl (2014). Jung's Evolving Views of Nazi Germany: From 1936 to the End of World War II, p. 261. *Journal of Analytical Psychology*, *59*, 245–262.

JUST 1/802 (Staffs. 1272), m. 46 dorse (n.d.). Cited in Zefira Entin Rokeah (1990). Unnatural Child Death Among Christians and Jews in Medieval England, p. 216, n. 65. *Journal of Psychohistory*, *18*, 181–226.

Kahr, Brett (1993). Ancient Infanticide and Modern Schizophrenia: The Clinical Uses of Psychohistorical Research. *Journal of Psychohistory*, *20*, 267–273.

Kahr, Brett (1994a). The Historical Foundations of Ritual Abuse: An Excavation of Ancient Infanticide. In Valerie Sinason (Ed.). *Treating Survivors of Satanist Abuse*, pp. 45–56. London: Routledge.

Kahr, Brett (1994b). R.D. Laing's Missing Tooth: Schizophrenia and Bodily Disintegration. *Journal of the Society for Existential Analysis*, *4*, 64–79.

Kahr, Brett (1995). Lecture on "Mucus, Saliva, Urine, Faeces, Semen, Menstrual Blood, Flatus, Vomitus, and Phlegm: On Patients Who Evacuate Bodily Fluids in Psychotherapy". Tavistock Clinic Mental Handicap Workshop. Child and Family Department, Tavistock Clinic, Tavistock Centre, Tavistock and Portman NHS Trust, Belsize Park, London. 16th June.

Kahr, Brett (1996). Interview with Ruth Brook Klauber. 29th June.

Kahr, Brett (1997a). Lecture on "Patients Who Evacuate Bodily Fluids During Psychotherapy". Tavistock Clinic Mental Handicap Workshop. Child and Family Department, Tavistock Clinic, Tavistock Centre, Tavistock and Portman NHS Trust, Belsize Park, London. 10th November.

Kahr, Brett (1997b). Interview with "Edmund Fothergill". 3rd January.

Kahr, Brett (1998a). Setting Up the Treatment: First Steps in Psychotherapy with Handicapped People. In *The Association for Psychotherapies in Learning Disability (A.P.I.L.D.): Proceedings of First Conference. "Psychodynamic Approaches in Learning Disability". Sheffield. March 1997*, pp. 1–14. Sheffield, South Yorkshire: Association for Psychotherapies in Learning Disability.

Kahr, Brett (1998b). An Unpublished Fragment by Donald Winnicott. *NewSquiggle*, *2*, 7.

Kahr, Brett (2000a). Academic Recognition for Forensic Psychotherapy. *Psychotherapy Review*, *2*, 261.

Kahr, Brett (2000b). 'A Harley Street for the Anxious Poor': The Tavistock Clinic in the 1930s. *Psychotherapy Review*, *2*, 397–399.

Kahr, Brett (Ed.). (2001a). *Forensic Psychotherapy and Psychopathology: Winnicottian Perspectives*. London: H. Karnac (Books), and New York: Other Press.

Kahr, Brett (2001b). *Exhibitionism*. Duxford, Cambridgeshire: Icon Books.

Kahr, Brett (2001c). Winnicott's Contribution to the Study of Dangerousness. In Brett Kahr (Ed.). *Forensic Psychotherapy and Psychopathology: Winnicottian Perspectives*, pp. 1–10. London: H. Karnac (Books), and New York: Other Press.

Kahr, Brett (2001d). The Legacy of Infanticide. *Journal of Psychohistory*, *29*, 40–44.

Kahr, Brett (2002). Lecture on "Male Genital Exhibitionism". Conference on "Indecent Exposure?: Exhibitionism, Art, Media and Psychoanalysis". Starr Auditorium, Tate Modern, London. 9th February.

Kahr, Brett (2004a). Juvenile Paedophilia: The Psychodynamics of an Adolescent. In Charles W. Socarides and Loretta R. Loeb (Eds.). *The Mind of the Paedophile: Psychoanalytic Perspectives*, pp. 95–119. London: H. Karnac (Books).

Kahr, Brett (2004b). Interview with Pearl King. 23rd September.

Kahr, Brett (2005a). On Practicing Therapy at 1:45 A.M. *American Imago*, *62*, 125–131.

Kahr, Brett (2005b). Why Freud Turned Down $25,000: Mental Health Professionals in the Witness Box. *American Imago*, *62*, 365–371.

Kahr, Brett (2007a). *Sex and the Psyche*. London: Allen Lane / Penguin Books, Penguin Group.

Kahr, Brett (2007b). Why Freud Turned Down $25,000. In Jane Ryan (Ed.). *Tales of Psychotherapy*, pp. 5–9. London: Karnac Books.

Kahr, Brett (2007c). The Infanticidal Attachment. *Attachment: New Directions in Psychotherapy and Relational Psychoanalysis*, *1*, 117–132.

Kahr, Brett (2007d). The Infanticidal Attachment in Schizophrenia and Dissociative Identity Disorder. *Attachment: New Directions in Psychotherapy and Relational Psychoanalysis*, *1*, 305–309.

Kahr, Brett (2008). *Who's Been Sleeping in Your Head?: The Secret World of Sexual Fantasies*. New York: Basic Books / Perseus Books Group.

Kahr, Brett (2010). Four Unknown Freud Anecdotes. *American Imago, 67*, 301–312.

Kahr, Brett (2011a). Winnicott's "*Anni Horribiles*": The Biographical Roots of "Hate in the Counter-Transference". *American Imago, 68*, 173–211.

Kahr, Brett (2011b). Lecture on "Dr. Estela Welldon's Contribution to Humanity". Closing Session, "Tribute to Dr. Estela Welldon: Twenty Years of the I.A.F.P.". Conference on "Murder in Mind", Twentieth International Conference, International Association for Forensic Psychotherapy, London, at the Apex International Hotel, Edinburgh, Scotland. 30th April.

Kahr, Brett (2012a). The Infanticidal Origins of Psychosis: The Role of Trauma in Schizophrenia. In Judy Yellin and Kate White (Eds.). *Shattered States: Disorganised Attachment and its Repair. The John Bowlby Memorial Conference Monograph 2007*, pp. 7–126. London: Karnac Books.

Kahr, Brett (2012b). Foreword. In Andrew Balfour, Mary Morgan, and Christopher Vincent (Eds.). *How Couple Relationships Shape Our World: Clinical Practice, Research, and Policy Perspectives*, pp. xvii–xxi. London: Karnac Books.

Kahr, Brett (2014a). Series Editor's Foreword: Towards Forensic Disability Psychotherapy. In Alan Corbett. *Disabling Perversions: Forensic Psychotherapy with People with Intellectual Disabilities*, pp. xiii–xxii. London: Karnac Books.

Kahr, Brett (2014b). Lecture on "The Intra-Marital Affair: From Erotic Tumour to Conjugal Aneurysm". Conference on "The Couple in the Room, the Couple in Mind: Reflections from an Attachment Perspective", the 21st John Bowlby Memorial Conference 2014. The Bowlby Centre, London, at The Kennedy Lecture Theatre, Wellcome Trust Building, Institute of Child Health, University College London, University of London, Holborn, London. 4th April.

Kahr, Brett (2014c). Lecture on "Sexual Cruelty in the Marital Bed: Unconscious Sadism in Non-Forensic Couples". Series on "Working Psychotherapeutically with Sadism: A Seminar Series for Psychotherapists and Psychologists". Confer, Tunstall, Woodbridge, Suffolk, at the Portland Suite [Seminar Suite], Grange Fitzrovia Hotel, London. 10th October.

Kahr, Brett (2015a). Winnicott's *Anni Horribiles*: The Biographical Roots of "Hate in the Counter-Transference". In Margaret Boyle Spelman and Frances Thomson-Salo (Eds.). *The Winnicott Tradition: Lines of Development – Evolution of Theory and Practice Over the Decades*, pp. 69–84. London: Karnac Books.

Kahr, Brett (2015b). "Led Astray by Their Half-Baked Pseudo-Scientific Rubbish": John Bowlby and the Paradigm Shift in Child Psychiatry. *Attachment: New Directions in Psychotherapy and Relational Psychoanalysis, 9*, 297–317.

Kahr, Brett (2016). "Happy Birthdeath to Me": Surviving Death Wishes in Early Infancy. In Stella Acquarone (Ed.). *Surviving the Early Years: The Importance of Early Intervention with Babies at Risk*, pp. 57–84. London: Karnac Books.

Kahr, Brett (2017). From the Treatment of a Compulsive Spitter: A Psychoanalytical Approach to Profound Disability. *British Journal of Psychotherapy, 33*, 31–47.

Kahr, Brett (Ed.). (2018a). *New Horizons in Forensic Psychotherapy: Exploring the Work of Estela V. Welldon*. London: Karnac Books.

Kahr, Brett (2018b). Introduction: Estela at La Scala. In Brett Kahr (Ed.). *New Horizons in Forensic Psychotherapy: Exploring the Work of Estela V. Welldon*, pp. 1–14. London: Karnac Books.

Kahr, Brett (2018c). "No Intolerable Persons" or "Lewd Pregnant Women": Towards a History of Forensic Psychoanalysis. In Brett Kahr (Ed.). *New Horizons in Forensic Psychotherapy: Exploring the Work of Estela V. Welldon*, pp. 17–87. London: Karnac Books.

Kahr, Brett (2018d). Committing Crimes without Breaking the Law: Unconscious Sadism in the "Non-Forensic" Patient. In Brett Kahr (Ed.). *New Horizons in Forensic Psychotherapy: Exploring the Work of Estela V. Welldon*, pp. 239–261. London: Karnac Books.

Kahr, Brett (2018e). Sexual Cruelty in the Marital Bed: Unconscious Sadism in Non-Forensic Couples. In Amita Sehgal (Ed.). *Sadism: Psychoanalytic Developmental Perspectives*, pp. 93–117. London: Routledge / Taylor and Francis Group, and Abingdon, Oxfordshire: Routledge / Taylor and Francis Group.

Kahr, Brett (2018f). Book Review of Alisa Roth. *Insane: America's Criminal Treatment of Mental Illness*. In Brett Kahr. Brett Kahr's Top Five Books for 2018: A Mid-Year Round-Up. *Autumn Programme 2018: Celebrating 20 Years of Confer*, p. 31. London: Confer.

Kahr, Brett (2018g). Book Review of Alisa Roth. *Insane: America's Criminal Treatment of Mental Illness*. In Brett Kahr. Top 10 Books: Brett Kahr's Top Ten Psychotherapy Books – 2018. Confer. [www.confer.uk.com/booksof2018.html].

Kahr, Brett (2018h). Lecture on "On Patients Who Explode: Surviving Petrifying Psychotherapeutic Experiences". Conference on "Bombs in the Consulting Room: How to Survive Hostile Transference and Relational Dynamics". Confer, Tunstall, Woodbridge, Suffolk, at N.C.V.O., Society Building, London. 9th June.

Kahr, Brett (2018i). Lecture on "Castration Anxiety in Men Who Murder". Panel on "Criminal Minds". Seminar Series on "Spotlight on the Archive: Film and Psychoanalysis in Focus". *The International Journal of Psychoanalysis*, London, and Media and the Inner World, School of Arts, University of Roehampton, London, and Faculty of Media and Communication, Bournemouth University, Ferne Barrow, Poole, Dorset, at the Sigmund Freud Room, Institute of Psychoanalysis, Byron House, Maida Vale, London. 11th December.

Kahr, Brett (Ed.). (2019a). *Forensic Psychotherapy and Psychopathology: Winnicottian Perspectives*. London: Routledge / Taylor and Francis Group, and Abingdon, Oxfordshire: Routledge / Taylor and Francis Group.

Kahr, Brett (Ed.). (2019b). *New Horizons in Forensic Psychotherapy: Exploring the Work of Estela V. Welldon*. [Hardback Edition]. London: Routledge / Taylor and Francis Group, and Abingdon, Oxfordshire: Routledge / Taylor and Francis Group.

Kahr, Brett (2019c). A Neglected Work of Genius: John Bowlby on "Hysteria in Children". *Attachment: New Directions in Psychotherapy and Relational Psychoanalysis*, *13*, 144–151.

Kahr, Brett (2019d). John Bowlby and the Birth of Child Mental Health. *Attachment: New Directions in Psychotherapy and Relational Psychoanalysis*, *13*, 164–180.

Kahr, Brett (2019e). Penile Trauma and Genital Exhibitionism: From Castration Anxiety to Verbal Potency. *International Journal of Forensic Psychotherapy*, *1*, 93–108.

Kahr, Brett (2019f). Professor Estela V. Welldon: Recipient of the Lifetime Achievement Award of the British Psychoanalytic Council. Presented on Saturday, 16th November, 2019, at the British Library, London. *International Journal of Forensic Psychotherapy*, *1*, 171–172.

Kahr, Brett (2019g). Professor Estela V. Welldon: Recipient of the Lifetime Achievement Award of the British Psychoanalytic Council. Presented on Saturday, 16th November, 2019, at the British Library, London. International Association for Forensic Psychotherapy. [https://www.forensicpsychotherapy.org/news-events-1].

Kahr, Brett (2019h). Foreword. In Andrew Balfour, Christopher Clulow, and Kate Thompson (Eds.). *Engaging Couples: New Directions in Therapeutic Work with Families*, pp. xv–xvii. London: Routledge / Taylor and Francis Group, and Abingdon, Oxfordshire: Routledge / Taylor and Francis Group.

Kahr, Brett (2019i). Lecture on "On Patients Who Explode: Surviving Petrifying Psychotherapeutic Experiences". Conference on "Working with Hostility in the Consulting Room: A Special One-day Event with Brett Kahr and Dr. Carine Minne". Confer, Woodbridge, Suffolk, and Confer Ireland, Dublin, Ireland, at the Palatine Room / Seomra Palatine, National Museum of Ireland – Decorative Arts and History / Ard Mhúsaem na hÉireann, Collins Barracks, Dublin, Ireland. 7ᵗʰ December.

Kahr, Brett (2020a). *Bombs in the Consulting Room: Surviving Psychological Shrapnel*. London: Routledge / Taylor and Francis Group, and Abingdon, Oxfordshire: Routledge / Taylor and Francis Group.

Kahr, Brett (2020b). *Dangerous Lunatics: Trauma, Criminality, and Forensic Psychotherapy*. London: Confer / Confer Books.

Kahr, Brett (2020c). *Banged Up*: A Chilling Glimpse into British Prisons. *International Journal of Forensic Psychotherapy*, *2*, 173–176.

Kahr, Brett (2020d). Professor Estela V. Welldon: Recipient of the Lifetime Achievement Award of the British Psychoanalytic Council. Presented on Saturday 16 November 2019, at the British Library, London. *New Associations*, Number *30*, pp. 10–11.

Kahr, Brett (2020e). Lecture on "Sub-Clinical Psychopathy". Course on "Diploma in Psychopathology: Theory and Practice", Course on "Certificate in Psychopathology: Theory and Practice", and Deep C.P.D. [Continuing Professional Development] Course in "Psychopathology: Theory and Practice". Confer, Woodbridge, Suffolk, at the Theatre Showroom, October Gallery, Lundonia House, Holborn, London. 5ᵗʰ March.

Kahr, Brett (2021a). *Freud's Pandemics: Surviving Global War, Spanish Flu, and the Nazis*. London: Karnac / Karnac Books, Confer.

Kahr, Brett (2021b). "The Piggle Papers": An Archival Investigation, 1961–1977. In Corinne Masur (Ed.). *Finding the Piggle: Reconsidering D.W. Winnicott's Most Famous Child Case*, pp. 41–100. Bicester, Oxfordshire: Phoenix Publishing House.

Kahr, Brett (2021c). Insults and Spears: The Tribulations of Forensic Disability Psychotherapy. In Nigel Beail, Patricia Frankish, and Allan Skelly (Eds.). *Trauma and Intellectual Disability: Acknowledgement, Identification and Intervention*, pp. 175–188. Shoreham by Sea, West Sussex: Pavilion / Pavilion Publishing and Media.

Kahr, Brett (2021d). On Patients Who Explode: Surviving Petrifying Psychotherapeutic Experiences. *International Journal of Forensic Psychotherapy*, *3*, 93–112.

Kahr, Brett (2021e). Professor Sir Michael Peckham: A Memorial Tribute. *International Journal of Forensic Psychotherapy*, *3*, 163–165.

Kahr, Brett (2021f). Lecture on "On Patients Who Explode: Surviving Petrifying Psychotherapeutic Experiences". Rafan House, London. 9ᵗʰ June. [Via Zoom].

Kahr, Brett (2021g). Lecture on "Взрывоопасные пациенты: как пережить шокирующее психотерапевтическое взаимодействие" ["On Patients Who Explode: Surviving Petrifying Psychotherapeutic Experiences"]. "35 конференция, Общество психоаналитической психотерапии, 125-летию со дня рождения Дональда Винникотта и полувековому юбилею его работы "Игра и реальность" " ["35th Conference of The Society of Psychoanalytic Psychotherapy: Playing and Reality: For Donald Woods Winnicott's 125th Birthday"], Общество психоаналитической психотерапии [Society of Psychoanalytic Psychotherapy], Moscow, Russia. 19ᵗʰ June. [Via Zoom].

Kahr, Brett (2021h). Lecture on "On Patients Who Explode: Surviving Petrifying Psycho-therapeutic Experiences". "Clinical Paper", Conference on "A Day with Professor Brett Kahr: Bombs in the Consulting Room. Surviving Attacks and Facilitating Cures", Basingstoke Counselling Service, Basingstoke, Hampshire. 6th November. [Via Zoom].

Kahr, Brett (2022a). The Spitting Patient: Speaking with Sputum and Free-Associating with Saliva. In Raffaella Hilty (Ed.). *Primitive Bodily Communications in Psychotherapy: Embodied Expressions of a Disembodied Psyche*, pp. 1–49, 201–207. London: Karnac / Karnac Books, Confer.

Kahr, Brett (2022b). Chapter 1. In Raffaella Hilty (Ed.). *Primitive Bodily Communications in Psychotherapy: Embodied Expressions of a Disembodied Psyche*, pp. 201–207. London: Karnac / Karnac Books, Confer.

Kahr, Brett (2022c). Sigmund Freud as the Father of Attachment Theory. *Attachment: New Directions in Psychotherapy and Relational Psychoanalysis*, *16*, 123–151.

Kahr, Brett (2022d). "Let the great axe fall": From Ancient Babylonian Torture to Modern Forensic Psychotherapy. Freud, Welldon, and the Humanisation of Criminality. *International Journal of Forensic Psychotherapy*, *4*, 89–118.

Kahr, Brett (2022e). Lecture on "The Case of Joseph Kallinger: My Reminiscences of a Multiple Murderer". Sohn Seminar, British Psychoanalytical Society, Byron House, London. 8th March. [Via Zoom].

Kahr, Brett (2022f). Lecture on " "Let the Great Axe Fall": From Ancient Babylonian Torture to Modern Forensic Psychotherapy. Freud, Welldon, and the Humanization of Criminality". Plenary 1, Conference on "Violence as a Public Health Emergency: Preventing, Treating and Humanizing the Dangerous Mind. Exploring the Past, Present and Future of Forensic Psychotherapy", Thirtieth Annual Conference (1992–2022), International Association for Forensic Psychotherapy, London, in association with the Violence Committee, International Psychoanalytical Association, and the Psychoanalysis and Law Committee, International Psychoanalytical Association, at the Paget Room, B.M.A. House, British Medical Association, London. 13th May, 2022. [In-Person and Via Remote Access, simultaneously].

Kahr, Brett (2023a). *How to Be Intimate with 15,000,000 Strangers: Musings on Media Psychoanalysis*. London: Routledge / Taylor and Francis Group, and Abingdon, Oxfordshire: Routledge / Taylor and Francis Group.

Kahr, Brett (2023b). Jeffrey Dahmer: From Neurocriminology to Castration Anxiety. Netflix Series Released on 21 September 2022. *International Journal of Forensic Psychotherapy*, *5*, 71–76.

Kahr, Brett (2024a). *Hidden Histories of British Psychoanalysis: From Freud's Death Bed to Laing's Missing Tooth*. Bicester, Oxfordshire: Karnac / Karnac Books.

Kahr, Brett (2024b). Castration Anxiety: A Neglected Aetiological Factor in the Male Murderer. *International Journal of Forensic Psychotherapy*, *6*, 1–15.

Kahr, Brett (2025a). (Ed.). *Expanding Psychoanalysis: The Contributions of Susie Orbach*. London: Routledge / Taylor and Francis Group, and Abingdon, Oxfordshire: Routledge / Taylor and Francis Group.

Kahr, Brett (2025b). *Winnicott's* Anni Horribiles: *The Creation of 'Hate in the Counter-Transference'*. [In Preparation].

King, Pearl (2002). Personal Communication to the Author. 8th November.

Kirtchuk, Gabriel; Gordon, John; Doctor, Ronald, and Ingram, Richard (2016). A Fertile Matrix: The Birth of the Forensic Psychotherapy Society. *Psychoanalytic Psychotherapy*, *3*, 182–195.

Klein, Melanie (1932a). *Die Psychoanalyse des Kindes*. Vienna: Internationaler Psychoanalytischer Verlag.

Klein, Melanie (1932b). *The Psycho-Analysis of Children*. Alix Strachey (Transl.). London: Hogarth Press and the Institute of Psycho-Analysis.

Klein, Melanie (1946). Notes on Some Schizoid Mechanisms. *International Journal of Psycho-Analysis, 27*, 99–110.

Koskenniemi, Erkki (2009). *The Exposure of Infants Among Jews and Christians in Antiquity*. Sheffield: Sheffield Phoenix Press.

Kupfermann, Kerstin (1977). A Latency Boy's Identity as a Cat. *Psychoanalytic Study of the Child, 32*, 363–385. New Haven, Connecticut: Yale University Press.

Kurdek, Lawrence A. (2008). Pet Dogs as Attachment Figures. *Journal of Social and Personal Relationships, 25*, 247–266.

Laing, Adrian C. (1991). R.D. Laing: The First Five Years. *Journal of the Society for Existential Analysis, 2*, 24–29.

Laing, Ronald D. (1960). *The Divided Self: A Study of Sanity and Madness*. London: Tavistock Publications.

Laing, Ronald D. (1964). Is Schizophrenia a Disease? *International Journal of Social Psychiatry, 10*, 184–193.

Laing, Ronald D. (1971). *The Politics of the Family and Other Essays*. London: Tavistock Publications.

Laing, Ronald D. (1976). A Critique of Kallmann's and Slater's Genetic Theory of Schizophrenia. In Richard I. Evans. *Dialogue with R.D. Laing: The Man and His Ideas*, pp. 97–156. New York: E.P. Dutton and Company.

Laing, Ronald D. (1981). A Critique of Kallmann's and Slater's Genetic Theory of Schizophrenia. In Richard I. Evans. *Dialogue with R.D. Laing*. [Revised Edition], pp. 97–156. New York: Praeger Publishers / CBS Educational and Professional Publishing, Division of CBS.

Laing, Ronald D. (1985). *Wisdom, Madness and Folly: The Making of a Psychiatrist. 1927–1957*. London: Macmillan London.

Lake, Peter, and Questier, Michael (2011). *The Trials of Margaret Clitherow: Persecution, Martyrdom and the Politics of Sanctity in Elizabethan England*. London: Continuum / Continuum International Publishing Group.

Langer, Walter C. (1972). *The Mind of Adolf Hitler: The Secret Wartime Report*. New York: Basic Books.

Large, David Clay (2015). *The Grand Spas of Central Europe: A History of Intrigue, Politics, Art, and Healing*. Lanham, Maryland: Rowman and Littlefield / Rowman and Littlefield Publishing Group.

Lazar-Geroe, Clara (1942). First Annual Report of the Melbourne Institute for Psychoanalysis for the Year 1941, pp. 613–615. In Notes. *Psychoanalytic Quarterly, 11*, 611–617.

Levenson, Jon D. (1993). *The Death and Resurrection of the Beloved Son: The Transformation of Child Sacrifice in Judaism and Christianity*. New Haven, Connecticut: Yale University Press.

Levy, John (1932). A Mental Hygiene Study of Juvenile Delinquency: Its Causes and Treatment. *American Journal of Psychiatry, 12*, 73–142.

Lewis, Brenda Ralph (2001). *Ritual Sacrifice: An Illustrated History*. Thrupp, Stroud, Gloucestershire: Sutton Publishing.

Lewis, Dorothy Otnow (1998). *Guilty by Reason of Insanity: A Psychiatrist Explores the Minds of Killers*. New York: Fawcett Columbine / Ballantine Publishing Group, Random House.

Lewis, Dorothy Otnow; Pincus, Jonathan H., Bard, Barbara; Richardson, Ellis; Prichep, Leslie S., Feldman, Marilyn, and Yeager, Catherine (1988). Neuropsychiatric, Psychoeducational, and Family Characteristics of 14 Juveniles Condemned to Death in the United States. *American Journal of Psychiatry*, *145*, 584–589.

Lewis, Dorothy Otnow; Yeager, Catherine A., Swica, Yael; Pincus, Jonathan H., and Lewis, Melvin (1997). Objective Documentation of Child Abuse and Dissociation in 12 Murderers with Dissociative Identity Disorder. *American Journal of Psychiatry*, *154*, 1703–1710.

Little, Margaret I. (1985). Winnicott Working in Areas Where Psychotic Anxieties Predominate: A Personal Record. *Free Associations*, Number *3*, 9–42.

Lombroso, Cesare (1876). *L'Uomo delinquente: Studiato in rapporto alla antropologia, alla medicina legale ed alle discipline carcerarie*. Milan: Ulrico Hoepli, Libraio-Editore.

Lorand, Sandor (1933). The Psychology of Nudism. *Psychoanalytic Review*, *20*, 197–207.

Lucas, Christopher (1990). Exhibitionism. *British Journal of Psychotherapy*, *7*, 15–24.

Lyons, Lewis (2003). *The History of Punishment*. London: Amber Books.

MacCarthy, Brendan (2002). Personal Communication to the Author. 29th May.

Mackintosh, James M. (1944). *The War and Mental Health in England*. New York: Commonwealth Fund, and London: Humphrey Milford / Oxford University Press.

MacLean, George (1986). A Brief Story About Dr. Hermine Hug-Hellmuth. *Canadian Journal of Psychiatry / Revue Canadienne de Psychiatrie*, *31*, 586–589.

MacLean, George, and Rappen, Ulrich (1991). *Hermine Hug-Hellmuth: Her Life and Work*. New York: Routledge / Routledge, Chapman and Hall.

Mackwood, John C. (1949). The Psychological Treatment of Offenders in Prison. *British Journal of Psychology: General Section*, *40*, 5–22.

Mackwood, John C. (1954). Psychotherapy in Prisons and Corrective Institutions: [*Abridged*]. *Proceedings of the Royal Society of Medicine*, Section of Psychiatry, *47*, 220–221.

Maeder, Alphonse (1909). Sexualität und Epilepsie. *Jahrbuch für psychoanalytische und psychopathologische Forschungen*, *1*, 119–154.

Maimonides (c. 1170–c. 1180). *The Code of Maimonides: Book Fourteen. The Book of Judges*. Abraham M. Hershman (Transl.). (1949). New Haven, Connecticut: Yale University Press, and London: Geoffrey Cumberlege / Oxford University Press.

Maletzky, Barry M. (1997). Exhibitionism: Assessment and Treatment. In D. Richard Laws and William O'Donohue (Eds.). *Sexual Deviance: Theory, Assessment, and Treatment*, pp. 40–74. New York: Guilford Press.

Mandeville, Bernard (1725). *An Enquiry into the Causes of the Frequent Executions at* Tyburn*: And A Proposal* for ʃome *Regulations* concerning *Felons* in *Prison,* and the good *Effects to be Expected from them. To which is Added, A* Diʃcourʃe *on Transportation, and a Method to render that* Puniʃhment *more Effectual*. London: J. Roberts.

Masters, Brian (1985). *Killing for Company: The Case of Dennis Nilsen*. London: Jonathan Cape.

Masters, Brian (1993). *The Shrine of Jeffrey Dahmer*. London: Hodder and Stoughton, and Dunton Green, Sevenoaks, Kent: Hodder and Stoughton, Hodder and Stoughton Limited.

Memorandum Submitted by the Institute of Psycho-Analysis to the Royal Commission on Capital Punishment (1950). G10/BA/F01/09. Archives of the British Psychoanalytical Society, British Psychoanalytical Society, Byron House, Maida Vale, London.

Menninger, Karl (1968). *The Crime of Punishment*. New York: Viking Press.

Mezey, Gillian; Vizard, Eileen; Hawkes, Colin, and Austin, Richard (1991). A Community Treatment Programme for Convicted Child Sex Offenders: A Preliminary Report. *Journal of Forensic Psychiatry*, *2*, 11–25.

Miles, Richard (2010). *Carthage Must be Destroyed: The Rise and Fall of an Ancient Mediterranean Civilization.* London: Allen Lane / Penguin Books, Penguin Group.

Miller, Alice (1988). *Der gemiedene Schlüssel.* Frankfurt am Main: Suhrkamp Verlag.

Miller, Alice (1998). The Political Consequences of Child Abuse. *Journal of Psychohistory, 26,* 573–585.

Millot, Catherine (2016). *La Vie avec Lacan.* Paris: Gallimard / Éditions Gallimard.

Minne, Carine (2008). The Dreaded and Dreading Patient and Therapist. In John Gordon and Gabriel Kirtchuk (Eds.). *Psychic Assaults and Frightened Clinicians: Countertransference in Forensic Settings,* pp. 27–40. London: Karnac Books.

Minne, Carine (2009). Infanticide, Matricide or Suicide. *British Journal of Psychotherapy, 25,* 194–202.

Minne, Carine, and Kassman, Paul (2018). Working with Gangs and within Gang Culture: A Pilot for Changing the Game. In Brett Kahr (Ed.). *New Horizons in Forensic Psychotherapy: Exploring the Work of Estela V. Welldon,* pp. 183–201. London: Karnac Books.

Moellenhoff, Fritz (1966). Hanns Sachs. 1881–1947: The Creative Unconscious. In Franz Alexander, Samuel Eisenstein, and Martin Grotjahn (Eds.). *Psychoanalytic Pioneers,* pp. 180–199. New York: Basic Books.

Mohr, George J. (1966). August Aichhorn: 1878–1949. Friend of the Wayward Youth. In Franz Alexander, Samuel Eisenstein, and Martin Grotjahn (Eds.). *Psychoanalytic Pioneers,* pp. 348–359. New York: Basic Books.

Molnar, Michael (1996). Of Dogs and Doggerel. *American Imago, 53,* 269–280.

Motz, Anna (2008). Women Who Kill: When Fantasy Becomes Reality. In Ronald Doctor (Ed.). *Murder: A Psychotherapeutic Investigation,* pp. 51–64. London: Karnac Books.

Motz, Anna (2009). Thinking the Unthinkable: Facing Maternal Abuse. *British Journal of Psychotherapy, 25,* 203–213.

Motz, Anna (2014). *Toxic Couples: The Psychology of Domestic Violence.* London: Routledge / Taylor and Francis Group, and Hove, East Sussex: Routledge / Taylor and Francis Group.

Murphy, William D. (1997). Exhibitionism: Psychopathology and Theory. In D. Richard Laws and William O'Donohue (Eds.). *Sexual Deviance: Theory, Assessment, and Treatment,* pp. 22–39. New York: Guilford Press.

Mush, John (1849). *Life and Death of Margaret Clitherow, The Martyr of York.* William Nicholson (Ed.). London: Richardson and Son.

Myers, Wayne A. (1991). The Course of Treatment of a Case of Photoexhibitionism in a Homosexual Male. In Charles W. Socarides and Vamik D. Volkan (Eds.). *The Homosexualities and the Therapeutic Process,* pp. 241–249. Madison, Connecticut: International Universities Press.

Natterson, Joseph M. (1966). Theodor Reik: b. 1888. Masochism in Modern Man. In Franz Alexander, Samuel Eisenstein, and Martin Grotjahn (Eds.). *Psychoanalytic Pioneers,* pp. 249–264. New York: Basic Books.

Newth, Alfred H. (1884). The Value of Electricity in the Treatment of Insanity. *Journal of Mental Science, 30,* 354–359.

Nilsen, Dennis (1983). *Nilsen Papers: Volume IXB,* p. 33. Quoted in Brian Masters (1985). *Killing for Company: The Case of Dennis Nilsen,* p. 142. London: Jonathan Cape.

O'Donnell, James P. (1978). *The Bunker: The History of the Reich Chancellery Group.* Boston, Massachusetts: Houghton Mifflin Company.

Ogden, Thomas H. (1982). *Projective Identification and Psychotherapeutic Technique.* New York: Jason Aronson.

Ortmann, David M., and Sprott, Richard A. (2013). *Sexual Outsiders: Understanding BDSM Sexualities and Communities*. Lanham, Maryland: Rowman and Littlefield Publishers / Rowman and Littlefield Publishing Group.

Overholser, Winfred (1952). Vernon C. Branham, M.D.: 1889–1951. *American Journal of Psychiatry*, *108*, 640.

Pailthorpe, Grace W. (1932). *Studies in the Psychology of Delinquency*. London: His Majesty's Stationery Office.

Perkins, David (1998). Compassion for Animals and Radical Politics: Coleridge's "To a Young Ass". *ELH*, *65*, 929–944.

Pfäfflin, Friedemann (1996). The Out-Patient Treatment of the Sex Offender. In Christopher Cordess and Murray Cox (Eds.). *Forensic Psychotherapy: Crime, Psychodynamics and the Offender Patient. Volume II. Mainly Practice*, pp. 261–271. London: Jessica Kingsley Publishers.

Pincus, Jonathan H. (2001). *Base Instincts: What Makes Killers Kill?* New York: W.W. Norton and Company.

Plvtarchi [Plutarch] (n.d.). *Vitarvm Parallelarvm: Volvmen Primvm, Thesevm, Romvlvm, Lycvrgvm, Nvmam, Solonem, Poplicolam, Themistoclem, Camillvm, Periclem, Fabivm Maximvm Tenens*. Ionnes Iacobvs Reiske [Johann Jakob Reiske] (Ed.). (1774). Leipzig: Gotth. Theoph. Georgi.

Preventing Suicide in Community and Custodial Settings: NICE Guideline (2018). National Institute for Health and Care Excellence. London: National Institute for Health and Care Excellence, Public Health England. [https://www.nice.org.uk/guidance/ng105/resources/preventing-suicide-in-community-and-custodial-settings-pdf-66141539632069; Accessed on 9th March, 2019].

Prichard, James Cowles (1835). *A Treatise on Insanity and Other Disorders Affecting the Mind*. London: Sherwood, Gilbert, and Piper.

Puri, Basant K., Baxter, Richard, and Cordess, Christopher C. (1995). Characteristics of Fire-Setters: A Study and Proposed Multiaxial Psychiatric Classification. *British Journal of Psychiatry*, *166*, 393–396.

Radzinowicz, Leon (1978). John Howard. In John C. Freeman (Ed.). *Prisons Past and Future*, pp. 7–13. London: Heinemann / Heinemann Educational Books.

Rafter, Nicole (2008). *The Criminal Brain: Understanding Biological Theories of Crime*. New York: New York University Press.

Raine, Adrian (2013). *The Anatomy of Violence: The Biological Roots of Crime*. New York: Pantheon Books / Random House.

Raine, Adrian; Buchsbaum, Monte, and LaCasse, Lori (1997). Brain Abnormalities in Murderers Indicated by Positron Emission Tomography. *Biological Psychiatry*, *42*, 495–508.

Raine, Adrian; Buchsbaum, Monte S., Stanley, Jill; Lottenberg, Steven; Abel, Leonard, and Stoddard, Jacqueline (1994). Selective Reductions in Prefrontal Glucose Metabolism in Murderers. *Biological Psychiatry*, *36*, 365–373.

Raine, Adrian; Lencz, Todd; Bihrle, Susan; LaCasse, Lori, and Colletti, Patrick (2000). Reduced Prefrontal Gray Matter Volume and Reduced Autonomic Activity in Antisocial Personality Disorder. *Archives of General Psychiatry*, *57*, 119–127.

Ramzy, Ishak (1953). Letter to William Gillespie. 14th July. Box 6. Folder 16. Papers of Princess Marie Bonaparte, Sigmund Freud Collection. Manuscript Reading Room, Room 101, Manuscript Division, James Madison Memorial Building, Library of Congress, Washington, D.C., U.S.A.

Ramzy, Ishak (1977). Editor's Foreword. In Donald W. Winnicott. *The Piggle: An Account of the Psychoanalytic Treatment of a Little Girl.* Ishak Ramzy (Ed.), pp. xi–xvi. New York: International Universities Press.

Rank, Otto (Ed.). (1907a). Vortragsabend: Am 6. Februar 1907. In Herman Nunberg and Ernst Federn (Eds.). (1976). *Protokolle der Wiener Psychoanalytischen Vereinigung: Band I. 1906–1908*, pp. 97–104. Frankfurt am Main: S. Fischer / S. Fischer Verlag.

Rank, Otto (Ed.). (1907b). Scientific Meeting on February 6, 1907. In Herman Nunberg and Ernst Federn (Eds.). (1962). *Minutes of the Vienna Psychoanalytic Society: Volume I: 1906–1908*. Margarethe Nunberg (Transl.), pp. 103–110. New York: International Universities Press.

Rank, Otto (Ed.). (1907c). Vortragsabend: Am 10. April 1907. In Herman Nunberg and Ernst Federn (Eds.). (1976). *Protokolle der Wiener Psychoanalytischen Vereinigung: Band I. 1906–1908*, pp. 150–156. Frankfurt am Main: S. Fischer / S. Fischer Verlag.

Renard, Simon (1551). Letter to Carlos. 21st March. In Royall Tyler (Ed.). (1914). *Calendar of Letters, Despatches, and State Papers, Relating to the Negotiations Between England and Spain, Preserved in the Archives at Vienna, Brussels, Simancas, and Elsewhere: Vol. X. Edward VI. 1550–1552*, pp. 248–250. Hereford: Hereford Times.

Rexford-Welch, Samuel C. (Ed.). (1958). *The Royal Air Force Medical Services: Volume III. Campaigns.* London: Her Majesty's Stationery Office.

Ribton-Turner, Charles J. (1887). *A History of Vagrants and Vagrancy and Beggars and Begging.* London: Chapman and Hall.

Romm, Sharon (1983). *The Unwelcome Intruder: Freud's Struggle with Cancer.* New York: Praeger Publishers / CBS Educational and Professional Publishing, Division of CBS / Praeger Special Studies / Praeger Scientific.

Rooth, F. Graham (1970). Some Historical Notes on Indecent Exposure and Exhibitionism. *Medico-Legal Journal*, *38*, 135–139.

Rosen, Ismond (Ed.). (1964a). *The Pathology and Treatment of Sexual Deviation: A Methodological Approach.* London: Oxford University Press.

Rosen, Ismond (1964b). Exhibitionism, Scopophilia and Voyeurism. In Ismond Rosen (Ed.). *The Pathology and Treatment of Sexual Deviation: A Methodological Approach*, pp. 293–350. London: Oxford University Press.

Rosenberg, Elizabeth (1943). A Clinical Contribution to the Psychopathology of the War Neuroses. *International Journal of Psycho-Analysis*, *24*, 32–41.

Roth, Alisa (2018). *Insane: America's Criminal Treatment of Mental Illness.* New York: Basic Books / Perseus Books, Hachette Book Group.

Rumney, David (1992). Origin and Early Struggles. In Eve Saville and David Rumney. *'Let Justice Be Done!': Your National and International Crime Forum After its Diamond Jubilee Year. A History of the I.S.T.D. A Study of Crime and Delinquency from 1931 to 1992*, pp. 1–9. London: Institute for the Study and Treatment of Delinquency.

Saunders, Jessica Williams (Ed.). (2001). *Life within Hidden Walls: Psychotherapy in Prisons.* London: H. Karnac (Books).

Schreiber, Flora Rheta (1973). *Sybil.* Chicago, Illinois: Henry Regnery Company.

Schreiber, Flora Rheta (1983). *The Shoemaker: The Anatomy of a Psychotic.* New York: Simon and Schuster.

Schur, Max (1972). *Freud: Living and Dying.* New York: International Universities Press.

Segal, Hanna (1973). *Introduction to the Work of Melanie Klein: New, Enlarged Edition.* London: Hogarth Press and the Institute of Psycho-Analysis.

Sehgal, Amita (Ed.). (2018). *Sadism: Psychoanalytic Developmental Perspectives*. London: Routledge / Taylor and Francis Group, and Abingdon, Oxfordshire: Routledge / Taylor and Francis Group.

Seldes, George (1953). *Tell the Truth and Run*. New York: Greenberg: Publisher.

Seneca, Lucius Annaeus (n.d. [c. 40s C.E.]). De Ira: Ad Novatum. In L. Annaei Senecae [Lucius Annaeus Seneca] (1797). *Opera Omnia: Qvae Svpersvnt. Volvmen Primvm*. Fridericvs Ernestvs Rvhkopf [Friedrich Ernst Ruhkopf] (Transl.), pp. 1–154. Leipzig: Libraria Weidmannia.

Serpell, James (1986). *In the Company of Animals: A Study of Human-Animal Relationships*. Oxford: Basil Blackwell.

Serpell, James (1991). Beneficial Effects of Pet Ownership on Some Aspects of Human Health and Behaviour. *Journal of the Royal Society of Medicine, 84*, 717–720.

Seruca, Tânia, and Silva, Carlos F. (2015). Recidivist Criminal Behaviour and Executive Functions: A Comparative Study. *Journal of Forensic Psychiatry and Psychology, 26*, 699–717.

Seward, Desmond (2014). *The Demon's Brood*. London: Constable / Constable and Robinson.

Shapiro, David (2000). *Dynamics of Character: Self-Regulation in Psychopathology*. New York: Basic Books.

Shea, Steven J. (1993). Personality Characteristics of Self-Mutilating Male Prisoners. *Journal of Clinical Psychology, 48*, 576–585.

Sheard, Michael H., Marini, James L., Bridges, Carolyn I., and Wagner, Ernest (1976). The Effect of Lithium on Impulsive Aggressive Behavior in Man. *American Journal of Psychiatry, 133*, 1409–1413.

Shelton, Jo-Ann (2014). Spectacles of Animal Abuse. In Gordon Lindsay Campbell (Ed.). *The Oxford Handbook of Animals in Classical Thought and Life*, pp. 461–477. Oxford: Oxford University Press.

Sheppard, Edgar (1867). On the Treatment of a Certain Class of Destructive Patients. *Journal of Mental Science, 13*, 65–75.

Shore, Heather (1999). *Artful Dodgers: Youth and Crime in Early Nineteenth-Century London*. Woodbridge, Suffolk: Royal Historical Society / Boydell Press, Boydell and Brewer.

Sims, Henry Marion (1893). Hystero-Epilepsy: A Report of Seven Cases Cured by Surgical Treatment. *American Journal of Obstetrics and Diseases of Women and Children, 28*, 80–88.

Sinason, Valerie (1986). Secondary Handicap and its Relationship to Trauma. *Psychoanalytic Psychotherapy, 2*, 131–154.

Sinason, Valerie (1988). Smiling, Swallowing, Sickening and Stupefying: The Effect of Sexual Abuse on the Child. *Psychoanalytic Psychotherapy, 3*, 97–111.

Sinason, Valerie (1992). *Mental Handicap and the Human Condition: New Approaches from the Tavistock*. London: Free Association Books.

Sinason, Valerie (1999). Psychoanalysis and Mental Handicap: Experience from the Tavistock Clinic. In Johan De Groef and Evelyn Heinemann (Eds.). *Psychoanalysis and Mental Handicap*. Andrew Weller (Transl.), pp. 194–206. London: Free Association Books.

Sinason, Valerie (2001). Children Who Kill Their Teddy Bears. In Brett Kahr (Ed.). *Forensic Psychotherapy and Psychopathology: Winnicottian Perspectives*, pp. 43–49. London: H. Karnac (Books), and New York: Other Press.

Sinason, Valerie (2012). Infanticide and Paedophilia as a Defence Against Incest: Work with a Man with a Severe Intellectual Disability. In John Adlam, Anne Aiyegbusi, Pam Kleinot, Anna Motz, and Christopher Scanlon (Eds.). *The Therapeutic Milieu Under Fire: Security and Insecurity in Forensic Mental Health*, pp. 175–185. London: Jessica Kingsley Publishers.

Smith, John M. Powis (1931). *The Origin and History of Hebrew Law*. Chicago, Illinois: University of Chicago Press.

Smith, Maurice Hamblin (1924). The Mental Conditions Found in Certain Sexual Offenders. *The Lancet*. 29th March, pp. 643–646.

Socarides, Charles W. (1988). *The Preoedipal Origin and Psychoanalytic Therapy of Sexual Perversions*. Madison, Connecticut: International Universities Press.

Southwood, Martin (1958). *John Howard: Prison Reformer. An Account of His Life and Travels*. London: Independent Press.

Stahl, Stephen M., and Morrissette, Debbi Ann (2014). *Stahl's Illustrated Violence: Neural Circuits, Genetics and Treatment*. Cambridge: Cambridge University Press.

Stansky, Peter (2007). *The First Day of the Blitz: September 7, 1940*. New Haven, Connecticut: Yale University Press.

Starchild, Adam (1990). Rape of Youth in Prisons and Juvenile Facilities. *Journal of Psychohistory*, *18*, 145–150.

Sterba, Richard F. (1982). *Reminiscences of a Viennese Psychoanalyst*. Detroit, Michigan: Wayne State University Press.

Steward, Jill (2012). Travel to the Spas: The Growth of Health Tourism in Central Europe, 1850–1914. In Gemma Blackshaw and Sabine Wieber (Eds.). *Journeys into Madness: Mapping Mental Illness in the Austro-Hungarian Empire*, pp. 72–89. New York: Berghahn Books.

Stewart, Lynn A. (1993). Profile of Female Firesetters: Implications for Treatment. *British Journal of Psychiatry*, *163*, 248–256.

Stewart, Pamela Windham (2016a). Interventions with Mothers and Babies in Prisons: Collision of Internal and External Worlds. In Stella Acquarone (Ed.). *Surviving the Early Years: The Importance of Early Intervention with Babies at Risk*, pp. 101–111. London: Karnac Books.

Stewart, Pamela Windham (2016b). Creating Mother and Baby Therapy Groups in Prison: Emotional Valuation. *Psychoanalytic Psychotherapy*, *30*, 152–163.

Stewart, Pamela Windham (2019). Twenty Years in Prison: Reflections on the Birth of the Born Inside Project and Psychotherapy in HMP Holloway. In Pamela Windham Stewart and Jessica Collier (Eds.). *The End of the Sentence: Psychotherapy with Female Offenders*, pp. 23–40. London: Routledge / Taylor and Francis Group, and Abingdon, Oxfordshire: Routledge / Taylor and Francis Group.

Stoller, Robert J. (1975). *Perversion: The Erotic Form of Hatred*. New York: Pantheon Books.

Stoller, Robert J. (1979). Centerfold: An Essay on Excitement. *Archives of General Psychiatry*, *36*, 1019–1024.

Stoller, Robert J. (1985). *Observing the Erotic Imagination*. New Haven, Connecticut: Yale University Press.

Strauss, Eric B. (1939). Psycho-Therapy in Prison. *Howard Journal*, *5*, 166–168.

Sugarman, Philip; Dumughn, Catherine; Saad, Karim; Hinder, Stephen, and Bluglass, Robert (1994). Dangerousness in Exhibitionists. *Journal of Forensic Psychiatry*, *5*, 287–296.

Temperley, Jane (1984). Settings for Psychotherapy. *British Journal of Psychotherapy*, *1*, 101–111.

Terranova, Claudio, and Rocca, Gabriele (2016). Homicide Committed by Psychiatric Patients: Psychiatrists' Liability in Italian Law Cases. *Medicine, Science and the Law*, *56*, 58–64.

Thomson, J. Bruce (1870a). The Hereditary Nature of Crime. *Journal of Mental Science*, *15*, 487–498.

Thomson, J. Bruce (1870b). The Psychology of Criminals. *Journal of Mental Science*, *16*, 321–350.

Tierney, Patrick (1989). *The Highest Altar: The Story of Human Sacrifice*. New York: Viking / Penguin Group / Viking Penguin, Penguin Books USA.

Toynbee, Jocelyn M.C. (1973). *Animals in Roman Life and Art*. London: Thames and Hudson.

van Leeuwen, Mirjam E., and Harte, Joke M. (2017). Violence Against Mental Health Care Professionals: Prevalence, Nature and Consequences. *Journal of Forensic Psychiatry and Psychology*, *28*, 581–598.

Vickers, Hugo (2000). *Alice: Princess Andrew of Greece*. London: Hamish Hamilton.

Vizard, Eileen (1997). Adolescents Who Sexually Abuse. In Estela V. Welldon and Cleo Van Velsen (Eds.). *A Practical Guide to Forensic Psychotherapy*, pp. 48–55. London: Jessica Kingsley Publishers.

Vizard, Eileen; Monck, Elizabeth, and Misch, Peter (1995). Child and Adolescent Sex Abuse Perpetrators: A Review of the Research Literature. *Journal of Child Psychology and Psychiatry and Allied Disciplines*, *36*, 731–756.

Vizard, Eileen; Wynick, Sarah; Hawkes, Colin; Woods, John, and Jenkins, Jill (1996). Juvenile Sex Offenders: Assessment Issues. *British Journal of Psychiatry*, *168*, 259–262.

von Krafft-Ebing, Richard (1895). *Nervosität und neurasthenische Zustände*. In Hermann Nothnagel (Ed.). *Specielle Pathologie und Therapie: XII. Band, II. Theil. Nervosität und neurasthenische Zustände von Prof. Dr. R. v. Krafft-Ebing*, pp. [v]–210. Vienna: Alfred Holder.

von Winterstein, Alfred Freiherr (1912). Zur Psychoanalyse des Reisens. *Imago*, *1*, 489–506.

Walker, Zuzana, and Seifert, Ruth (1994). Violent Incidents in a Psychiatric Intensive Care Unit. *British Journal of Psychiatry*, *164*, 826–828.

Walker-Meikle, Kathleen (2011). *Medieval Cats*. London: British Library.

Ward, Laurence (2015). *The London County Council: Bomb Damage Maps. 1939–1945*. London: Thames and Hudson.

Warren, Muriel Prince (2001). *Behavioral Management Guide: Essential Treatment Strategies for Adult Psychotherapy*. Northvale, New Jersey: Jason Aronson.

Weitzman, Susan (2000). *"Not to People Like Us": Hidden Abuse in Upscale Marriages*. New York: Basic Books / Perseus Books Group.

Welldon, Estela (n.d. [1985]). Application of Group Analytic Psychotherapy to Those with Sexual Perversions. In Terence E. Lear (Ed.). *Spheres of Group Analysis*, pp. 96–108. n.p.: n.p.

Welldon, Estela V. (1988). *Mother, Madonna, Whore: The Idealization and Denigration of Motherhood*. London: Free Association Books.

Welldon, Estela V. (1991). Psychology and Psychopathology in Women: A Psychoanalytic Perspective. *British Journal of Psychiatry*, *158*, Supplement *10*, 85–92.

Welldon, Estela V. (1993). Forensic Psychotherapy and Group Analysis. *Group Analysis*, *26*, 487–502.

Welldon, Estela V. (1996). Contrasts in Male and Female Sexual Perversions. In Christopher Cordess and Murray Cox (Eds.). *Forensic Psychotherapy: Crime, Psychodynamics and the Offender Patient. Volume II. Mainly Practice*, pp. 273–289. London: Jessica Kingsley Publishers.

Welldon, Estela (2001). Babies as Transitional Objects. In Brett Kahr (Ed.). *Forensic Psychotherapy and Psychopathology: Winnicottian Perspectives*, pp. 19–25. London: H. Karnac (Books), and New York: Other Press.

Welldon, Estela V. (2002). *Sadomasochism*. Duxford, Cambridge: Icon Books.

Welldon, Estela V. (2011). *Playing with Dynamite: A Personal Approach to the Psychoanalytic Understanding of Perversions, Violence, and Criminality*. London: Karnac Books.

Welldon, Estela (2012). Couples Who Kill: The Malignant Bonding. In John Adlam, Anne Aiyegbusi, Pam Kleinot, Anna Motz, and Christopher Scanlon (Eds.). *The Therapeutic Milieu Under Fire: Security and Insecurity in Forensic Mental Health*, pp. 162–172. London: Jessica Kingsley Publishers.

Welldon, Estela (2015). Forensic Psychotherapy. *Psychoanalytic Psychotherapy*, *29*, 211–227.

Welldon, Estela V. (2016). *Sadomasochism in Art and Politics*. n.p.: n.p.

Welldon, Estela V. (2017). *Sex Now Talk Later*. London: Karnac Books.

Welldon, Estela (2021). Personal Communication to the Author. 4th December.

Welldon, Estela V., and Van Velsen, Cleo (Eds.). (1997). *A Practical Guide to Forensic Psychotherapy*. London: Jessica Kingsley Publishers.

Westwick, Atwell (1940). Criminology and Psychoanalysis. *Psychoanalytic Quarterly*, *9*, 269–282.

Widom, Cathy Spatz (1977). A Methodology for Studying Noninstitutionalized Psychopaths. *Journal of Consulting and Clinical Psychology*, *45*, 674–683.

Williams, Arthur Hyatt (1964). The Psychopathology and Treatment of Sexual Murderers. In Ismond Rosen (Ed.). *The Pathology and Treatment of Sexual Deviation: A Methodological Approach*, pp. 351–377. London: Oxford University Press.

Winnicott, Donald W. (1943). Delinquency Research. *New Era in Home and School*, *24*, 65–67.

Winnicott, Donald W. (1945). The Return of the Evacuated Child. In Donald W. Winnicott (1957). *The Child and the Outside World: Studies in Developing Relationships*. Janet Hardenberg (Ed.), pp. 88–92. London: Tavistock Publications.

Winnicott, Donald W. (1949a). Hate in the Counter-Transference. *International Journal of Psycho-Analysis*, *30*, 69–74.

Winnicott, Donald W. (1949b). Letter to the Editor of *The Times*. 10th August. In Donald W. Winnicott (1987). *The Spontaneous Gesture: Selected Letters of D.W. Winnicott*. F. Robert Rodman (Ed.), pp. 15–16. Cambridge, Massachusetts: Harvard University Press.

Winnicott, Donald W. (1949c). Letter to S.H. Hodge. 1st September. In Donald W. Winnicott (1987). *The Spontaneous Gesture: Selected Letters of D.W. Winnicott*. F. Robert Rodman (Ed.), pp. 17–19. Cambridge, Massachusetts: Harvard University Press.

Winnicott, Donald W. (1956). The Antisocial Tendency. In Donald W. Winnicott (1958). *Collected Papers: Through Paediatrics to Psycho-Analysis*, pp. 306–315. London: Tavistock Publications.

Winnicott, Donald W. (1958). Psycho-Analysis and the Sense of Guilt. In Donald W. Winnicott, John Bowlby, Ilse Hellman, Marion Milner, Roger Money-Kyrle, Elliott Jaques, and Joan Riviere. *Psycho-Analysis and Contemporary Thought*. John D. Sutherland (Ed.). pp. 15–32. London: Hogarth Press and the Institute of Psycho-Analysis.

Winnicott, Donald W. (1962a). The Development of a Child's Sense of Right and Wrong. In Donald W. Winnicott (1993). *Talking to Parents*. Clare Winnicott, Christopher Bollas, Madeleine Davis, and Ray Shepherd (Eds.), pp. 105–110. Reading, Massachusetts: Addison-Wesley Publishing Company.

Winnicott, Donald W. (1962b). Introduction. In Robert W. Shields. *A Cure of Delinquents: The Treatment of Maladjustment*, pp. 9–10. London: Heinemann Educational Books.

Winnicott, Donald W. (1962–1963). The Antisocial Tendency Illustrated by a Case. *A Criança Portuguesa*, *21*, 195–209.

Winnicott, Donald W. (1964). This Feminism. In Donald W. Winnicott (1986). *Home is Where We Start From: Essays by a Psychoanalyst*. Clare Winnicott, Ray Shepherd, and Madeleine Davis (Eds.), pp. 183–194. Harmondsworth, Middlesex: Penguin Books / Pelican Books.

Winnicott, Donald W. (1966). A Psychoanalytic View of the Antisocial Tendency. In Ralph Slovenko (Ed.). *Crime, Law and Corrections*, pp. 102–130. Springfield, Illinois: Charles C Thomas, Publisher.

Winnicott, Donald W. (1968). Delinquency as a Sign of Hope. *Prison Service Journal*, *7*, Number *27*, 2–7.

Winnicott, Donald W. (1969a). The Use of an Object. *International Journal of Psycho-Analysis*, *50*, 711–716.

Winnicott, Donald W. (1969b). Letter to Richard Balbernie. 18th March. Box 7. File 10. Donald W. Winnicott Papers. Archives of Psychiatry, The Oskar Diethelm Library, The DeWitt Wallace Institute of Psychiatry: History, Policy, and the Arts, Department of Psychiatry, Joan and Sanford I. Weill Medical College, Cornell University, The New York Presbyterian Hospital, New York, New York, U.S.A.

Winnicott, Donald W. (1970). The Place of the Monarchy. In Donald W. Winnicott (1986). *Home is Where We Start From: Essays by a Psychoanalyst*. Clare Winnicott, Ray Shepherd, and Madeleine Davis (Eds.), pp. 260–268. New York: W.W. Norton and Company.

Winnicott, Donald W. (1971). The Concept of a Healthy Individual. In John D. Sutherland (Ed.). *Towards Community Mental Health*, pp. 1–15. London: Tavistock Publications.

Winnicott, Donald W. (1977). *The Piggle: An Account of the Psychoanalytic Treatment of a Little Girl*. Ishak Ramzy (Ed.). New York: International Universities Press.

Winnicott, Donald W., and Britton, Clare (1944). The Problem of Homeless Children. *New Era in Home and School*, *25*, 155–161.

Winnicott, Donald W., and Britton, Clare (1947). Residential Management as Treatment for Difficult Children: The Evolution of a Wartime Hostels Scheme. *Human Relations*, *1*, 87–97.

Winnicott, Violet (1943). Letter to Alice Winnicott. 23rd November. PP/DWW/B/D/3. Donald Woods Winnicott Collection. Archives and Manuscripts, Rare Materials Room, Wellcome Library, Wellcome Collection, The Wellcome Building, London.

Wolf [Anna Freud] (1926). 6. Mai 1926. Typescript. Freud Museum London, Swiss Cottage, London.

Woods, John (1997). Breaking the Cycle of Abuse and Abusing: Individual Psychotherapy for Juvenile Sex Offenders. *Clinical Child Psychology and Psychiatry*, *2*, 379–392.

Woon, Basil (1941). *Hell Came to London: A Reportage of the Blitz During 14 Days*. London: Peter Davies.

Wortis, Joseph (1934a). Diary Entry. 10th October. In Joseph Wortis (1954). *Fragments of an Analysis with Freud*, pp. 23–25. New York: Simon and Schuster.

Wortis, Joseph (1934b). Diary Entry. 1st November. In Joseph Wortis (1954). *Fragments of an Analysis with Freud*, pp. 54–59. New York: Simon and Schuster.

Wortis, Joseph (1940). Fragments of a Freudian Analysis. *American Journal of Orthopsychiatry*, *10*, 843–849.

Wray, George A., and Eldridge, Harold W. (1970). A Knife Swallowed in Prison Retrieved at Oesophagoscopy. *Medicine Science and the Law*, *10*, 85.

Yang, Yaling; Raine, Adrian; Narr, Katherine L., Colletti, Patrick, and Toga, Arthur W. (2009). Localization of Deformations within the Amygdala in Individuals with Psychopathy. *Archives of General Psychiatry*, *66*, 986–994.

Young-Bruehl, Elisabeth (1988). *Anna Freud: A Biography*. New York: Summit Books / Simon and Schuster.

Yukhnenko, Denis; Sridhar, Shivpriya, and Fazel, Seena (2019). A Systematic Review of Criminal Recidivism Rates Worldwide: 3-Year Update. *Wellcome Open Research*, *4:28*, 1–12. Wellcome Open Research. [https://wellcomeopenresearch.org/articles/4-28; Accessed on 24th November, 2022].

Zavitzianos, George (1971). Fetishism and Exhibitionism in the Female and Their Relationship to Psychopathy and Kleptomania. *International Journal of Psycho-Analysis*, *52*, 297–305.

Zavitzianos, George (1972). Homeovestism: Perverse Form of Behaviour Involving Wearing Clothes of the Same Sex. *International Journal of Psycho-Analysis*, *53*, 471–477.

Zavitzianos, George (1977). More on Exhibitionism in Women. *American Journal of Psychiatry*, *134*, 820.

Zilboorg, Gregory (1931). Translator's Note. In Franz Alexander and Hugo Staub. *The Criminal, the Judge, and the Public: A Psychological Analysis*. Gregory Zilboorg (Transl.), pp. v–x. New York: Macmillan Company.

Index